THE DEVELOPING MIND

THE DEVELOPING MIND

Toward a Neurobiology of Interpersonal Experience

DANIEL J. SIEGEL, MD

THE GUILFORD PRESS
New York   London

© 1999 Daniel J. Siegel

Published by The Guilford Press
A Division of Guilford Publications, Inc.
72 Spring Street, New York, NY 10012
http://www.guilford.com

Printed in the United States of America

This book is printed on acid-free paper.

Last digit is print number: 9   8   7   6   5   4   3   2   1

Library of Congress Cataloging-in-Publication Data

Siegel, Daniel J., 1957–
    The developing mind: toward a neurobiology of interpersonal
experience / Daniel J. Siegel.
        p.   cm.
    Includes bibliographic references and index.
    ISBN 1-57230-453-7 (hardcover)
    1. Developmental psychology.   2. Interpersonal relations.
3. Intellect.   4. Brain—Physiological aspects.   I. Title.
    [DNLM: 1. Human Development.   2. Interpersonal Relations.
3. Brain—physiology.   4. Psychological Theory.   BF 713 S571d 1999]
BF713.S525 1999
153.6—dc21
DNLM/DLC   98-50993
for Library of Congress   CIP

About the Author

Daniel J. Siegel received his medical degree from Harvard University and completed his postgraduate medical education at the University of California, Los Angeles, with training in pediatrics, general adult psychiatry, and child and adolescent psychiatry. He has served as a National Institute of Mental Health Research Fellow at UCLA, where he studied family interactions, with an emphasis on how attachment experiences influence emotions, behavioral regulation, autobiographical memory, and narrative processes.

Dr. Siegel's clinical activities include work as a child, adolescent, adult, and family psychiatrist. An award-winning educator, he formerly directed the UCLA training program in child psychiatry and is the recipient of the departmental teaching award and several honorary fellowships. He is currently the medical director of the Infant and Preschool Service at UCLA and associate clinical professor of psychiatry at the UCLA School of Medicine. He also serves as the director of interdisciplinary studies for the international nonprofit Children's Mental Health Alliance Foundation in New York.

Dr. Siegel's integrated developmental approach has led him to be invited to local, national, and international organizations to address audiences of educators, lawmakers, parents, public administrators, medical and mental health practitioners, and neuroscientists.

Preface

What is the mind? How does the mind develop? This book synthesizes information from a range of scientific disciplines to explore the idea that the mind emerges at the interface of interpersonal experience and the structure and function of the brain.

Like many adolescents, as a teenager I became filled with a particular intellectual passion: I was fascinated with people and the nature of the mind. Through a series of journeys, I eventually became a psychiatrist, specializing in the care of children and families. Along the way have been encounters with a wide variety of people and the stories of their lives. Trained in science and immersed in human struggles, I found myself naturally trying to understand the process of human development—of how people become who they are—by investigating what was known from research and getting as close as possible to the subjective experience at the core of people's lives. This book presents the integration of this effort to gain insights into the mind and human development.

From mountaintops and quiet conversations to lecture halls and the bustling discussions of a weekend conference, this exploration of the nature of the developing mind has come to involve people from many walks of life. At recent seminars, I have met with a range of professionals—in child development, education, medicine, neuroscience, psychology, public administration, and social work—to discuss basic questions regarding the mind and the ways experience shapes development. These experiences as an educator have motivated me to synthesize this work into a framework that provides an integrated scientific foundation regarding the interpersonal and neurobiological basis of the developing mind.

This book may be useful for those working in a variety of disciplines. Understanding these processes can enable clinicians to help patients heal. Academicians may find such an interdisciplinary effort useful in gaining insight into how their own work relates to independent fields of research. Educators can benefit from insights into how emotion and interpersonal relationships are fundamental motivational aspects of learning and memory. For child development specialists and others who care for children, knowing how forms of communication directly shape a child's developing brain can be essential in creating programs that are scientifically based and that can optimize the care of children. For many other people, learning about how the mind emerges from the substance of the brain and the processes of interpersonal relationships can provide useful insights that can improve their professional as well as personal lives. Interpersonal experience shapes the mind as it continues to develop throughout the lifespan. This book is about *how* these interpersonal processes occur and how we can utilize ideas about neurobiology to help others, and ourselves, to grow and develop.

In my own field of psychiatry, the tremendous expansion of neuroscientific research seems to have been interpreted in the extreme by some as a call to "biological determinism"—that is, to a view of psychiatric disorders as a result of biochemical processes, most of which are genetically determined and little influenced by experience. This impression may sound reductionistic, but I wish that the sense of demoralization expressed by many educators and students in psychiatry didn't support the notion that the field has been losing its mind in favor of the brain. What is ironic, and what up until now has not been well known, is that recent findings of neural science in fact point to just the opposite: Interactions with the environment, especially relationships with other people, directly shape the development of the brain's structure and function. There is no need to choose between brain or mind, biology or experience, nature or nurture. These divisions are unhelpful and inhibit clear thinking about an important and complex subject: the developing human mind.

As I was finishing up the last chapter revisions for this book, an article by a renowned neuroscientist who is also trained as a psychiatrist appeared in the *American Journal of Psychiatry*. Eric Kandel's paper "A New Intellectual Framework for Psychiatry"[1] suggests that the field of psychiatry in recent times has suffered from a series of damaging divisions within its ranks. These divisions have blocked the ability to integrate a wide range of information about human experience, mind, and brain. It is my hope that presenting a scientifically grounded synthesis focusing on these domains will enable such professional divisions to give way to a new conceptual foundation that will be useful for clinicians and others who help people develop.

Although it is important to be aware of the significant and very real contributions of genetic and constitutional factors to the outcome of development, it is equally crucial that we examine what in fact is known about how experience shapes development. Such a balanced view enables us as parents, for example, to have a sense of responsibility for the experiences we provide without the unnecessary burden of guilt generated by the belief that our actions are solely responsible for the outcome of our children's development.

One factor turning some mental health care providers' attention away from the role of experience in human development may be our attempt to avoid some of the devastating errors of the past. Not so long ago, the mothers of children with autism were accused of being "refrigerators"; the families of patients with schizophrenia were said to be giving "double binds"; individuals with bipolar disorder were given thousands of hours of therapy, in search of the "psychological cause" of their mood swings; and people with obsessive–compulsive disorder were thought to be repressing some early trauma that may have produced their worries. In each of these painful examples, we as professionals looked toward experience to explain the causes of our patients' anguish and dysfunction. Despite the goodness of our intentions, these views were misguided and not helpful to our patients. They produced accusations of blame and a sense of guilt that were unfounded. They did not lead to growth or healing in our patients or their families.

Many people have been spared devastating amounts of pain and suffering because of our modern understanding of psychiatric illness and the appropriate use of pharmacological agents. Psychiatry has had to embrace the notion that the brain contributes to mental dysfunction, in order to pursue these extremely important avenues of medical care. But losing sight of the important role of experience, especially social experience, in shaping the mind does not help us to understand development or to help our patients.

If social factors—that is, human relationships—shape the development of the brain and thus the mind, *how* does this occur? The purpose of this book is to explore this question by examining some ways in which interpersonal experience shapes the developing mind and fosters emotional well-being.

An exciting challenge in writing this book has been to attempt to deepen an understanding of subjective everyday life, of the mind and human relationships, by drawing on the objective views of science. The benefit of this approach is that we can learn much more about what creates human experience than is possible with only everyday logic or self-reflection. For example, by learning how the circuits in the brain develop during the first years of life, we can gain insights into why older children or adults generally cannot consciously recall their experiences before the preschool years. By learning about the nature of how the brain creates an awareness of other minds, we can begin to understand the biological basis for emotional communication and what may be occurring when empathy is not a part of human relationships. In addition, understanding how trauma affects the developing brain can yield insights into the subsequent impairments in memory processing and the ability to cope with stress. Using science to understand the mind has provided a powerful tool for deepening our comprehension of subjective mental life and interpersonal relationships. These insights have proven tremendously useful in helping others grow and develop.

To see how these neurobiological ideas help others develop and heal not only has fueled my enthusiasm, but has generated the energy required for the completion of this book. This task would not have been possible without the loving support of my family. How many times they heard the excited call "It's finished!", only to find me working on the next draft a few weeks later. Their continuing encouragement is of immeasurable importance to me.

When The Guilford Press initially asked me to write this book, its focus was to be on memory and psychotherapy. Since that time, the topic of the book has broadened; it has come to include, with the helpful assistance of my patient editor, Kitty Moore, the much wider topic of these fundamental questions about the mind, the brain, and human relationships. I thank her for her belief in the work and her skillful help with the process of bringing it to completion. I would also like to express my appreciation to the efficient and responsive publication staff at Guilford, and especially to Anna Brackett and Marie Sprayberry, for their thoughtful attention to the text.

In my professional life, it can't be overstated that my patients have had the largest impact on my clinical education. In ways both professional and personal, they have taught me more than I ever dreamed I'd learn in a lifetime. I have also had the good fortune of having had several clinical teachers who have been especially supportive and helpful in my development as a psychotherapist, including Jim Grotstein, MD, Chris Heinicke, PhD, Regina Pally, MD, Arnold Scheibel, MD, and Don Schwartz, MD. Also along the journey have been many students—especially those in the Infant and Preschool Service, which I direct with Mary O'Connor, PhD, at UCLA—whose questions keep an investigating and conceptualizing mind reflective and excited about trying both to understand and to communicate complex ideas. One of the most moving teaching experiences has come from the opportunity to work with many teams of psychotherapists from over a dozen nations in Eastern Europe who have been struggling to deal with the ravages of political wars and childhood abuse. The Children's Mental Health Alliance Foundation, directed by Pamela Sicher, MD, and Owen Lewis, MD, has developed a novel educational program to teach these devoted and sacrificing therapists the basic elements of evaluating, treating, and (we all hope) preventing child abuse in their developing nations. It is inspiring to see their dedication, and exhilarating to hear that the ideas of this book have been accessible and useful across cultures.

These issues about how experiences shape the brain and thus organize the mind have been topics of passionate discussion for a local study group called, affectionately, the ID-CNS (Institute for Developmental and Clinical Neural Science). My thanks to its members—Lou Cozolino, PhD, Allan Schore, PhD, Judith Schore, PhD, and John Schumann, PhD—for our intellectual companionship on this journey into mind and brain. My childhood friend and longtime conversation partner in matters of the mind, Jonathan Fried, has offered valuable comments on the text and has been especially helpful in pointing out the abundance of "thuses" in the original manuscript; thus I thank him. Others who have read this work at various stages in its evolution and have provided immensely useful comments and questions include Daniel Attias, Lisa Capps, PhD, Leston Havens, MD, Erik Hesse, Althea Horner, PhD, Mary Main, PhD, Eleanor Ochs, PhD, Sarah Steinberg, Caroline Welch, and several anonymous reviewers through the editing process at The Guilford Press.

Several other people also need to be acknowledged. In medical school, Tom Whitfield III, MD, was my pediatric mentor and friend who taught me early on that "the way to care for patients is to care about them." The initial version of what was to become this book was begun on a trip to visit Tom and his wife, Peg, in the Berkshires before his death in 1996. The lessons I have learned from trying to make sense of the process of losing such an important attachment figure in my life are contained within these pages. Another person in those years who "saved my life" in medical school is Leston Havens, MD, who gave me the strength to hold on to my own experience in the confusing Boston psychiatric climate at the time. During my years of adult and child psychiatric residency, Joel Yager, MD, and the late Dennis Cantwell, MD, supported my explorations of different directions and my efforts to organize my professional passions. In my National Institute of Mental Health research training years at UCLA, Marian Sigman, PhD, and Robert Bjork, PhD, were extremely supportive in guiding me through the wonderful interdisciplinary learning that the research fellowship allowed.

During many of those years as a trainee in psychiatry, I had the honor of being supervised by Robert Stoller, MD, who devoted much of his professional life to exploring the ways in which early life experiences shape development. We would spend hours discussing patients, the mind, and our own experiences as therapists. One of our topics was about human communication. As Bob wrote in one of his last books before his tragic accidental death:

> Still, yearning for clarity contains a pleasure of which I am only now fully aware. Sometimes, on paring a sentence down to its barest minimum, I find it transforms into a question, paradox, or joke (all three being different states of the same thing, like ice, water and steam). That is a relief: clarity asks; it does not answer. Maybe then, in a hundred years, sitting on my haunches like a Zen master, I shall finally write a clear sentence. But it will have no words.[2]

I have tried my best to use simple language, to avoid unnecessary jargon, and to make sentences concise and clear. Though words are limited in their ability to convey exactly what we mean, they are one of our only ways of sharing information about complex ideas, as well as about simple truths. Words enable us to communicate across the boundaries of time and space that separate one mind from another. Words allow us to tell the stories of our lives and relate the scientific explorations that reflect our drive to understand ourselves and the world in which we live. I hope that the stories and science in the book will help people to understand the social brain more fully and to focus our attention on the many intriguing and important unanswered questions about interpersonal experience and the developing mind across the lifespan.

Contents

THE DEVELOPING MIND

CHAPTER 1

—

Introduction

Mind, Brain, and Experience

THE DEVELOPING MIND
AND HUMAN RELATIONSHIPS

The mind emerges from the activity of the brain, whose structure and function are directly shaped by interpersonal experience. This book explores how recent findings from the study of human development and neurobiology can bring us to a new understanding of the developing mind.

There are many views from science on how the mind functions, providing in-depth but distinct perspectives on human experience. For example, neuroscience can inform us about how the brain gives rise to mental processes such as memory and perception. Developmental psychology offers us a view of how children's minds grow within families across time. Psychiatry gives us a clinical view of how individuals may suffer from emotional and behavioral disturbances that profoundly alter the course of their lives. Often these disciplines function in isolation from one another. Yet, when one attempts to synthesize their recent findings, an incredible convergence of many of these independent fields of study is revealed. These findings shed light on how the mind emerges from the substance of the brain as it is shaped by interpersonal relationships. My aim is to provide an overview and integration of some of these scientific perspectives, in order to build a foundation for a neurobiology of interpersonal experience.

The ideas of this framework are organized around three funda-mental principles:

1. The human mind emerges from patterns in the flow of energy and information within the brain and between brains.
2. The mind is created within the interaction of internal neuro-physiological processes and interpersonal experiences.
3. The structure and function of the developing brain are deter-mined by how experiences, especially within interpersonal relationships, shape the genetically programmed maturation of the nervous system.

In other words, human connections shape the neural connections from which the mind emerges.

What is the mind? There is an entity called the "mind" that is as real as the heart or the lungs or the brain, though it cannot be seen with or without a microscope. The foundation of the mind parallels a dictionary definition of the psyche: "1. the human soul; 2. the intellect; 3. psychiatry—the mind considered as a subjectively per-ceived, functional entity, based ultimately upon physical processes but with complex processes of its own: it governs the total organism and its interaction with the environment."[1]

Because it reveals the connection between brain structure and function, current neuroscience provides us with new insights into how experience shapes mental processes.[2] By altering both the activ-ity and the structure of the connections between neurons, experience directly shapes the circuits responsible for such processes as memory, emotion, and self-awareness. We can use an understanding of the impact of experience on the mind to deepen our grasp of how the past continues to shape present experience and influence future actions. Insights into the mind, brain, and experience can provide a window into these connections across time, allowing us to see human development in a four-dimensional way.

This book attempts to synthesize concepts and findings from a range of scientific disciplines, including those studying attachment, child development, communication, complex systems, emotion, evo-lution, information processing, memory, narrative, and neurobiology. I have attempted to provide enough of an introduction for those who may be totally unfamiliar with these domains to be able to under-stand the material and apply the relevant findings in their profes-sional work and personal lives. When we examine what is known about how the mind develops, we can gain important insights into the ways in which people can continue to grow throughout life. The mind does not stop developing even as we grow past childhood and adolescence. Through understanding the connections between mental processes and brain functioning, we can build a neurobiological foundation for the ways in which interpersonal relationships—both early in life and throughout adulthood—continue to play a central role in shaping the emerging mind.

ENERGY AND INFORMATION

The mind—the patterns in the flow of energy and information—can be described as emanating from the activity of the neurons of the brain.[3] Several different measures of forms of energy can be used to study these. Brain imaging studies examine the metabolic, energy-consuming processes in specific neural regions, or the blood flow to certain areas that are thought to be a clustering of localized neuronal activity. Electroencephalograms (EEGs) assess the electrical activity across the surface of the brain as measured by electrodes on the head. These assessments of "energy flow" are not popularized, unscientific views of the flow of some mysterious energy through the universe. Neuroscience studies the way in which the brain functions through the energy-consuming activation of neurons. The degree and localization of this arousal and activation within the brain—this flow of energy—directly create our mental processes.

But the mind is more than the flow of energy across time within the brain. The mind is also about the flow of information.[4]

The mind has distinct modes of processing information. For example, our sensory systems can respond to stimuli from the outside world, such as sights or sounds, and can "represent" this information as patterns of neural firing that serve as mental symbols. The activity of the brain creates "representations" of various types of information about the outer and inner worlds. For example, we have representations of sensations in the body, of perceptions from our five senses, of ideas and concepts, and of words. Each of these forms of representation is thought to be created in different circuits of the brain. These information-processing modes can act independently, and also have important interactions with one another that directly affect their processing. We can have complex representations of sensations, perceptions, ideas, and linguistic symbols as we think, for example, of some time in the past. The integration of these distinct modes of information processing into a coherent whole may be a central goal for the developing mind across the lifespan.

Interpersonal relationships may facilitate or inhibit this drive to integrate a coherent experience. Relationships early in life may shape the very structures that create representations of experience and allow a coherent view of the world: Interpersonal experiences directly influence how we mentally construct reality. This shaping process occurs throughout life, but is most crucial during the early years of childhood. Patterns of relationships and emotional communication directly affect the development of the brain. Studies in animals, for example, have demonstrated that even short episodes of maternal deprivation have powerful neuroendocrine effects on the ability to cope with future stressful events.[5] Studies of human subjects reveal that different patterns of child–parent attachment are associated with differing physiological responses, ways of seeing the world, and interpersonal relationship patterns. The communication of emotion may be the primary means by which these attachment experiences shape the developing mind. Research suggests that emotion serves as a central organizing process within the brain. In this way, an individual's abilities to organize emotions—a product, in part, of earlier attachment relationships—directly shapes the ability of the mind to integrate experience and to adapt to future stressors.

THE ORGANIZATION OF THE BOOK

The book is composed of two general forms of information. The scientific findings from a range of disciplines are summarized and synthesized to construct a conceptual foundation for an "interpersonal neurobiology" of the developing mind. This scientific foundation creates a new, interdisciplinary view of established knowledge. Conceptual implications and new proposals that are derived from data, clinical experience, and synthetic reasoning across disciplines can then be drawn from this framework.

Each chapter explores a major domain of human experience: memory, attachment, emotion, representation, states of mind, self-regulation, interpersonal connection, and integration. Presenting the information in this sequence allows for an overview of how experience shapes the mind in the discussions of memory and attachment before the related topics of emotion and representation are addressed. The more elaborated processes of states of mind and complex systems naturally follow and prepare us for a detailed discussion of the ways in which the mind develops the capacity to organize its functioning within self-regulation, patterns of interpersonal connection, and mental integration.

Memory

In Chapter 2, research in various forms of memory is summarized in order to help us understand how our earliest experiences in life shape not only what we remember, but how we remember and how we shape the narrative of our lives. Memory can be seen as the way the mind encodes elements of experience into various forms of representation. As a child develops, the mind begins to create a sense of continuity across time, linking past experiences with present perceptions and anticipations of the future. Within these representational processes, generalizations or mental models of the self and the self with others are created; these form an essential scaffold in which the growing mind interacts with the world.

One way in which the mind attempts to integrate these varied representations and mental models is within the narrative process. Autobiographical narratives are reviewed, in order to explore how the mind creates coherence within its own processes and how this central integrative function influences the nature of interpersonal relationships. In part, such an integrative function reveals the capacity of the mind to represent and process the activity of the minds of both self and others. Such a capacity appears to be central to secure attachment relationships.

Attachment

This overview of the mind, memory, and autobiographical narrative sets the stage for examining attachment in children as well as in adults in Chapter 3. Repeated patterns of children's interactions with their caregivers become "remembered" in the various modalities of memory and directly shape not just what children recall, but how the representational processes develop. Behavior, emotion, perceptions, sensations, and models of others are engrained by experiences that occur before children have autobiographical memory processes available to them. These implicit elements of memory also later influence the structure of autobiographical narratives, which have been found to differ dramatically across the various attachment patterns.

A profound finding from attachment research is that the most robust predictor of a child's attachment to parents is the way in which the parents narrate their own recollections of their childhood experiences. This implies that the structure of an adult's narrative process—not merely *what* the adult recalls, but *how* it is recalled—is the most powerful feature in predicting how an adult will relate to a child. Studies of couples expecting their first child can predict how each parent will relate to their yet-to-be-born infant by examining the nature of the narratives of their own childhoods. The practical relevance of this finding is explored, along with other important discoveries from the field of adult attachment. These attachment studies provide a framework for understanding how communication within relationships facilitates the development of the mind.

Emotion

The primary ingredient of secure attachment experiences is the pattern of emotional communication between child and caregiver. This finding raises the fundamental question of why emotion is so important for the evolving identity and functioning of a child, as well as in the establishment of adult relationships.

Chapter 4 further explores the role of emotion in shaping interpersonal relationships and the human mind. What is emotion? Why does a child require emotional communication and the alignment of emotional states in order to allow for healthy development? To attempt to answer these questions fully, we need to synthesize a number of independent perspectives. The way the mind establishes meaning—the way it places value or significance on experience—is closely linked to social interactions. This connection between meaning and interpersonal experience occurs because these two processes appear to be mediated via the same neural circuits responsible for initiating emotional processes. Research into the nature of emotion serves as the foundation of a synthetic framework for understanding its central role in creating our subjective and our interpersonal experiences.

Representations

In Chapter 5, the way the mind creates mental representations of experience is reviewed in detail. Emotion can be seen as the fundamental process of the mind that links states of arousal with the appraisal of the value or the meaning of its own representational processes. In this way, the mind's creation of representations provides us with insight into how reality is shaped by emotional and interpersonal processes. Our internal experiences are constructive processes; our interpersonal relationships help shape the ways in which these representational processes develop. Emotion can thus be seen as an integrating process that links the internal and interpersonal worlds of the human mind.

From the beginning of life, the brain has an asymmetry in its circuitry, which leads to the specialization of functions on each side of the brain. The ways in which the mind creates representations of experience is shaped by this lateralization of function. The capacities to sense another person's emotions, to understand others' minds, and even to express one's own emotions via facial expressions and tone of voice are all mediated predominantly by the right side of the brain. In certain insecure attachment patterns, communication between parent and child may lack these aspects of emotions and mental experience. In contrast, secure attachments seem to involve the sharing of a wide range of representational processes from both sides of the brain. In essence, such balanced interpersonal communication allows the activity of one mind to sense and respond to the activity of another. Such sharing of activity can be seen as the sharing of states of mind, the topic of the next chapter.

States of Mind

Chapter 6 examines how different mental processes are organized within a state of mind. These states allow disparate activities of the brain to become cohesive at a given moment in time. A single brain functions as a system that can be understood by examining the "theory of nonlinear dynamics of complex systems," or, more briefly, "complexity theory." This perspective has been applied to a range of inanimate and living systems in an attempt to understand the often unpredictable but self-organizing nature of complex clusters of entities functioning as a system. The human brain has recently been examined by a number of theoreticians as one such system. Chapter 6 reviews these ideas and then proposes how the laws of such complex systems can be applied not only to the single mind, but to the functioning of two or more minds acting as a single system. This new application allows us to deepen our earlier discussion of states of mind and their fundamental importance in both creating internal subjective experience and shaping the nature of human relationships.

Self-Regulation

Chapter 7 then explores self-regulation—the way the mind organizes its own functioning—by examining how complex systems, such as the mind and interpersonal relationships, regulate the flow of their states by various means. Self-regulation is fundamentally related to the modulation of emotion. As we'll see, this process involves the regulation of the flow of energy and information via the modulation of arousal and the appraisal of meaning of cognitive representations of experience. Emotion regulation is initially developed from within interpersonal experiences in a process that establishes self-organizational abilities.

Interpersonal Connection

Chapter 8 examines the nature of the connections between minds. Interpersonal relationships shape the mind by allowing new states to emerge within interactions with others. Though relationships early in life shape the structural development of the brain, the mind appears to be open to ways in which interpersonal experience continues to facilitate development throughout the lifespan. Examples from families and individual patients in psychotherapy are offered to illustrate these ideas by examining how patterns of communication between parent and child help determine the ways in which self-regulation emerges early in development. These patterns can help us to understand how relationships throughout life may facilitate emotional well-being. Self-organization thus emerges out of self–other interactions.

Integration

At a given time, a state of mind creates cohesion within the various mental processes that define it. Mental states reflect specific patterns of activity, such as states of anger or shame. Some of these states become engrained over time with characteristic patterns of activity. These states can be seen as "self-states." How the self creates a sense of coherence across time as various self-states become active is reflected in the concept of integration, the central topic of Chapter 9. "Integration" refers to the way the mind establishes a functional flow in the states of mind across time. An important means of assessing integration is in the coherence of the structure of autobiographical narratives. Narrative coherence is reflected in both the way a life story is told and the manner in which life activities are lived. These linguistic and behavioral outputs are generated from a proposed central integrative process. Developing the capacity to integrate mental coherence is profoundly influenced by experience. In this way, attachment histories revealed in adult attachment narratives reflect the capacity of the individual to integrate a coherent sense of self.

By organizing the self across past, present, and future, the integrating mind creates a sense of coherence and continuity. In various forms of mental dysfunction, integration may be impaired, leading to a sense of paralysis or chaos. The ways in which human relationships foster resilience and emotional well-being by facilitating an integrative capacity are explored as part of the developmental framework of mind, brain, and interpersonal experience.

APPROACHING NEUROBIOLOGY

What are the mechanisms by which human relationships shape brain structure and function? How is it possible for interpersonal experience—the interactions between two people—to affect something so inherently different as the activity of neurons? Though this book is organized by a focus on the mental processes described above, exploring insights from neuroscience will greatly enhance our ability to address these basic questions. For this reason, this introductory chapter offers a brief overview of some relevant aspects of neurobiology—the study of the way neurons work and how the brain functions.

(A brief note for those new to thinking about the brain: The aim of the book is to help you to understand the developing mind by providing an integration of mental processes [such as memory and emotion] with both neurobiology [such as neural activity in specific circuits] and interpersonal relationships [such as patterns of communication]. This integration is indeed the challenge of the book, both in the writing and in the reading. My concern is that those who are new to neurobiology—like many of my students in the past—may initially feel too overwhelmed at the unfamiliar ideas and vocabulary to continue. Numerous teaching experiences, however, have demonstrated that the outcome is worth the effort. There are many readily accessible concepts and much useful information just below the surface of these sometimes new names and ideas. A shared understanding of neurobiology from the beginning will help you in making

sense of the intricate and exciting findings about interpersonal relationships and the developing mind. I have tried to include enough of
a background as the chapters evolve that each domain can be understood by those who may be totally unfamiliar with a given area.
New concepts and vocabulary are inevitable, but I have tried to
incorporate information throughout the book in a "user-friendly"
manner, summarizing the significance of certain findings and including reminders of certain trends as they recur in the book. For those
who are charting new waters, I welcome you to the exciting world of
interdisciplinary study!)

What follows is a brief overview of some relevant highlights
from neurobiology. This information may be useful as a resource
later in the book and is offered here as an introductory frame of ref-
erence.

The Organization of the Brain

The brain is a complex system of interconnected parts. The "lower
structures" include those circuits of the brainstem deep within the
skull that mediate basic elements of energy flow, such as states of
arousal and alertness and the physiological state of the body (temperature, respiration, heart rate). At the top of the brainstem is the
thalamus, an area that serves as a gateway for incoming sensory
information and has extensive connections to other regions of the
brain, including the neocortex, just above it. As we shall see, one theory considers the activity of the thalamocortical circuit to be a central process for the mediation of conscious experience. The "higher
structures," such as the neocortex at the top of the brain, mediate
"more complex" information-processing functions such as perception, thinking, and reasoning. These areas are considered to be the
most evolutionarily "advanced" in humans and mediate the complex
perceptual and abstract representations that constitute our associational thought processes. The centrally located "limbic system"—
including the regions called the orbitofrontal cortex, anterior cingulate, and amygdala—plays a central role in coordinating the activity
of higher and lower brain structures. The limbic regions are thought
to mediate emotion, motivation, and goal-directed behavior. Limbic
structures permit the integration of a wide range of basic mental processes, such as the appraisal of meaning, the processing of social
experience (called "social cognition"), and the regulation of emotion.
This region also houses the medial temporal lobe (toward the mid-

dle, just to the sides of the temples), including the hippocampus, which is thought to play a central role in consciously accessible forms of memory. The brain as a whole functions as an interconnected and integrating system of subsystems. Although each element contributes to the functioning of the whole, regions such as the limbic system, with extensive input and output pathways linking widely distributed areas in the brain, may be primarily responsible for integrating brain activity. When we look to understand how the mind develops, we need to examine how the brain comes to regulate its own processes. Such self-regulation appears to be carried out in large part by these limbic regions.

The limbic and lower regions of the brain also house the hypothalamus and the pituitary, which are responsible for physiological homeostasis, or bodily equilibrium, established by way of neuroendocrine activity (neuronal firing and hormonal release). Stress is often responded to by the "hypothalamic–pituitary–adrenocortical (HPA) axis," and this system can be adversely affected by trauma. This neuroendocrine axis, along with the autonomic nervous system (regulating such things as heart rate and respiration) and the neuroimmune system (regulating the body's immunological defense system) are ways in which the function of the brain and body are intricately intertwined.

To gain a visual grasp of some of this brain structure, it may be helpful to use a readily available, three-dimensional model that will enable you to have neuroanatomy in the palm of your hand, so to speak. If you make a fist with your thumb bent toward the center of your palm and your fingers curled around it and resting on the lower part of your hand, you'll have a model of the brain: Your lower arm represents the location of the spinal cord inside the backbone and your wrist is at the base of the skull; the various parts of your hand represent the three major regions we've discussed above—lower, limbic, and neocortical areas. Looking directly at your fist from the palmar side, the orbits of the eyes would emerge around the areas of the fingernails of your third and fourth fingers. The ears would extend from either side of your fist. Your fingers represent the neocortex: Facing you are its frontal lobes; at the top are the neocortical areas that mediate motor control and somatosensory representations; to the sides and back of your hand are the posterior parts that mediate perceptual processing. The lower parts of the brain are represented by the midline portion of your lower palm. Just below your knuckles, deep inside your fist where the end of your thumb rests, is the limbic system. Most of the brain is split into the left and right hemispheres, which are connected with bands of tissue called the corpus callosum and the anterior commissures, thought to serve as direct sources of information transfer between the two sides of the brain. The cerebellum, which would be located at the back of your hand near its connection to your wrist, may also indirectly transfer information across the division that separates the two halves of the brain. The cerebellum itself may carry out a number of informational and integrating processes.

The areas of your fist jutting out from the front of your palm are the frontal lobes. The very front of this anterior region is called the prefrontal cortex, an area we will be exploring throughout the book. We will examine two important aspects of this frontal neocortical region: the ventral medial (also known as the orbitofrontal cortex, the term we shall use in this book) and the lateral prefrontal cortex. The lateral prefrontal cortex rests to the sides (thus "lateral") and is represented by your index finger on one side and your fifth finger on the other. The lateral prefrontal cortex is thought to play a major role in working memory and the focusing of conscious attention. On your fist model, the orbitofrontal area lies, as you may have guessed, just behind and above the orbits of the eyes, especially where your last knuckles bend and the tips of your fingers push inward toward your palm. Notice that in this position the orbitofrontal region is adjacent to a number of areas from which it receives and to which it sends pathways carrying information: the deeper structures of the brain that process sensory and bodily data, the limbic system itself, and the neocortex just above it. In this manner, the orbitofrontal region can be seen, in fact, as the uppermost part of the limbic system as well as a part of the frontal lobes of the neocortex. Some call this area a part of the "paralimbic" cortex. This three-dimensional model thus gives you a direct experiential/ visual example of neural interconnections and the relevance of anatomy for coordinated function.

The brain is highly interconnected, and controversy exists in academic circles about how distinct these regions actually are in anatomy and function.[6] The notion of a limbic "system," for example, has been challenged, in that defining its limits (where it starts and where it ends) has been scientifically difficult. Nevertheless, the limbic regions appear to utilize specific neurotransmitters, to have highly interconnected circuitry, to carry out complementary functions, and to have similarities in their evolutionary history. For example, the orbitofrontal cortex, sitting at the top of the limbic system and anatomically connected to a wide array of areas in the neocortex and the deeper structures of the brain, carries out a vital role in the coordination of the activity from all three regions.[7] As we shall see, recent studies from neuroscience suggest that this orbitofrontal region may play a major role in many of the integrating processes we will be examining, such as memory, emotion, and attachment.

The brain has an estimated one hundred billion neurons, which are collectively over two million miles long. Each neuron has an average of ten thousand connections that directly link itself to other neurons.[8] Thus there are thought to be about one million billion of these connections, making it "the most complex structure, natural or artificial, on earth."[9] A neuron sends an electrical impulse down its long axons; this releases a neurotransmitter at the space at the end, called a "synapse," which then excites or inhibits the downstream neuron. A synapse is the connection that functionally links neurons to one another. Because of the spider-web-like interconnections, activation of one neuron can influence an average of ten thousand neurons at the receiving ends! The number of possible "on–off" patterns of neuronal firing is immense, estimated as a staggering ten times ten one million times (ten to the millionth power). The brain is obviously capable of an imponderably huge variety of activity; the fact that it is often organized and functional is quite an accomplishment!

Brain Development

The activation of neural pathways directly influences the way connections are made within the brain. Though experience shapes the activity of the brain and the strength of neuronal connections throughout life, experience early in life may be especially crucial in organizing the way the basic structures of the brain develop. For example, traumatic experiences at the beginning of life may have more profound effects on the "deeper" structures of the brain, which are responsible for basic regulatory capacities and enable the mind to respond later to stress. Thus we see that abused children have elevated baseline and reactive stress hormone levels. More common, everyday experiences also shape brain structure. The brain's development is an "experience-dependent" process, in which experience activates certain pathways in the brain, strengthening existing connections and creating new ones. Lack of experience can lead to cell death in a process called "pruning." This is sometimes called a "use-it-or-lose-it" principle of brain development. An infant is born with a genetically programmed excess in neurons, and the postnatal establishment of synaptic connections is determined by both genes and experience. Genes contain the information for the general organization of the brain's structure, but experience determines which genes become expressed, how, and when. The expression of genes leads to the production of proteins that enable neuronal growth and the formation of new synapses. Experience—the activation of specific neural pathways—therefore directly shapes gene expression and leads to the maintenance, creation, and strengthening of the connections that form the neural substrate of the mind. Early in life, interpersonal relationships are a primary source of the experience that shapes how genes express themselves within the brain.

At birth, the infant's brain is the most undifferentiated organ in the body. Genes and early experience shape the way neurons connect to one another and thus form the specialized circuits that give rise to mental processes. In this way, experiences early in life have a tremendously important impact on the developing mind. The differentiation of circuits within the brain involves a number of processes including (1) the growth of axons into local and widely distributed regions; (2) the establishment of new and more extensive synaptic connections between neurons; (3) the growth of myelin along the lengths of neurons, which increases the speed of nerve conduction and thus "functionally" enhances the linkage among synaptically connected nerve cells; (4) the modification of receptor density and sensitivity at the postsynaptic "receiving" cell making connections more efficient; and (5) the balance of all of these factors with the dying away or pruning of neurons and synapses resulting from disuse or toxic conditions such as chronic stress. In experimental animals, enriched environments have been shown to lead to increased density of synaptic connections and especially to an increased number of neurons and actual volume of the hippocampus, a region important for learning and memory.[10] Experiences lead to an increased activity of neurons, which enhances the creation of new synaptic connections. This experience-dependent brain growth and differentiation is thus referred to as an "activity-dependent" process.

Interpersonal experiences continue to influence how our minds function throughout life, but the major structures—especially those that are responsible for self-regulation—appear to be formed in the early years. It is for this reason that we will look closely at the early years of life to understand the ways in which the mind develops and comes to regulate its own processes. An open question in neuro-biology is how "plastic," or open to further development, the brain remains throughout the lifespan. We can look toward the lessons from studies of early interpersonal experience to try to understand the ways in which relationships may continue to foster the develop-ment of the mind throughout life.

Information Processing and Neurobiology

From an information-processing perspective, brain anatomy and neu-ral circuit functioning can be understood as follows. Signals from the deep structures representing physiological data from the body are received and processed by the centrally located limbic structures. More elaborately processed data from the activities of the limbic sys-tem itself are integrated by limbic regions, including the orbitofrontal cortex and anterior cingulate. These areas send emotional and somatosensory input to the neocortex, which also processes percep-tual representations from the sensory cortices, conceptual from the associational cortices, and linguistic representations from the lan-guage-processing centers. The information-processing task of inte-grating regions such as the associational cortices and orbitofrontal cortex is to take in the different neural "codes," coordinate the infor-mation contained within these signals, and "translate" them into transformed neural activity, which then is sent as output to the vari-ous regions. Such neural translation of the various forms of represen-tations allows for information to be both processed and then com-municated in different codes to the relevant regions. This translation process allows for a type of neural integration of complex informa-tion within the mind.

An analogy is this: We can transmit an electronic mail message with a file containing the twenty-six letters of the alphabet, spacing, and a handful of punctuation marks. With electrical flow through wires in a pattern of impulses, we can send a detailed written note. Through the same wires, we can send an entire photograph or even a video. Though the message contains different information (note, photo, video), the fundamental form in which the data is transmitted is identical—electrical impulses flowing as patterns of energy through a wire. The information contained within the different messages var-ies in its patterns and its complexity. Without the proper receiving device to translate these electrical impulses into words, pictures, or video, the complex representation has no meaning.

The same is true with the brain. Neural activity is the fundamental form in which information is transmitted. The sending area is capable of transmitting a certain kind of information as neural codes. The receiving circuits or systems must be capable of processing such signals for them to have any meaning. The brain is genetically programmed to be able to differentiate its regions, which carry different forms of information. These forms vary in pattern and complexity from the most "simple" signals of the deeper structures (such as heart rate) to the more complex ones of the neocortex (such as ideas about freedom or about the mind itself). Experience not only provides the input that serves to activate (give the information to) these regions; it is necessary for the proper development of the brain itself. Experience-dependent maturation is a part of even the basic sensory systems of our brains. The brain must "use it or lose it" in many cases of brain specialization. For example, studies in animals reveal that the lack of exposure to certain types of visual information, such as vertical lines, during a critical period early in life leads to loss of the capacity for perceiving such lines later in life. Specific forms of experience are necessary for the normal development of information-processing circuits in the visual cortex.[11] The same process may occur for other systems in the brain, such as the attachment system. Children who have had no experience with an attachment figure (not merely suboptimal attachment, but a lack of attachment) for the first several years of life may suffer a significant loss of the capacity to establish intimate interpersonal relationships later on.[12]

In this way, we can reexamine one of our initial questions: How does experience shape the mind? A general principle can be proposed here: *Experiences can shape not only what information enters the mind, but the way in which the mind develops the ability to process that information.* How this occurs can be seen as the modification of the actual circuits of the brain responsible for processing that particular type of information. Experience creates representations, as well as stimulating the capacity for specific forms of information processing.

The Brain as a System

At the most basic level, the brain can be considered as a living system that is open and dynamic. It is an integrated collection of component subsystems that interact together in a patterned and changing way to create an irreducible quality of the system as a whole.[13] A living system must be open to the influences of the environment in order to survive, and the brain is no exception. The system of the brain becomes functionally linked to other systems, especially to other brains. The brain is also dynamic, meaning that it is forever in a state of change. An open, dynamic system is one that is in continual emergence with a changing environment and the changing state of its own activity.

Furthermore, the brain is a complex system, meaning that there are multiple layers of component parts capable of chaotic behavior.[14] These parts can be conceptualized at various levels of analysis, and include the single neuron and its sending and receiving functions; neuronal groups; circuits; systems; regions; hemispheres; and the whole brain. The basic components, the neurons, are the simplest. As we move up the levels of components, the units become more and more elaborate. Some authors use the terms "lower-order" to refer to the basic level of organizational unit and "higher-order" to refer to the more intricate level of organization. For the most part, each subsystem can be considered to have both lower and higher orders of systems with which it relates. For example, the activity of the visual cortex is made up of the lower-level input from the eyes, but itself contributes to the higher-level processing of the entire perceptual system.[15]

From the point of view of the brain as an open system, each region of the brain may take in unique input from outside of itself. The deeper structures of the brain receive sensory input from the body and from the external world; the limbic system receives input from the deeper structures and from the neocortex; and the neocortex receives data from the limbic system itself. Neuroanatomic studies reveal that the neocortical regions are also intricately interwoven with the "lower" levels of the system, and thus our "higher thinking" is actually directly dependent upon activity of the entire brain. The regions coordinating the state of activation of the subcomponents of the brain, however, are not in the "most evolved," higher-level neocortex. For this reason, the limbic system is more effective in the regulation of the body and emotions than the "higher" neocortex. This finding also demonstrates how emotions, generated and regulated by the activity of the limbic system, are integral parts of our neocortically derived "rational thoughts" as well as the overall functioning of our minds.[16]

These issues also suggest that specific circuits within the brain may function as somewhat distinct "subsystems" that create their own predominant states of processing. For example, the left and right sides of the brain have distinct circuits that become predominant early in life, even in the embryo. Each of these pathways has its dominant neurotransmitters and involves distinct evaluative components that serve to direct each hemisphere to process information in distinct manners. How each hemisphere is activated will directly shape our subjective sensations and the ways in which we communicate with others.

Genes and Experience

In an era when science is enabling us to understand human experience in new ways, it is important to examine the common debate about how much of development and personality can be attributed to "nature" or genetics, as opposed to "nurture" or experience. Misinterpretations of genetic studies have lead to beliefs such as "What parents do has no effect on their children's development." Although it is certainly true that temperament and other constitutional variables play a huge, and perhaps previously underrecognized, role in child development,[17] riding the swing of the "What shapes development?" pendulum to either the genetics end or the experience end can lead to erroneous conclusions.[18]

A wide range of studies[19] has in fact now clarified that development is a product of the effect of experience on the unfolding of genetic potential. Genes encode the information for how neurons are to grow, make connections with each other, and die back as the brain attains differentiation of its circuitry. These processes are genetically preprogrammed *and* experience-dependent. Genes have two major functions.[20] First, they act as "templates" for information that is to be passed on to the next generation; second, they have a "transcription" function based on the information encoded within their DNA, which determines which proteins will be synthesized. Transcription is directly influenced by experience. Experience determines when genes express themselves via the process of protein synthesis. For the brain, this means that experience directly influences how neurons will connect to one another—creating new synaptic connections, altering their strengths, and allowing others to die away.[21]

Genes do not act in isolation from experience. Genes and experience interact in such a way that certain biological tendencies can create characteristic experiences. For example, certain temperaments may produce characteristic parental responses.[22] These responses in turn shape the way in which neuronal growth, interconnections, and pruning (dying back) occur. Embracing this approach to the nature–nurture issue can allow us to move on scientifically solid grounds toward understanding human development and the growth of the mind. The question isn't "Is it heredity *or* experience?", but "How do heredity *and* experience interact in the development of an individual?"

Allan Schore addresses the issue of how child–caregiver interactions shape the development of the brain:

> In such transactions the primary caregiver is providing experiences which shape genetic potential by acting as a psychobiological regulator (or dysregulator) of hormones that directly influence gene transcription. This mechanism mediates a process by which psychoneuroendocrinological changes during critical periods initiate permanent effects at the genomic level. The final developmental outcome of early endocrine–gene interactions is expressed in the imprinting of evolving brain circuitry.[23]

The development of the mind has been described as having "recursive" features.[24] That is, what an individual's mind presents to the world can reinforce the very things that are presented. A typical environmental/parental response to a child's behavioral output may reinforce that behavior. Therefore, the child plays a part in shaping the experiences to which the child's mind must adapt. In this way, behavior itself alters genetic expression, which then creates behavior. In the end, changes in the organization of brain function, emotional regulation, and long-term memory are mediated by alterations in neural structure. These structural changes are due to the activation or deactivation of genes encoding information for protein synthesis. Experience, gene expression, mental activity, behavior, and continued interactions with the environment (experience) are tightly linked in a transactional set of processes.[25] Such is the recursive nature of development and the way in which nature and nurture, genes and experience, are inextricably part of the same process.

Genetic studies of behavior commonly note that fifty percent of each of the personality features measured is attributable to heredity. The majority of the other half of the variability is thought to be due to "nonshared" aspects of the environment, such as school experiences and peer relationships.[26] But siblings—including even identical twins, who are raised by the same parents at the same time—actually have a "nonshared" environment, in that parental behavior is not identical for each child.[27] The recursive quality of mental development magnifies initial individual differences and creates a challenge to the sometimes held opinion that growing up in the same family is a shared (statistically identical) experience. This reminds us that each individual's history reflects an inseparable blend of how the environment, random events, and the person's temperament all contribute to the creation of experiences in which adaptation and learning recursively shape the development of the mind.

The importance of "epigenetic factors"—the ways in which experience directly influences how genes are expressed—is also revealed in the study of the inheritance of certain psychiatric disorders, such as schizophrenia.[28] In identical twins, who share all of their genetic information, there is less than a fifty percent concordance in the behavioral expression of the illness. This implies that many factors determine how a "genotype" (genetic template or information) becomes expressed as a "phenotype" (genetic transcription function leading to protein synthesis and external manifestation as physical or behavioral features).

For the growing brain of a young child, the social world supplies the most important experiences influencing the expression of genes, which determines how neurons connect to one another in creating the neuronal pathways which give rise to mental activity. The function of these pathways is determined by their structure; thus alterations in genetic expression change brain structure and shape the developing mind. The functioning of the mind—derived from neural activity—in turn alters the physiological environment of the brain, and thus itself can produce changes in gene expression. This is clearly seen in the production of corticosteroids as a response to stress, which directly influences gene function.[29] In children with shy temperaments, for example, there is a huge physiological response to even mild environmental changes.[30] Such individuals create their own internal world of stress responses that heighten their brains' reactivity to novelty.[31] Likewise, a child traumatized early in life will have an alteration in physiological response, such that small stressors lead to large hormonal responses.[32] Thus both constitutional and experientially "acquired" reactivity can lead to further physiological features that maintain the hypervigilant response over time. Jerome Kagan and his colleagues have demonstrated that parenting behavior makes a large difference for the trajectory of development.[33] In their research, those parents who supportively encouraged their shy children to explore new situations enabled the children to develop more outgoing behaviors than those parents who did not help their children with their fears. These and other intervention studies clearly demonstrate that parenting has a direct effect on developmental outcome, even in the face of significant inherited features of physiological reactivity.[34] Throughout the book we will return to discussions of shy and traumatized children as examples of the interactions between constitutional and experiential variables in development.

Interpersonal Experience and the Brain

In this book, I am proposing that the mind develops at the interface of neurophysiological processes and interpersonal relationships. Relationship experiences have a dominant influence on the brain because the circuits responsible for social perception are the same as or tightly linked to those that integrate the important functions controlling the creation of meaning, the regulation of bodily states, the modulation of emotion, the organization of memory, and the capacity for interpersonal communication. Interpersonal experience thus plays a special organizing role in determining the development of brain structure early in life and the ongoing emergence of brain function throughout the lifespan.

One fundamental finding relevant for developing this "interpersonal neurobiology" of the mind comes from numerous studies across a wide variety of cultures: Attachment is based on collaborative communication. Secure attachment involves contingent communication, in which the signals of one person are directly responded to by the other. Sounds simple. But why is this type of reciprocal communication so important? Why doesn't it happen in all families? During early development, a parent and child "tune in" to each other's feelings and intentions in a dance of connection that establishes the earliest form of communication. Mary Ainsworth's early studies suggest that healthy, secure attachment requires that the caregiver have the capacity to perceive and respond to the child's mental state.[35]

We will review recent findings from neuroscience that can help us to understand the mechanisms underlying how these early reciprocal communication experiences are remembered and how they allow a child's brain to develop a balanced capacity to regulate emotions, to feel connected to other people, to establish an autobiographical story, and to move out into the world with a sense of vitality. The capacity to reflect on mental states, both of the self and of others, emerges from within attachment relationships that foster such processes.[36] These patterns of communication literally shape the structure of the child's developing brain. These important early interpersonal experiences are encoded within various forms of memory. But the need for this type of communication and connection may not end with childhood. As adults, we need not only to be understood and cared about, but to have another individual simultaneously experience a state of mind similar to our own. With this shared, collaborative experience, life can be filled with an integrating sense of connection and meaning.

CHAPTER 2

Memory

A GENERAL DEFINITION OF MEMORY

We often think of "memory" as what we can consciously recall about what happened in the past. If you think about what you did last weekend or last year, for example, you may begin to visualize some event or interaction with other people. How are experiences remembered? How does recollection actually happen? In this chapter, we explore answers to these questions by looking at what is known about the mechanisms of memory. Although people have been fascinated with memory for thousands of years of recorded history, reflecting on past experiences and telling the stories of major events, it is only recently that we have been able to understand in a scientific way what some of the basic elements of memory actually are.[1]

As we explore the remembering mind, try to keep an eye on your everyday basic assumptions about memory. You may be surprised to find that many of them are helpful, but that some of them may be in need of revision. Common misconceptions about memory include the following: that we are always aware of what we have experienced; that when we remember something, we have the feeling of recollection; and that the mind is somehow able to make a sort of photograph of experiences, which is stored without further modification. Recollection is thus often seen as the presentation of some bits of information, independent of elements present at the time of recall or of bias by prior experiences. As we'll see, the structure of memory is quite complex and sensitive to both external and internal factors as it constructs the past, the present, and the anticipated future.[2]

23

Memory is more than what we can consciously recall about events from the past. A broader definition is that *memory is the way past events affect future function*. Memory is thus the way the brain is affected by experience and then subsequently alters its future responses. In this view, the brain experiences the world and encodes this interaction in a manner that alters future ways of responding. What we shall soon see is that this definition of memory allows us to understand how past events can directly shape how and what we learn, even though we may have no conscious recollection of those events. Our earliest experiences shape our ways of behaving, including patterns of relating to others, without our ability to recall consciously when these first learning experiences occurred.

As discussed in Chapter 1, the brain is composed of spider-web-like neural networks capable of firing in a myriad of patterns, called a "neural net profile."[3] Scientists studying the behavior of such networks have found that the structure of the neural net allows it to learn through an encoding process that initially activates a specific set of associated neuronal firing patterns, which are distributed throughout the brain.[4] Writers who explore this phenomenon describe what has been called "connectionist theory" and "parallel distributed processing." The essential feature of these studies is that the connection of neurons in an intricate network, the structure of the brain, allows for learning to occur.[5] It is the firing of the components of the network, the circuits of neurons, that alters the probabilities of certain patterns' firing in the future. If a certain pattern has been stimulated in the past, the probability of activating a similar profile in the future is enhanced. If the pattern is fired repeatedly, the probability of future activation is further increased. The increased probability is created by changes in the synaptic connections within the network of neurons. Changes at the level of the cell membrane thus alter the firing probability of specific combinations of neurons.[6] The process of "long-term potentiation" has been described as one way in which such alteration of connection strengths among neurons occurs.[7] The specific pattern of firing, the energy contained within a certain neural net profile of activated neurons, contains within it "information." Thus the network learns from its past experiences. *The increased probability of firing a similar pattern is how the network "remembers."* Information is encoded and retrieved through the synaptic changes that direct the flow of energy through the neural system, the brain.

In a direct way, experience shapes the structure of the brain. As we've seen in Chapter 1, this general process is called "experience-dependent" brain development and refers to the general processes by which neuronal connections are maintained, strengthened, or created during experience. As we continue to learn and remember throughout life, our brains and our minds can be seen as having ongoing development across the lifespan. The infant brain has an overabundance of neurons with relatively few synaptic connections at birth, compared to the highly differentiated and interconnected set of connections that will be established in the first few years of life. Experience and genetic information will determine to a large extent how those connections are established. Memory utilizes the processes by which chemical alterations strengthen associations among neurons for short-term encoding and actually activate the genetic machinery required for the establishment of new synaptic connections for long-term memory storage.

As Milner, Squire, and Kandel have noted, "recent work on plasticity in the sensory cortices has introduced the idea that the structure of the brain, even in sensory cortex, is unique to each individual and dependent on each individual's experiential history."[8] Thus the structure and function of the brain are shaped by experience. Developmental and memory processes may actually be based on similar neural and molecular mechanisms underlying synapse formation.[9] These changes in synaptic connection alter the ways in which the brain functions. What we usually think of as "memory" refers to the way in which events can influence the brain in a way that allows for future activity to be altered in a specific manner. As we'll see, the brain has a wide array of direct mechanisms by which it "remembers" experience.

How we recall the past will be determined by which components of the massive network of the brain is activated in the future. For example, if you see the Eiffel Tower on a trip to Paris, your visual system (and other parts of your brain) will respond to the sight with activation of its circuitry, creating a representation or image of the Tower within your mind. This is called "encoding" a memory. The next stage is the "storage" of memory, which is the increased probability that a similar profile will be activated again in the future. Note that there is no "storage closet" in the brain in which something is placed and then taken out when needed. *Memory storage is the change in probability of activating a particular neural network pattern in the future.* Your brain will have the potential to reactivate the visual circuitry, the neural net profile, similar to the initial encoding. Memory, then, is a process which is based on altering the probabilities of neuronal firing. "Retrieval" is the actual activation of that potential neural net profile, which resembles—but is not identical with—the profile activated in the past. Thus, when you intentionally try to recall the Eiffel Tower, you may experience an internal visual image of the structure, as well as other aspects of your Paris journey.

The neural net of the brain can activate a set of anatomically and chronologically associated firings in response to the environment. This profile is encoded, stored, and retrieved on the basis of a simple axiom defined by Donald Hebb: Neurons which fire together at one time will tend to fire together in the future.[10] Another way of phrasing Hebb's law is this: Neurons that fire together wire together. As Donald Hebb pointed out, in 1949, "The general idea is an old one, that any two cells or systems of cells that are repeatedly active at the same time will tend to become 'associated,' so that activity in one facilitates activity in the other."[11] This neural association that functionally links the activity of neurons is now understood to involve transient metabolic changes for short-term memory and more stable structural changes for long-term memory storage. The principle of linkage involves both anatomic and temporal association of neuronal activity. As we'll see, this temporospatial integration of function at the neural level means that it is fundamentally through memory that the complex neural network creates anatomically distributed and functionally clustered assemblies of activation across time. The alteration of synaptic connections, or "synaptic strengths," either by the creation of new connections or the modification of existing ones (for example, by way of changes in neurotransmitter release or receptor sensitivity) directly changes the probabilities of neuronal firing. This associational process is called Hebb's Axiom, in honor of his foresight into these basic processes. This is the essence of how the neural net remembers.

Let's continue with the example of the Eiffel Tower. You may be able—if you've actually seen the Tower or a picture of it—to "see" an image of the Tower in your mind's eye. What does this actually mean? Recent brain studies suggest that, given the task to visualize an object, the parts of your brain responsible for visual processing will become active.[12] What is believed to be occurring is that a neural net profile similar to the one activated at the time you actually saw the object is now being reactivated in the same parts of the brain. This is called a "visual representation." Thus the mind is able to generate a pattern of neural firing at the time of seeing with your eyes, as well as to generate an image independently in the process of imagining with your mind. Representations come in many forms, including perceptual ones (like visualizing the Eiffel Tower), semantic ones (like seeing the words "Eiffel Tower" and knowing their meaning), and multiple sensory ones (such as having a feeling of hunger because when you were at the Tower you had to wait for a picnic, and now your mind is bringing up the associated sensation of hunger).[13]

Our memories are based on the binding together of various aspects of these neuronal activation patterns. These "associational linkages" make it more likely that items will be activated simultaneously during the retrieval process. Representations are linked together via a wide range of internal mental processes unique to each individual. Brain imaging studies suggest that the representation of an experience may be stored in particular regions of the brain, such as the perceptual areas in the posterior part of the neocortex (at the back of the head), which initially were activated in response to the experience. Encoding and retrieval processes may be mediated via separate regions (such as the orbitofrontal cortex, just in back of and above the eyes).[14] Thus specific regions may actively mediate a process whereby neural activation patterns (representations) are activated and then bound together in the act of encoding or during recollection.[15] What are stored are the probabilities of neurons' firing in a specific pattern—not actual "things." Your recollection of the Eiffel Tower will differ from mine for many reasons: the unique aspects of several factors such as the nature of our experiences, the ways in which our brains create representations, and the manner in which the encoding and retrieval process may function. For example, if you were bitten by a dog during that Parisian picnic, you may begin to feel a sense of fear or even pain (emotional and bodily representations, respectively) when you think of the Tower. If you loved France, your sensory representations may be quite different than they would be if you disliked France when you first visited. How you feel at the time you are remembering will also profoundly influence which elements become associated with this complexly bound representation during retrieval.

In memory research, the initial impact of an experience on the brain has been called an "engram."[16] If you visited the Eiffel Tower with a friend and were talking about existential philosophy and Impressionist paintings as you were having your picnic, your engram might include the various levels of experience: semantic (factual—something about philosophy or art or knowledge about the Tower), autobiographical (your sense of yourself at that time in your life), somatic (what your body felt like at the time), perceptual (what things looked like, how they smelled), emotional (your mood at the time), and behavioral (what you were doing with your body). Your original Eiffel Tower engram would include linkages connecting each of these forms of representations. Scientists have named the first two types of consciously accessible memory "explicit" or "declarative" memory. The other forms of memory are quite distinct and are grouped together as "implicit" or "nondeclarative" memory. Researchers have used various names such as "early" versus "late," "nondeclarative" versus "declarative," "procedural" versus "semantic/episodic," and "implicit" versus "explicit."[17] For the purposes of this book, the terms "implicit" and "explicit" are used to identify these functionally distinct systems.

Some authors use the notion of "trace theory" to describe the encoding, storage, and retrieval processes of memory. In this view, your engram or memory trace has both a "gist" (the general notion that you were in France at the Tower) and specific details.[18] With time, the details of an experience may begin to fade away and become less tightly bound together. The gist, however, may remain easily accessible for retrieval and quite accurate. When we try to retrieve an "original memory," in fact, we may be calling up the gist at first ("I was at the Eiffel Tower when I was in my early twenties") and then later trying to reconstruct the details. This reconstruction process may be profoundly influenced by the present environment, the questioning context itself, and other factors, such as current emotions and our perception of the expectations of those listening to the response. Memory is not a static thing, but an active set of processes. Even the most "concrete" experiences, such as recalling an architectural structure, are actually dynamic representational processes. Remembering is not merely the reactivation of an old engram; *it is the construction of a new neural net profile with features of the old engram and elements of memory from other experiences, as well as influences from the present state of mind.*

IMPLICIT MEMORY: MENTAL MODELS, BEHAVIORS, IMAGES, AND EMOTIONS

From the first days of life, infants perceive the environment around them. Research has shown that infants are able to demonstrate recall for experiences in the form of behavioral, perceptual, and emotional learning.[19] Examples of these forms of memory are numerous and demonstrate how active infants are in perceiving and learning about their environment. Babies can turn their heads to a learned stimulus. They can perceive visual patterns and can even relate these to other perceptual modalities, such as touch or sound. If they become frightened by a loud noise associated with a particular toy, they will get upset when shown that toy in the future. These forms of memory are called "implicit." They are available early in life and, when retrieved, are not thought to carry with them the internal sensation that something is being recalled. An infant who sees that toy just gets upset; the infant doesn't sense, "Oh, yes, I remember that toy. It made a loud noise before. Perhaps it will make one again. Oh, no!" Instead, the neural net/Hebbian associations automatically link the visual input of the toy with an internal emotional response of fear.

Implicit memory involves parts of the brain that do not require conscious processing during encoding or retrieval.[20] When implicit memory is retrieved, the neural net profiles that are reactivated involve circuits in the brain that are a fundamental part of our everyday experience of life: behaviors, emotions, and images. These implicit elements form part of the foundation for our subjective sense of ourselves: We act, feel, and imagine without recognition of the influence of past experience on our present reality.

Implicit memory relies on brain structures that are intact at birth and remain available to us throughout life. These structures include the amygdala and other limbic regions for emotional memory, the basal ganglia and motor cortex for behavioral memory, and the perceptual cortices for perceptual memory. Though research has not explored somatosensory (bodily) memory as a part of implicit processes, one could imagine that this form of nonverbal recall might meet the criteria for implicit memory and possibly be mediated by the somatosensory cortex, the orbitofrontal cortex, and the anterior cingulate—regions responsible for bodily representations.

With repeated experiences, the infant's brain—functioning with its rapidly developing neural net/parallel processor—is able to detect similarities and differences across experiences. From these comparative processes, the infant's mind is able to make "summations" or generalized representations from repeated experiences as encoded in these areas of the brain. This is a fundamental aspect of learning. These generalizations form the basis of "mental models" or "schemata," which help the infant (in fact, each of us) to interpret present experiences as well as to anticipate future ones. *Mental models are basic components of implicit memory.* Our minds use mental models of the world in order to assess a situation more rapidly and to determine what the next moment in time is most likely to offer.

The brain creates multimodal models—models that span perceptual modalities. For example, if infants are allowed to feel the shape of a nipple with their mouths in a darkened room, they later will be able to pick out the familiar nipple from a visual display.[21] Their minds have created a mental image from touch, which then can be used to sense a familiar pattern by sight. The brain can also average across different experiences. Infants can be shown an array of facial images and then later pick out the ones that are summations of those seen earlier. From the first days of life, the infant's brain is capable of creating a multimodal model of the world. These capacities further suggest that the mind is capable from the very beginning of creating generalizations from experience.

These mental models are derived from encounters with the world. Mental models in turn help the mind to seek out familiar objects or experiences and to know what to expect from the environment. Deviations from the usual can be ascertained, and the world becomes a familiar and negotiable place to live. Studies of children and adults suggest that here-and-now perceptual biases are based on these nonconscious mental models.[22] For example, if you've seen numerous city streets before, you may be more likely to see the next one from a similar viewpoint, without examining subtle differences in detail. On the other hand, if you have never been to a city before, you will see each street as unique "for what it is" rather than making automatic perceptual presumptions. *The brain can be called an "anticipation machine," constantly scanning the environment and trying to determine what will come next.*[23] Mental models of the world are what allow our minds to carry out this vital function which has enabled us as a species to survive. Prior experiences shape our anticipatory models, and thus the term "prospective memory" has been used to describe how the mind attempts to "remember the future," based on what has occurred in the past.[24] Each moment, the brain automatically tries to determine what is going on; it classifies an experience by activating a mental model, which helps bias present perceptions to allow for more rapid processing of the immediate environment. Readiness for response is enhanced by anticipating the next moment in time—what the world may offer next and what behavior to initiate in response.

Let's look at an example. If prior encounters with animals with large teeth have shown that they present a danger, then the association within the memory of such an animal will include a feeling of fear. The next time we encounter such a beast, we will be motivated by fear to run for safety. If we did not have the capacity to create a mental model that establishes the generalization "Large-toothed animals are dangerous," then encounters with a slightly different type of beast might not prompt us to run. We would have to learn anew with every experience. Mental models, the generalizations from past experiences, are the essence of learning. These models, derived from the past, shape our perceptual experience of the present and help us to anticipate and act in the future. As we'll see, *anticipating* the future may be a fundamental component of implicit memory, distinct from the capacity to *plan* for the future. The more complex and deliberate aspect of planning may depend upon the explicit memory processes discussed in the next section.

Parenthetically, the procedure of asking how a mental process was used adaptively in our evolutionary past is sometimes called "reverse-engineering the mind."[25] The brain, after all, is constructed by genetics, by aspects of the physiological internal environment (such as nutrients, hormones, toxins, drugs, or lack of oxygen), and by experience. The genetic contribution to brain functions and mental processes can be seen through the eyes of the evolutionary biologist: Those functions enhancing the probability that the genes would be replicated (passed on through the gametes [the eggs or sperm] in creating offspring) were most likely to be passed on through the generations. In this way, the genetic determination of mental processes may be in the direction of adaptations to past environments, not necessarily to our current ones. For the mind, what this means is that processes such as memory, attention, perception, and emotional responses may be understood (at least in part) by their past function in the evolutionary history of our species, as well as by how they are shaped by present conditions and earlier experiences of the individual.[26]

DEVELOPMENTAL IMPLICATIONS
OF IMPLICIT MEMORY

The following examples provide an introduction to some ideas about attachment, which will be explored in greater detail in the next chapter.[27] They are offered here to illustrate the ubiquitous role of implicit memory throughout the lifespan. (In these examples and throughout the book, incidentally, I alternate between "she" and "he" as the third-person singular pronoun, to avoid sexist usage.) An infant who has a healthy, secure attachment has had the repeated experience of nurturing, perceptive, sensitive, and predictable caregiving responses from her mother, which have been encoded implicitly in her brain. She has developed a generalized representation of that relationship— a mental model of attachment—which helps her know what to expect from her mother. Given that these repeated experiences have been predictable, and that when there have been disruptions in mother–infant communication the mother has been relatively quick and effective at repairing the ruptures, this fortunate infant has been able to develop a secure, organized mental model of their emotional relationship. Her implicit memory anticipates that the future will continue to provide such contingent communication.

An infant with an insecure attachment may have experienced his parents as less predictable, emotionally distant, or perhaps even frightening. These experiences, too, become encoded implicitly, and the infant's mind has a generalized representation of this relationship that can be filled with uncertainty, distance, or fear. With the stimulus cue of being alone with a parent who has been the source of confusion and terror, these implicit representations can become reactivated and create a very unpleasant, disorganizing, and frightening internal world for the infant. This state of mind, a part of his emotional memory, has been implicitly learned during the first year of his life.

By a child's first birthday, these repeated patterns of implicit learning are deeply encoded in the brain. Indeed, attachment studies at this time yield striking differences in infants' behavior when they are with each parent. An infant's states of mind when she is with the mother can affect her differently from those that are activated when she is with her father. As we'll see in the next chapter, this is the origin of the differences that can be seen in the infant's attachment to the two parents. By eighteen months, the maturation of various parts of the child's brain has allowed for the blossoming of her comprehension and expression of language. At about this time, frontal parts of the brain are developing rapidly and enable her to have evocative memory, in which it is believed she is able to bring forward in her mind a sensory image of a parent in order to help soothe herself and regulate her emotional state.[28] Infants are likely to be calmed by the image of a parent with whom they have a secure attachment, and to be anxious, distant, or fearful with a parent with whom they have an insecure attachment.

The patterns of particular states of mind in an infant can be seen as encoded as an implicit form of memory. Repeated experiences of terror and fear can be engrained within the circuits of the brain as states of mind. With chronic occurrence, these states can become more readily activated (retrieved) in the future, such that they become characteristic traits of the individual.[29] In this way, our lives can become shaped by reactivations of implicit memory, which lack a sense that something is being recalled. We simply enter these engrained states and experience them as the reality of our present experience.

Insights into the ways in which early experiences have shaped the implicit memory system can aid in the understanding of various aspects of human relationships. Being with a particular person can activate distinct mental models that affect our perceptions, emotions,

---

TABLE 1. Types and Characteristics of Memory

Forms of memory

Early, nondeclarative, procedural, implicit
   versus
Late, declarative, episodic/semantic, explicit

Developmental biology of memory

Implicit processing systems (early memory): Present at birth.
Explicit processing systems (late memory):
   Semantic: Develops initially by one to two years of age.
   Autobiographical: Progressive development with onset after second year of life.

Implicit memory

A form of memory devoid of the subjective internal experience of "recalling,"
   of self, or of time. Involves mental models and "priming."
Includes behavioral, emotional, perceptual, and perhaps somatosensory memory.
Focal attention *not* required for encoding.
Is mediated via brain circuits involved in the initial encoding and independent
   of the medial temporal lobe/hippocampus.

Explicit memory

A form of memory requiring conscious awareness for encoding and having
   the subjective sense of recollection (and, if autobiographical, of self and time).
Includes semantic (factual) and episodic (autobiographical) memory.
Focal attention needed for encoding.
Hippocampal processing required for storage.
Cortical consolidation makes selected events a part of permanent memory.

behaviors, and beliefs in response to this other person. The notion of implicit memory's influencing our experiences with others is one way of understanding the complex feelings and perceptions arising within interpersonal relationships. Each of us filters our interactions with others through the lenses of mental models created from patterns of experiences in the past. These models can shift rapidly outside of awareness, sometimes creating abrupt transitions in states of mind and interactions with others. In this way, "transference"—the activation of old mental models and states of mind from our relationships with important figures in the past—happens all the time, both inside and outside the psychotherapy suite. Knowing about implicit memory allows us the opportunity to free ourselves from the prison of the past.

EXPLICIT MEMORY: FACTS, EVENTS, AND AUTOBIOGRAPHICAL CONSCIOUSNESS

By the second birthday, toddlers have developed new capacities: to talk about their recollections of the day's events, and to remember more distant experiences from the past. These abilities reflect the maturation of the brain's medial temporal lobe (which includes a part called the hippocampus) and orbitofrontal cortex; this maturation process allows them to have "explicit" memory.[30] Explicit memory is what most people mean when they refer to the generic idea of memory. When explicit recollections are retrieved, they have the internal sensation of "I am remembering." Two forms of explicit memory are "semantic" (factual) and "episodic" (autobiographical or oneself in an episode in time). Table 1 provides an overview of the types and characteristics of memory.

The development of the unique aspects of explicit memory involves a number of domains in a child's experiencing. A sense of sequencing, thought to be a function of the hippocampus as a "cognitive mapper," develops during the child's second year of life.[31] Recalling the order in which events in the world occur allows the child to develop a sense of time and the sequence of things. Children come to expect, with at times intense and passionate reactions to deviations, what typically comes first and what comes next in a given situation. Associated with this hippocampal ability is the establishment of a spatial representational map of the locations of things in the world. Loss of hippocampal functioning in animals, for example, leads to loss of memory for running a maze.[32] What is interesting in this finding is the notion that this cognitive mapper is thus able to create a four-dimensional sense of the self in the world across time. The brain's ability to create such a temporal and spatial representation is clearly of great survival value. Explicit memory plays the important role of providing a sense of space and time, allowing people to remember where things are and when they were there.

As children grow into their second year, they begin to develop a more complex image of themselves in the world. This sense of self has been identified by studies examining how children respond to seeing themselves in the mirror with a red mark placed on their faces. They notice something different in their reflection, suggesting that they have a mental image in their minds of what they usually look like. By eighteen months they are able to touch themselves rather than the mirror in exploring the red mark. Taken together, the developmental phase of the second year suggests that a child is developing a sense of the physical world, of time and sequence, and of the self, all of which form the foundation of explicit autobiographical memory.[33] Before this time, events in the child's life may have been remembered ("event memory"), but it is thought that these are semantic recollections of experiences without an enriched sense of self across time, which is the hallmark of autobiographical (episodic) recollection.[34]

Wheeler, Stuss, and Tulving have summarized recent neuroimaging studies, which suggest that memory for facts (semantic memory)—including events—is functionally quite distinct from memory of the self across time (episodic memory).[35] Semantic memory allows for propositional representations—symbols of external or internal facts that can be declared with words or in graphic form and can be assessed as "true" or "false." Such semantic knowledge has been called "noesis" and allows us to know about facts in the world. In contrast, autobiographical or episodic memory requires a capacity termed "autonoesis" (self-knowing) and appears to be dependent upon the development of frontal cortical regions of the brain. These regions undergo rapid experience-dependent development during the first few years of life (continuing possibly into adulthood) and are postulated to mediate autonoetic consciousness. The ability of the human mind to carry out what Tulving and colleagues have termed "mental time travel"—to have a sense of recollection of the self at a particular time in the past, awareness of the self in the lived present, and projections of the self into the imagined future—is the unique contribution of autonoetic consciousness.[36] By the middle of the third year of life, a child has already begun to join caregivers in mutually constructed tales woven from their real-life events and imagining.[37] The richness of self-knowledge and autobiographical narratives appears to be mediated by the interpersonal dialogues in which caregivers co-construct narratives about external events and the internal, subjective experiences of the characters.[38] In this way, we can hypothesize that attachment experiences—that is, communication with parents and other caregivers—may directly enhance a child's capacity for autonoetic consciousness. This can be proposed to be one reason why shared communication about remembered events enhances recollection.[39] The details of such a view will be explored in the next chapter.

The encoding process for both forms of explicit memory (semantic and episodic) appears to require focal, conscious, directed attention to activate the hippocampus.[40] As encoding occurs, stimuli are placed initially in "sensory" memory, which lasts for about a quarter to half a second. This sensory "buffer" contains the initial neural activations of the perceptual system. Only selected items from this huge immediate sensory process are then placed in "working" memory, which lasts up to half a minute if there is no further rehearsal. If the mind rehearses or refreshes the activity of these activated circuits of working memory, then the items can be either maintained for longer periods of time in this process (such as practicing a phone number long enough to dial it repeatedly if the line is busy) or placed into longer-term storage.

Working memory has been called the "chalkboard of the mind." It is the mental process involved when we say that we are "thinking about something"; it allows us to reflect upon items perceived in the present and recalled from the past.[41] When we consciously think of a problem or an event, working memory allows us to link together various representations and manipulate them in our minds. The product of such cognitive processing can then enter a more stable component, "long-term" memory. In some individuals with disorders of attention, working memory appears to be unable to handle the amount of items for as long as the working memory of normal subjects. Imaging studies have supported this clinical finding by identifying abnormalities in the lateral prefrontal cortex, the site thought to be a primary mediator of working memory.[42]

Long-term explicit memory is thought to be the process by which items are stored for extended periods of time beyond working memory.[43] For example, recalling a close friend's phone number requires it to be placed in long-term storage. Remembering the phone number of a shop you need to call only once requires working memory to hold on to those digits just long enough to dial the number. After the call, the shop's number vanishes from any form of permanent storage. If working memory persisted, we would be bombarded by irrelevant information from the past. Placing a needed item into long-term memory allows us to recall important data. When we ask others to recall their experiences from the last month, we are in effect requesting them to activate a representational process that has been "stored" as an increased probability of firing within a neural net. This is mediated by genetically activated structural alterations in synaptic connections within the network. In contrast, working memory is thought to be independent of gene-activated protein synthesis. It involves functional (not structural) alterations in synaptic strengths, such as increases in synaptic excitability that temporarily enhance the probability of specific neuronal firing. Recollection can be viewed as the actual activation of a potential or latent representation. The hippocampus is essential for both encoding items into and retrieving them from long-term explicit memory. The linkage of this process to the circuits of the lateral prefrontal cortex is one view of the mechanism for having working memory activate the structurally embedded elements of long-term memory, where they can be consciously examined, manipulated, and reported to others.[44]

Long-term memory does not last forever. For these items to become a part of permanent explicit memory, a process called "cortical consolidation" is thought to occur.[45] Though the mechanism has not been elucidated thus far, some views suggest that cortical consolidation requires a nonconscious activation or rehearsal process that allows representations to be stored in the "associational cortex."[46] This region of the cerebral cortex appears to integrate representations from a variety of parts of the brain. Consolidation appears to involve the reorganization of existing memory traces, not the laying down of new engrams. In this manner, consolidation may make new associational linkages, condense elements of memory into new clusters of representations, and incorporate previously unintegrated elements into a functional whole. In cortical consolidation, information is finally free of the need for the hippocampus for retrieval. This consolidation process appears to depend on the rapid-eye-movement (REM) sleep stage, which is thought to be attempting to make sense of the day's activities.[47] Though filled with a combination of seemingly random activations, aspects of the day's experiences, and elements from the more distant past, dreams may be a fundamental way in which the mind consolidates the myriad of explicit recollections into a coherent set of representations for permanent, consolidated memory.

Research is still in its infancy regarding the details of the consolidation process.[48] Interestingly, cortical consolidation may take weeks, months, or perhaps years to occur. For example, if a man sustains a head injury in a motorcycle accident on the first of January, he may lose recollection of events from November and December of the prior year, but may be able to recall those from October and earlier without difficulty. This is called "retrograde" amnesia and involves impairment in the ability of the hippocampus to retrieve not-yet-consolidated memories. He may also experience severe difficulty recalling events after the accident, called "anterograde" amnesia. This involves damage to the hippocampus's ability to encode new items into long-term explicit memory. Working memory may remain unimpaired. Also, the man's ability to encode or retrieve items from implicit memory will be intact. He can learn new skills and have emotional associations to recent events, but he will be unable to recall when he acquired the new knowledge or to have any sense of time or self connected with the recollections.

Many forms of amnesia involve the impairment of explicit processing in the setting of intact implicit memory. Explicit recollections, as we've seen, require focal, conscious attention, and are processed through the initial phases of encoding in working memory and then into long-term memory on their way toward cortical consolidation. There are certain situations, however, in which there is a disassociation between implicit and explicit memory. "Infantile" or "childhood" amnesia is one such example we will discuss below, in which normal infants' and young children's implicit memory is intact, but their explicit recall, especially episodic memory, is impaired. Other examples include hypnotic amnesia; the effects of certain medications, such as the benzodiazepines (minor tranquilizers); surgical anesthesia; neurological conditions such as brain injury and Korsakoff's syndrome; and divided-attention phenomena, such as an experiment in dichotic listening. In this last case, a subject is asked to pay attention to only one ear while listening to two auditory lists on a set of headphones. For example, in the left ear is played a list of zoo animals, in the right a list of flowers. When asked to repeat what was heard in the focally attended ear (say, the left), most subjects have excellent recall of the animals. When asked what was heard in the right ear, subjects usually state that they don't know. When asked to fill in the blank spaces on partially spelled words, such as "r__ __e," they are much more likely than subjects exposed to a different list to fill in the word "rose." This is an example of indirect recall, a measure of implicit memory. A subject's brain has encoded the flowers implicitly, so that the brain is "primed" (that is, made more likely) to bring up a flower when given a cue. Subjects have no conscious recall of what they heard, or even a sense that what they are writing is a reflection of something they experienced. *Without focal attention, items are not encoded explicitly.* Implicit memory is intact, but explicit memory is impaired for that stimulus or event.[49]

THE SUBJECTIVE EXPERIENCE OF EXPLICIT AND IMPLICIT MEMORY

When either semantic or episodic explicit memory is retrieved, there is an internal sensation of "I am recalling something." This distinguishes explicit recollection from implicit ones, in which there is no such subjective sense of remembrance. Explicit memories take a number of forms. Semantic memory is a type in which we can recall factual information, such as the capitals of the major countries of Europe. If we recall that we were once in those cities but cannot summon the sensation of the self in time on the trip, then this reflects a semantic memory for a personally experienced event. In the past, this form of memory may have been considered by academicians as a part of autobiographical recall, but recent neuroscientific studies support the notion that semantic recall lacking a sense of self is in fact quite different from episodic recall.[50] Noetic consciousness (knowing the fact that one was once in Europe) is thought to be quite distinct from autonoetic consciousness (recalling the self's experience of the trip), both in subjective experience and in the involvement of the prefrontal cortices in the latter process. Episodic recall activates autobiographical memory representations and evokes a process of mental time travel—the sense of the self in time—which differentiates it from semantic recollections.

The distinct experiential aspects of memory are thought to involve different centers of activation within the brain.[51] For example, semantic recall appears to involve a dominance of left over right hippocampal activation. Autobiographical recall, in contrast, in-

volves more of the right hippocampus and right orbitofrontal cortex.[52] Here we see that structure and function within the brain correlate with our day-to-day encounters with subjective experience. This
distinction may reveal itself when we sense that a fact is known
without any feeling that it is a part of our experienced life. Though
semantic and episodic memory have much in common—they are
flexibly accessible, have virtually unlimited capacities for representing "data," are encoded with contextual features, and can be
retrieved in a declarative manner via language or drawing—they in
fact appear to be mediated by somewhat distinct mechanisms.[53]

For episodic memory, there appears to be a much larger process
involved than merely the autobiographical content of representations
of personally experienced events: Autonoetic awareness involves the
experience of mental time travel and is directly linked to the processes of the prefrontal regions of the brain. Autonoetic consciousness is created within the various layers of prefrontal function.[54]
These include an integrating capacity, in which more posteriorly
stored information can be organized and sequenced into a meaningful set of representations; executive functions, which provide a more
global control of widely distributed brain processes; and the mediation of self-reflection and social cognition.[55] We can see that mental
time travel is more than a subjective sense of feeling oneself in the
past, present, or future: It is an actively constructive mental process
that creates the self within a social world. It turns out that several
independent lines of research point to the frontal regions—especially
the orbitofrontal cortex in the right hemisphere—as a crucial area
for integrating memory,[56] attachment,[57] emotion,[58] bodily representation and regulation,[59] and social cognition.[60]

Within explicit autobiographical memory, we can find a number
of variations on these elements of self in time. For example, you may
recall a general sense of yourself from your senior year in high
school. This generic episodic recollection can be thought of as a general descriptor summating across your perceptions of a year of specific episodes. In a sense this is a self-concept, or a self-schema made
conscious, about yourself during that year. In contrast, you may be
able to recall a specific event during that time, such as your last day
of high school. In retrieving this memory, you may recall it as an
event you observed from a distance, as if you were taking an out-
sider's perspective. This is an "observer" recollection, which some
might consider a distanced form of episodic retrieval, but others
would label an event memory within semantic recall.[61] In contrast,
you may recall the event as if you were actually there; this is a "par-

ticipant" or "field" recollection. In this case, you would be able to see things from your actual perspective. Observer recollections appear to involve less emotional intensity than field recollections do. Autonoesis thus evokes elements of the self's lived experience, rather than merely the propositional (factual) representations of noetic consciousness.

The process of reactivating representations from explicit memory is often dependent on the features of the internal and external environment. When there is a match between retrieval cue and memory representation, the process is called "ecphory."[62] Ecphory depends upon the features of the eliciting stimulus and the form in which the representation has been stored in memory. This effect of the context on the retrieval of explicit memory reveals how retrieval is enhanced when conditions have similarities in the physical world (sights, sounds, smells) or in one's state of mind (emotions, mental models, states of general arousal) to those that were present at the time of the initial encoding. In this way, explicit memory is said to be "context dependent." The hippocampus is able to encode its cognitive mapping on experiences, giving them a context in which they are both registered and stored. The actual representations of such experiences are thought to be stored in more posterior portions of the brain. The prefrontal regions are thought to carry out the process of creating an episodic "retrieval state" in which a match between retrieval cue and stored representation (ecphory) can occur.[63]

Individuals may have recollections in which they may lack an understanding of how the contextual cues have led to specific events' being recalled. They may explore these memories by searching for a match between the features present at the time of retrieval and at the time of the original event. Such a search can sometimes reveal the underlying emotional meaning or gist of a particular recollection. However, the sense of mental time travel by itself does not mean that the recollection is accurate. It merely implies that the prefrontally mediated autonoetic awareness circuits are involved in the activation of stored or internally generated representations, not that ecphory has occurred. In this manner, the prefrontal region may serve to attempt to create accurate assemblies of representations—but, accurate or not, they may contain a sense of the self recalling the past. This can be viewed as what we can call an "ecphoric sensation," which has a sense of conviction that the recalled memory is indeed accurate. We can have a clear sense that something happened when in fact it did not. Such subjective sensations may be a part of imagination, dreaming, or inaccurate as well as accurate recollection.

The richness of recollection we may feel in reflecting on past experiences is shaped in part by internal or external context cues, which can then initiate a cascade of further related recollections. Initial ecphory (the retrieval cue's matching the stored memory representation) is followed by a series of sometimes unpredictable associative linkages influenced by both memory and present experience. These associated recollections and retrieval cues can be woven into the process of remembering and can become a part of the "reconstructed" memory. Representations resembling those of the past are reassembled anew during the process of recollection. Retrieval is thus, as Robert Bjork has suggested, a "memory modifier": The act of reactivating a representation can allow it to be stored again in a modified form.[64] The frontal lobes, in carrying out the integrative, executive, and socially constructive remembering of the self, can directly shape the nature of autobiographical recollections and life stories. These processes explain one way in which our memories—things we may regard as facts—can actually change over time and evolve over the lifespan.

Often cues will activate both explicit and implicit elements of memory. The initial subjective experience of this frequent process can often be the emergence of nonverbal sensations or behavioral impulses (implicit recollections), which initiate the beginning of an explicit recollection. These elements may not feel as if something is actually being recalled, but may be experienced as a wave of internal sensations and images. As explicit memory retrieval becomes linked to these implicit counterparts, one may begin to get a sense of some factual elements or images that begin to have the sensation of "I am remembering something now." On a daily basis, we actively reconstruct neural net profiles that have encoded both implicit and explicit circuits establishing representations derived from past experiences. The internal, subjective sensations of these distinct forms of memory parallel their anatomic distinction within the brain.[65]

Explicit memory is often communicated to ourselves and to others in the form of descriptive words or pictures communicating a story or sequence of events. If these involve the sense of self at some time in the past, then they are a part of explicit autobiographical memory. We listen to the words and receive a linguistic message, or see the pictures and have a conscious sense of the story being told. But recollections usually involve the association of these explicit elements with their implicit counterparts. To sense these, it is important to recall (explicitly) that the activation of implicit memory does not have a sense of "something is being remembered." We sense, perceive, or filter our explicit memory through the mental models of implicit memory. We can watch for the shadows that such implicit "recollections" cast on the stories we tell, as well as on nonverbal aspects of behavior and communication.

For example, a thirty-five-year-old woman began to recount her experiences of being raised by a violent, alcoholic father. When she began to tell her story, her eyes became filled with tears, her hands began to tremble, and she turned away from her therapist. She stopped speaking and seemed to become frozen, with a look of terror on her face. For the therapist, the feeling in the room was intense and consuming. The patient began to speak again, but this time spoke of her father's "positive attributes." Her nonverbal communication remained, though she wiped away her tears and tried to "compose" herself and not "worry so much about the past." In this case, the patient was being flooded by the implicit elements of her early experiences, evoked in part by her recounting the story of her father's rages. As she began to divert the narrative she was relating, only parts of the implicit memories were able to be diffused. Despite this diversion, for the remainder of the session she continued to feel frightened and humiliated.

The challenge in cases like this one is to listen to the words as well as the nonverbal elements of communication that let us know what others are experiencing and remembering. We must keep in mind that only a part of memory can be translated into the language-based packets of information people use to tell their life stories to others. Learning to be open to many layers of communication is a fundamental part of getting to know another person's life.

CHILDHOOD AMNESIA

For over a century, clinicians have been aware of an impairment in the ability of older children or adults to recall the first years of their lives. Initial impressions suggested that this "memory barrier" is for the period before the ages of five to seven years. Psychoanalytic writings from the past suggested that infantile amnesia is due to some traumatic, overwhelming experiences that are being blocked, and that one focus of treatment should be to uncover this "repression barrier."[66] Modern analytic thinking does not support this notion, however.

Developmental psychologists view childhood amnesia differently, suggesting that immaturities in the sense of self, in the sense of time, in verbal ability, and in narrative capacity may be the factors limiting recall for the period before the age of about two to three years.[67] Neurobiologists investigating this form of amnesia have looked at the development of the hippocampus/medial temporal lobe and the orbitofrontal region during the first years of life as a possible mediator of the phenomenon of childhood amnesia.[68] This view supports the developmental psychologists' observations in providing the likely neurobiological underpinnings to this normal developmental form of amnesia. In this way, explicit memory may require the neural maturation of the hippocampus to allow for the full expression of first semantic and then later episodic memory.

Let's explore the nature of the development of explicit memory by examining the experiences of a young girl. A one-year-old is able to have implicit recollection of all sorts of experiences: becoming excited when she hears the car pull into the garage, knowing emotionally on some level that her mother is coming home; learning to walk; or generating mental models for repeated experiences. She has already developed the capacity for generalized recollections, called "general event knowledge."[69] Before the age of eighteen months, she has begun to develop the ability to recall the sequence of events in her world.[70] She thus can encode and retrieve facts from specific experiences. This can be considered a form of semantic memory, in which knowledge of specific events can be recalled after a long delay.[71]

After about eighteen months, the child develops self-referential behaviors which reveal a sense of continuity of the self through time. By her second birthday, she can now begin to talk about events that have happened to her. As she continues to mature, her sense of self develops more fully and may allow for the gradual emergence of episodic memory and the capacity for mental time travel—for remembering herself in specific experiences in the past. As her prefrontal regions develop, this capacity becomes increasingly complex and sophisticated. These regions may continue to develop into adulthood and may explain the deepening capacity for self-awareness and autonoetic consciousness throughout the lifespan. At this early age, the child can say that she saw a dog that morning, or that she went to visit her grandfather at the park. She can narrate her ongoing experience and can verbalize and plan for her anticipations of future events. Though now she can talk about her recent recollections, she cannot episodically remember when she was an infant. Some facts that she has learned during her second year of life, however, may be quite available to her within semantic memory, such as the names of objects and what things do. The work of Patricia Bauer and her colleagues suggests that even experiences that occurred after the child's first birthday but before the advent of spoken language may be recalled verbally with considerable accuracy after many months. These recollections are likely a part of explicit semantic memory and not derived from the yet-to-be-accessible autobiographical process.[72]

Some authors argue that childhood amnesia is not an impairment in general explicit recall, but rather is very specifically due to the developmental lag in the onset of episodic memory.[73] Support for this view comes from the more recent findings that children even in their second year of life have a remarkable ability to retain facts about novel experiences with great accuracy.[74] Thus these studies suggest that semantic explicit memory is intact from quite early on.

How does episodic memory develop? A few findings that explore the impact of experience on autobiographical memory may be useful in examining this question. Children who have more experiences of talking about their memories with their parents are able to recall more details about their lives later on.[75] "Memory talk" is a common process in which parents focus their attention on the contents of a child's memories. A similar observation is that parents who participate in an "elaborative" form of communication have children with a richer sense of autobiographical recall. Elaborative parents talk with their children about what they, the children, think about the stories they read together. In contrast, "factual" parents—the classification designating parents who are found to talk only about the facts of stories, not a child's imagination or response—have children with a less developed ability for recall.[76] There is probably a range of communication styles between the extremes of these two research categories. Nevertheless, these findings support the general principle that interpersonal experiences appear to have a direct effect on the development of explicit memory. As Bauer and colleagues have stated, "The talk in which children and parents engage prior to, during, and/or after an event works to organize, integrate, and, thereby, facilitate children's memory for it."[77]

Are these merely genetic findings revealing that parents give rise to offspring who naturally, genetically, will have their same traits? To be sure, one must await further studies, such as those that might examine the narratives of identical twins raised apart, to clarify the origin of these differences in narrative style. There is clearly a difference in narrative experience, whatever the origin: Some families participate in frequent co-construction of narrative and elaborative memory talk. In reinforcing this kind of experience, parents may facilitate their children's ability to describe their memories, as well as their imaginations. In a similar fashion, children raised in families that discussed people's emotional reactions tended to be more interested in and able to understand others' emotions.[78] These children are also taught that what they have to say about the contents of their minds is important. Each of these experiences may enhance the capacity for emotional regulation.[79] Could these effects be mediated by the experience-dependent growth of the orbitofrontal regions responsible for affect regulation and the encoding and retrieval of episodic memory? No studies exploring this possibility have been published yet.

In general, childhood amnesia raises the larger issue about remembering and forgetting. Our internal sense of who we are is shaped both by what we can explicitly recall, and by the implicit recollections that create our mental models and internal subjective experience of images, sensations, emotions, and behavioral responses. The inability to recall the first years of life explicitly reveals a differential development among several modalities of memory. The first year appears to enable implicit but not explicit encoding and retrieval. The circuits mediating the various forms of implicit memory are fairly well developed at birth. The second year has been shown to allow for a form of explicit recollection that is most likely to be semantic in nature. Such a capacity is likely mediated by the maturation of the medial temporal lobe, including areas of the hippocampus. By eighteen months to two or three years of age, episodic memory begins to emerge. The emergence of this process may be facilitated by the development of the prefrontal regions of the brain, especially the orbitofrontal cortex. As these regions develop actively during the preschool years, episodic memory undergoes significant maturation. The ongoing development of a sense of self during this time enables this form of autonoesis to grow rapidly and become more elaborate. As the sense of self continues to develop, the intricacies of self-experience evolve.

Nelson and Carver explain, "What makes possible the changes in explicit memory through the preschool period is the development of various prefrontal functions that can come to the assistance of the medial temporal lobe (explicit) memory system. For example, it is generally not until the preschool period that children begin to routinely employ strategies to help them remember things; the use of strategies, of course, is a quintessential prefrontal function." They further state that "the neural circuitry involved in long-term memory develop slowly over the infancy and preschool period. The relevant structures that are thought to develop during this interval include the circuits that pass along information from the medial temporal lobe, where initial encoding and consolidation is performed, and the cortex, where memory is stored. It is neural maturation, then, that likely accounts for the gradual 'recovery' from infantile amnesia."[80]

EMOTION, REMEMBERING, AND FORGETTING

Is everything that is experienced remembered? No. Forgetting is an essential aspect of explicit memory; if we were to have easy access to every experience we have encoded, our working memory would be flooded with extraneous facts and images, and normal functioning would become impaired.[81] Which events, then, are more likely to be remembered and which forgotten? It turns out that many studies of emotion and memory point to an inverted-U-shaped-curve effect.[82] Experiences that involve little emotional intensity seem to do little to arouse focal attention, and have a higher likelihood of being registered as "unimportant" and therefore not easily recalled later on. Events experienced with a moderate to high degree of emotional intensity seem to get labeled as "important" (probably by anatomic structures in the limbic system, such as the amygdala and orbitofrontal cortex, which we'll discuss later in the book) and are more easily remembered in the future. If events are overwhelming and filled with terror, a number of factors may inhibit the hippocampal processing of explicit memory, and therefore may block explicit encoding and subsequent retrieval.[83] Such factors include divided attention, amygdala discharge, and release of noradrenaline and corticosteroids in response to massive stress. Such conditions allow implicit memory to be encoded while explicit processing is impaired.[84]

Although even one-time occurrences can alter synaptic strengths, repeated experiences and emotionally arousing experiences have the greatest impact on the connections within the brain. In other words, not all encounters with the world affect the mind equally. Studies have demonstrated that if the brain appraises an event as "meaning-ful," it will be more likely to be recalled in the future.[85] The brain appraises the significance of stimuli in numerous ways, including the activation of areas such as the amygdala. If the amygdala is acti-vated, then the engram encoded at that particular time is thought to be marked as significant; this has been called a "value-laden" mem-ory.[86] The neuronal mechanism for this labeling is the pronounced increase in synaptic strengths at the time of that specific experience. As we'll see in Chapter 4, value systems in the brain may serve as neuromodulatory circuits with processes that (1) enhance neuronal excitability and activation; (2) enhance neuronal plasticity and the creation of new synaptic connections; and (3) have extensive innervation linking various brain regions. This emotionally charged value-laden memory is thus made more likely to be reactivated among the myriad of infinite engrams laid down throughout life.

The relationship between emotion and memory suggests that emotionally arousing experiences are more readily recalled later on. As James McGaugh has suggested, "the evidence suggests the possi-bility that the influences of several neuromodulatory systems on memory may be integrated by interactions occurring within the amygdala. ... The evidence thus strongly supports the general hypothesis that endogenous neuromodulatory systems activated by experience play a role in regulating memory storage." He goes on to suggest that "the strength of memories depends on the degree of emotional activation induced by learning. Highly emotional stimula-tion may well, as William James (1890) suggested, 'almost ... leave a scar on the cerebral tissue' in the form of lasting changes in synap-tic connectivity."[87] In other words, emotion involves a modulatory process that enhances the creation of new synaptic connections via increases in neuronal plasticity.

What are the mechanisms of this increased plasticity? The exact link between emotion and the activation of genes to initiate new syn-apse formation has not been clarified. However, there are some intriguing possibilities suggested by studies done on the molecules of memory in invertebrate animals.[88] A protein called CREB-1 (cyclic AMP response element-binding) appears to lead to the activation of genes that initiate the protein synthesis necessary to establish synap-tic connections. The growth of new synapses is normally constrained by inhibitory memory-suppressor genes that appear to regulate the transfer of information from short-term storage, such as working memory, into long-term memory. This suppression may be mediated by a protein called suppressor CREB-2. If this process studied in "lower" animals is found to be utilized by our own memory processes, then perhaps it is our brain's way to ensure that irrelevant stimuli are not encoded into long-term memory: Some active process would need to be initiated to produce structurally based encoding of events into long-term memory. While these are exciting findings, their relevance to human memory, and specifically to the emotional mechanisms by which the amygdala and other structures enhance memory encoding, must await future investigations.

The relationships among memory, emotion, and the self are complex. Looking toward neurobiology for some insights into these processes can be enlightening. As Robert Post and colleagues have suggested:

> The amygdala is thought to be involved with imparting the emotional significance to an object and linking it to other memory systems initially imparted by the hippocampus but then subserved by other complex cerebral pathways potentially involving many hundreds of thousands if not millions of synapses. Just the way the properties of objects are synthesized convergently by different pathways, we can surmise that the historical and emotional significance of objects are likewise "synthesized," but also edited, updated, and revised based on new experiences. In this fashion, the more complex associative experiential properties and cues may be attached to critical objects in the environment, such as one's parents, siblings, and even the concept of oneself.[89]

By creating meaning, our emotional neuromodulatory systems help organize and integrate our memories. Our lives are filled with implicit influences, the origins and impact of which we may not be aware. *In the case of childhood amnesia, this intact implicit memory in the presence of an impairment in explicit recall is a normal finding unrelated to trauma.* As children's lives unfold, they are able to recall more and more of the events in their lives as these are woven into a narrative picture of the self across time. This narrative emerges as value-laden memories are consolidated and become a part of the permanent explicit autobiographical memory system. Not every experience will be episodically recalled; this is a part of normal forgetting. Our minds must selectively inhibit the encoding, recollection, and consolidation of many events that have occurred. If we were to become bombarded by irrelevant explicit detail, we would become confused and overwhelmed.

STRESS, TRAUMA, AND MEMORY

Stressful experiences may take the form of highly emotional events or, when overwhelming, overtly traumatizing experiences. The degree of stress will have a direct effect on memory: Small amounts have a neutral effect on memory; moderate amounts facilitate memory; and large amounts impair memory. The effect of stress appears to be mediated by the characteristic neuroendocrine responses involving the immediate transient effects (lasting seconds to minutes) of noradrenaline release and the more sustained effects (lasting minutes to hours) of glucocorticoids such as cortisol, also known as "stress hormones." The mechanisms of these agents are complex. Recent studies suggest that the HPA axis involves the release of stress hormones that directly affect the hippocampus, a region with the highest density of receptors for these blood-borne agents. Chronic stress may produce elevated baseline levels of stress hormones and abnormal daily rhythms of hormone release. The effects of high levels of stress hormones on the hippocampus may initially be reversible and involve the inhibition of neuronal growth and the atrophy of cellular receptive components called dendrites.[90] High levels of stress not only transiently block hippocampal functioning, but excessive and chronic exposure to stress hormones may lead to neuronal death in this region, possibly producing decreased hippocampal volume, as found in patients with chronic posttraumatic stress disorder.[91] Activation of the autonomic nervous system leads to the release of epinephrine and norepineprhine (known as the catecholamines), which are thought to affect the amygdala directly. The amygdala, as we've seen, plays an important role in establishing the value of an experience and integrating elements of encoding with the hippocampal processing of the event. Excessive stress hormone or catecholamine release appears, respectively, to impair the hippocampal and amygdala contributions to memory processing.[92]

Highly emotional events may involve a certain degree of stress response. Particular cascades of physiological and cognitive reactions may reinforce the effects of stress on memory. As Bower and Sivers have noted:

> Several factors working in concert promote better memory for highly emotional events. Prominent among these are the personal significance of the event, its distinctiveness or rarity and selective rehearsal. . . . When emotionally aroused, the brain triggers reac-

tions from the autonomic nervous system and the endocrine system; the latter releases stress hormones into the blood stream, creating persistent arousal and reactivation of whatever thoughts are salient in the cognitive system. This arousal persists for several minutes and has an effect analogous to involuntary recycling of the stressful occurrence and the events leading up to it. Such rehearsal enhances the degree of learning of whatever aspects of the event were encoded. Beyond this physiological arousal that continues for several minutes, our minds have a tendency to return repeatedly over many hours or days to memories of emotionally upsetting events, perhaps triggered by external cues or ideational sequences that have been associated with the aversive event.[93]

In this manner, emotionally arousing experiences become better remembered by a combination of direct physiological effects (perhaps on the genetic activation leading to synapse formation, as discussed above) and complex cognitive effects on the encoding of memory via the retrieval, rehearsal, and reencoding process.

Under some conditions, explicit memory may be blocked from encoding at the actual time of an experience. Trauma may be proposed to be such a situation. Various factors may contribute to the inhibition of hippocampal functioning needed for explicit memory at the time of a severe trauma.[94] During a trauma, the victim may focus his attention on a nontraumatic aspect of the environment or on his imagination as a means of at least partial escape. Divided-attention studies suggest that this situation will lead to the encoding of parts of the traumatic experience implicitly but not explicitly. Furthermore, the release of large amounts of stress hormones and the excessive discharge of amygdala activity in response to threat may impair hippocampal functioning. The outcome for a victim who dissociates explicit from implicit processing is an impairment in autobiographical memory for at least certain aspects of the trauma (explicit blockage may refer to "psychogenic" amnesia). Implicit memory of the event is intact and includes intrusive elements such as behavioral impulses to flee, emotional reactions, bodily sensations, and intrusive images related to the trauma.[95] Individuals who dissociate during and after a traumatic experience have been found to be the most vulnerable to developing posttraumatic stress disorder.[96] As we've discussed, chronic stress may actually damage the hippocampus itself, as suggested by the finding of decreased hippocampal volume in patients suffering from chronic posttraumatic stress disorder.[97] Under such conditions, future explicit processing and learning may be chronically impaired. Furthermore, in addition to damaging the hippocampus, early child maltreatment may directly affect circuits that link bodily response to brain function: the autonomic nervous system, the HPA axis, and the neuroimmune process.[98] These ingrained ways in which adverse child experiences are "remembered," and directly affect the development of regulatory brain structures that govern basic brain–body processes, may explain the markedly increased risk for medical illness in adults with histories of childhood abuse and dysfunctional home environments.[99]

On the basis of this information, one can propose that psychological trauma involving the blockage of explicit processing also impairs the victim's ability to cortically consolidate the experience.[100] With dissociation or the prohibition of discussing with others what was experienced, as is so often the case in familial child abuse, there may be a profound blockage to the pathway toward consolidating memory. Unresolved traumatic experiences from this perspective may involve an impairment in the cortical consolidation process, which leaves the memories of these events out of permanent memory. But the person may be prone to experiencing continually intrusive implicit images of past horrors. Nightmares, occurring during the dream stage of sleep and involving active REM sleep disturbances, may reveal futile attempts of the brain to resolve and consolidate such blocked memory configurations. Dream stages of sleep are thought to play a central role in reorganizing memory and in reinforcing the connections between memory and emotion.[101]

Although not linked within their independent domains of study, dream research, memory investigations, and the study of adaptation to trauma may help us understand some important processes in memory and trauma. Endel Tulving and coworkers have proposed a model of "hemispheric encoding–retrieval asymmetry."[102] In brief, this model draws on a range of investigations suggesting that the left prefrontal cortex plays a dominant role in the *encoding* of episodic memory, whereas the right prefrontal cortex is essential in episodic *retrieval*. The dreams of REM sleep involve markedly increased brain activity. Eye movements have been associated with the activation of the opposite side of the brain (that is, movement to the left is associated with right-hemisphere activation).[103] (This finding explains why so many individuals look to the left during autobiographical recall— which, as we now know, activates right prefrontal regions.)

All of these findings taken together raise the following proposal, which remains to be substantiated by specific research. During the normal dreaming state, the left and right hemispheres are activated in an alternating, rhythmic, and synchronous fashion. Activation of the right orbitofrontal region of the prefrontal cortex mediates a "retrieval state" for the reactivation of episodic representations. Left orbitofrontal activation initiates an "encoding state" in which representations can be registered, linked together, and encoded into a reorganized or consolidated form. REM sleep is crucial for memory consolidation and has been suggested to facilitate long-term potentiation, allowing the strengthening of synaptic connections.[104] Consolidation may be mediated by a process involving the synchronous retrieval of autobiographical memory via the right orbitofrontal cortex with the encoding into episodic memory via the left orbitofrontal region of those right-hemisphere representations. Memory may be "reorganized" during dreaming via the simultaneous retrieval (right side) of information that is then encoded into new consolidated forms (left side) via the dream process. The prefrontal regions have extensive innervation to various parts of the brain, including the neocortical associative cortex. The newly reorganized episodic memory becomes consolidated within the associational cortex, where it is now independent of the hippocampus and available for later retrieval. Future access of these newly reorganized memory representations can occur within autonoetic consciousness as mediated by the right orbitofrontal regions. The essential feature of such a process is the synchronous activation of right and left hemispheres to synthetically retrieve and encode episodic memory into a consolidated form. Dreaming thus permits episodic memory representations to become the engrams for consolidative encoding. The result may be, literally, a "consolidation" of episodic memory into a coherent set of reprocessed and more fully integrated representations. The result of such a process, we can propose, is the stuff of our life narratives.

We can further propose that autonoetic consciousness of traumatic events is disturbed in individuals who have experienced trauma that remains "unresolved." As we'll see in future chapters, this unresolved state of mind has important implications for the mind's functioning and for interpersonal relationships. Some individuals may become flooded by excessive implicit recollections, in which they lose the self-monitoring features of episodic recall and feel not as if they are intensely recalling a past event, but rather that they are in the event itself.[105] Others have knowledge of a traumatic event but no sense of self: They have noetic but not autonoetic awareness of the experience. The capacity of the left prefrontal region to encode episodic memory may have been impaired by blocked explicit encoding as proposed above and/or by the flood of right-hemisphere representations of the overwhelming event. Various studies of trauma patients reveal a significant asymmetry in hemispheric activity, with unresolved traumatic memories being associated with an excessively right-dominant activation pattern.[106] Traumatized children have also been found to have asymmetric brain abnormalities and altered development of their corpus callosum, the band of tissue that allows for interhemispheric transfer of information.[107] These findings, combined with the clinical observation of REM sleep disturbances in those with posttraumatic stress disorder, support the proposal that bilateral cooperation of the hemispheres may be necessary for the consolidation of memory in general—and that failure to consolidate memories of traumatic events may be at the core of unresolved trauma. Such a view also points to the generalization that impairment in bilateral integration of information (the flow of energy and representations across the hemispheres) may be proposed as a marker of psychological impairment.

In individuals with chronic posttraumatic stress disorder, the damage documented in hippocampal structure and function may reveal one aspect of their difficulties in resolving traumatic experiences.[108] The resolution process can thus be proposed to involve the integration of the trauma into a larger associational matrix within the mind. Such an integration may result in a more coherent autobiographical narrative and a resolution of disturbances in REM sleep, and may depend upon the integration of various domains of the mind within the consolidation of memory. These possibilities will be explored in detail in the final two chapters.

As we shall also see in subsequent chapters, a lack of cortical consolidation may clinically be seen in the absence of a narrative version of a traumatic experience. Furthermore, there may be an inability to establish a sense of coherence and continuity across various states of mind. Traumatic states may remain isolated from the normal integrative functioning of the individual and thus impair development. Implicit elements of major and perhaps even minor traumatic events may continue to shape the individual's life without conscious awareness. In this view, negative influences on development may impair mental health by blocking the normally unrestricted flow of information within the mind.

This restricted flow may impair the creation of life stories that would otherwise allow for emotionally significant events to be placed in the larger associational network of permanent, consolidated memory. Schemata of the self and of others in the world help shape the structure of such a cognitive framework of memory. In other words, implicit mental models help shape the organization of explicit autobiographical memory. Traumatic memories that are unresolved do not reach this point of being consolidated into the larger framework of implicit–explicit consolidated narrative memory. They can be seen instead as remaining in an unstable state of potential implicit activations, which tend to intrude upon the survivor's internal experiences and interpersonal relationships.

THE ACCURACY OF MEMORY
AND THE IMPACT OF TRAUMA

Clinicians, educators, journalists, attorneys, and lawmakers all share concerns about answers to questions of remembering and forgetting, especially in cases involving allegations of childhood abuse. As one reviews the research findings and wades through the controversies and politics, a few simple truths become clear. Individuals can experience traumatic events and be unable to recall them explicitly later on; a wide range of research over the last hundred years supports this view.[109] Research in the last ten years has supplied a neuroscientific explanation for this old knowledge.[110] Years can go by before a contextual change in an individual's life occurs and the recollection of a traumatic event can become available to conscious recollection.[111] This has sometimes been referred to as "delayed recall." Although delayed recollection may be quite accurate, explicit memory is exquisitely sensitive to the conditions of recall. Recounting the elements of explicit autobiographical memory is a social experience that is profoundly influenced by social interaction. Thus what is recounted is not the same as what is initially remembered, and it is not necessarily completely accurate in detail.

The human mind is extremely suggestible throughout life, particularly in childhood.[112] This suggestibility allows us to attend schools and to permit our minds to become deeply influenced by the views of others. Often we maintain critical analyses of whether the information we are being supplied is trustworthy, and thus whether it should become a part of our memory systems. However, the accurate determination by such "metamemory" processes of the veridicality of a memory can be distorted by a number of factors, including drug states, hypnosis, and intense and repeated questioning within certain forms of interrogation. Some individuals may in general be more susceptible to suggestive influences than others. Suggestibility studies suggest that it is possible for an individual to be firmly convinced of the veridicality of a "recollection" when in fact the event being recalled has never occurred. Thus a person's degree of conviction about the accuracy of a memory may not correspond to its accuracy.[113] The use of internal corroborations, such as the structure of memory systems and the relationship between implicit and explicit components of the memory of an event, may be useful in understanding how past experiences have influenced a person's life. External corroborations, such as the reported experiences of other family members, police reports, photo albums, and journals, may be useful in creating a fuller picture. Knowing that memory is social and suggestible, and that the act of retrieving a memory can actually alter its form for subsequent storage, is important for interviewer and interviewee alike.

To put it simply, actual events can be forgotten, and non-experienced "recollections" can be deeply felt to be true memories. These findings leave us with several important principles. Patients are vulnerable to the suggestive conditions of psychotherapy. Clinicians must be careful to take a neutral stance with respect to their belief in the accuracy of recollections. Conditions that enhance suggestibility and the suspension of critical metamemory processes should be either avoided altogether or used only with extreme caution and informed consent. These conditions include hypnosis, amytal interviews, and intense, repeated questioning by an examiner. Clinicians should make special efforts to be aware of professional and personal biases that may directly influence their views about trauma and psychopathology. These views may manifest themselves in both the verbal and nonverbal behavior of a therapist. Excessive interest in a patient's traumatic experience versus interest in the patient himself can lead to a nonconscious pressure within the patient to keep the therapist involved by elaborating stories of trauma.

On the other hand, those who deny or are unaware of the effects of trauma on the functioning and development of the mind (such as the adaptations of dissociation and amnesia) are also likely to inhibit the elaboration of others' actual life histories, both verbally and nonverbally. If a person's history includes trauma, then a relationship with a nonaware friend, spouse, or therapist will not provide the safe haven in which the traumatized individual can begin to explore the often fragmented and frightening aspects of memory. Traumatized individuals may be extremely cautious about revealing the humiliating and painful past experiences they may have had. They may have a deep sense of shame regarding these traumatic events, which can make them exquisitely sensitive to the attitudes of others and vulnerable to a sense of being misunderstood or discounted. Victims of childhood abuse may be especially susceptible to feeling that they are "not being believed" and will be wary of revealing their hidden pain to a nonsupportive listener. For example, a therapist who is not able to entertain the possibility that a given individual may indeed have a quite accurate and perhaps delayed recall of a traumatic event may be inhibiting proper therapy from occurring.

There is great societal concern, controversy, and confusion about the accuracy of memories and the effects of trauma. Memory researchers have focused their efforts on how best to study the effects of trauma on memory, and can help bring our attention to the impact of trauma on us as individuals, communities, and a society. A special issue of the journal *Development and Psychopathology* has compiled the latest thinking about these issues.[114] To exemplify some of these academicians' concerns, what follows are a number of reflections on the impact of trauma by some of our leading investigators in the study of memory.

The investigation of trauma and memory is challenging because the laboratory setting of experiments, as well as available naturalistic experiences of highly stressful events such as visits to the doctor, invasive medical procedures, or even natural disasters, are in some ways inherently different from intrafamilial child maltreatment. As Robyn Fivush has stated:

> The research on traumatic memories conducted thus far, however, has focused on public events, events which may be painful or stressful, but do not involve secrecy or shame. But many traumas experienced by young children are silenced. The ability to discuss past events with others, and to verbally rehearse these events to oneself, may play an instrumental role in children's developing abilities to understand and interpret their experiences. Placing past events in the context of one's ongoing life history allows one to integrate past experiences into a cohesive sense of how the world works and who one is. Children experiencing traumatic experiences who are not given the opportunity to discuss these events with others may not be able to integrate these negative experiences, and thus may be left with recurring fragments of memory

that are associated with highly negative affect that cannot be resolved.[115]

Other memory researchers share this compassionate view of the impact of trauma and urge us to work toward alleviating the suffering that trauma produces both in individuals and in our societies. As Christianson and Lindholm suggest:

> Although there are documentation of forgotten, as well as of remembered, childhood trauma, it seems that most often the memory processes associated with traumas experienced in early age are not simply a matter of either/or, such that we either remember or forget them. Instead, both forgetting and remembering can occur selectively, and individuals may represent these memories in very different ways. . . . Children lack the experiences and resources to handle trauma on their own and therefore they need a lot of support from parents to overcome these experiences. Children who have been involved for example in accidents or catastrophes, usually process the experience by talking about it with their parents who help them come to terms with the event. If a close relative, on the other hand, is responsible for inflicting the trauma, such as in incest cases or domestic violence, a child is not in the same position to deal with the experience. . . . Unprocessed and disintegrated memories of a childhood trauma may not only cause problems and suffering for the individual him/herself, but can also constitute a serious threat for other people. Perpetrators of serious crimes, such as murder or rape, have often experienced severe traumas in childhood for which they have never received any help.[116]

Violence in our society has multiple causes.[117] The impact of violence on children may be complicated by the fact that their inherent mental models of the world as a safe place are directly affected by their witnessing of violence in the community. As Lynch and Cicchetti have noted:

> Children exposed to ongoing stress and trauma, such as that associated with exposure to community violence, may develop schemas of the world as a hostile place (Cicchetti and Lynch, 1993, Dodge, 1993) and experience changed attitudes about people, life, and the future (Terr, 1991). Significant figures such as children's caregivers may come to be viewed as incapable of keeping children safe from the dangers present in their environment. Likewise, children may

feel that they are not worthy of being kept safe. If such beliefs persist, then they may contribute to the development of insecure relationships with caregivers among children who live in threatening and violent environments (Lynch and Cicchetti, 1998[b]).[118]

These learning experiences in the community may thus have a direct effect on children's models of attachment to their caregivers. As we shall see in the next chapter, these models directly influence a wide range of mental processes, from memory to emotion regulation. Lynch and Cicchetti describe one aspect of the cascading effect of trauma on security of attachment by noting that

> secure children may attend to interpersonal information more flexibly, resulting in increased relationship success. If children who have been traumatized can develop and maintain representational models that are open and secure, then the likelihood that they will experience successful interpersonal relationships and more positive overall adaptation may be greater. Traumatized children with insecure representational models may be more likely to experience traumatic stress reactions, in part because they may be less able to engage in successful and supportive interpersonal relationships.[119]

In other words, attachment relationships that offer children experiences that provide them with emotional connection and safety, both in the home and in the community, may be able to confer resilience and more flexible modes of adaptation in the face of adversity.

The impact of trauma is also mediated by the direct toxic effects of chronic stress on the brain. As Bremner and Narayan have urged us to note:

> Findings of hippocampal atrophy and memory deficits in stress have broad implications for public policy. With recent data showing that 16% of women have a history of childhood sexual abuse, it is clear that childhood trauma is a major public health problem. If stress results in damage to the hippocampus, this could have far reaching effects on childhood development. Given the important role that the hippocampus plays in learning and memory, victimized children may suffer in terms of academic achievement. These deficits in academic achievement may plague them throughout the rest of their lives. An increased emphasis is needed to direct resources and attention to the prevention and treatment of childhood victimization as well as stress at other stages of development.[120]

Memory forms the foundation for both the implicit reality (behavioral responses, emotional reactions, perceptual categorizations, schemata of the self and others in the world, and possibly bodily memories) and explicit recollections of facts and of the self across time. In this way, we must understand the many layers of memory in order to comprehend other persons' present and past life experiences and the ways they anticipate and plan for the future. As we shall see, the disorganizing effects of trauma and its lack of resolution can be passed from generation to generation. The emotional suffering, the stress-induced damage to cognitive functioning, the internal chaos of intrusive implicit memories, and the potential interpersonal violence created as a result of trauma produce ripple effects of devastation across the boundaries of time and human lives. As we will explore in the chapters ahead, disruptive interpersonal relationships produce incoherent functioning of the individual mind. This connection between interpersonal and individual process is clearly seen in an important aspect of memory, the narrative telling of our life stories.

MEMORY AND NARRATIVE

The telling of stories has a central place in human cultures throughout the world and plays a crucial role in the interaction between adult and child.[121] From an early stage in development, children begin to narrate their lives—to tell the sequence of events and internal experiences of their daily existence.[122] What is so special about stories? Why are we as a species so consumed by the process of telling and listening to stories?

By the second year of life, children begin to develop the "later" form of memory, called declarative or explicit, which includes both semantic (factual) and episodic (remembering oneself in an episode in time) memory.[123] "Narrative" memory is a term referring to the way in which we may store and then recall experienced events in story form. "Co-construction of narrative" is a fundamental process, studied across cultures by anthropologists, in which families join together in the telling of stories of daily life.[124]

The developmental psychologist Lev Vygotsky said that a child's internalization of her experiences with parents creates thought.[125] In this view, children who narrate life events with their parents will begin to narrate to themselves. Their imaginings and the contents of their memories will become active parts of their internal and conscious worlds. This view also reveals the possibility that some of our most cherished personal processes, such as thought or even self-reflection, may have their origins as interpersonal communication.

As fundamental creations of social experience, stories embody shared cultural rules and expectations, exploring the reasons for human behavior and the consequences of deviations from the cultural norm. Stories also captivate our attention, in that they require us to participate in the active construction of the mental lives and experiences of the characters. In this way, a story is created by both teller and listener.

The hippocampus and prefrontal (including orbitofrontal) regions mediate explicit autobiographical memory, and thus this form of memory is directly related to an integrated spatial and temporal map. As the millions of traces of perception within explicit encoding are laid down through working memory, only a selected portion will be brought into long-term memory. Of this selected set of memory traces, much fewer will survive the translation of these into permanent memory. This latter process of cortical consolidation, as discussed above, may be fundamentally related to dreams and to the narrativization of episodic memory. Dreaming is a multimodal narrative process containing various elements of our daily experience, past events, mental models, and present perceptual experience. The unit of a day, marked by the consolidation process of REM sleep, may thus be seen as a form of chapter in a life story. Each day is literally the opportunity to create a new episode of learning, in which recent experience will become integrated with the past and woven into the anticipated future.

Stories involve the perspective of the teller (first or third person, past or present), various characters' activities and mental states (emotions, perceptions, beliefs, memories, intentions), and the depiction of conflicts and their resolution.[126] Several genres of narrative are present from early life on: fictional, schematic (general descriptors of events), and factual. These stories can be about others, or they can be autobiographical. Stories of each type may actually overlap to varying degrees with the other genres. For example, fictional stories often involve elements of the teller's own life story, even if this is unintentional on the part of the teller. Autobiographical accounts may often incorporate generalizations from repeated experiences or aspects of imagined events. Thus the emergence of a story may involve multiple layers of narrative genres.

Stories, in the form of bedtime routines, myths, films, plays, novels, diary entries, dinner conversations, or psychotherapy sessions, are present throughout our lives. Many forms of human interaction—from children's play and drawing to adults' joint attention to autobiographical reflections—involve the co-construction of narrative around the memory talk between individuals.

Narrative can be seen as a fundamental process that reveals itself in various ways. It creates shareable stories (often called "narratives"), determines patterns of behavior (called "narrative enactment" or "performance"), and may influence our internal lives (in the form of dreams, imagery, sensations, and states of mind). As discussed in later chapters, we can also propose that the narrative process directly influences emotional modulation and self-organization.

The storytelling and story-listening process often involves the essential features of social interaction and discourse. The teller produces verbal and nonverbal signals that are received by the listener, and then similar forms of communication are sent back to the teller. This intricate dance requires that both persons have the complex capacity to read social signals, to share the concept of the existence of a subjective experience of mind, and to agree to participate in culturally accepted rules of discourse. Stories are thus socially co-constructed. One can argue that even writers working in "isolation" have an imagined audience with whom they are engaged in active discourse. It is no wonder that the story process requires an intact social system of the brain to mediate this exquisite circle of communication.[127]

The creation of narrative coherence can be facilitated by social experiences. It is by focusing on this narrative system that we can begin to see the relationship between narrative co-construction and the acquisition of more adaptive self-organization, leading to coherent functioning. In the next chapter, we will explore the ways in which attachment relationships promote narrative processing, emotional communication, and the development of the mind.

The influence of narrative on internal experience is revealed most dramatically in dreams, guided imagery, and journal writing. The myriad of representations in each of these processes may often surprise the conscious mind. Dreams weave elaborate stories incorporating a wide array of images from various points in time. Guided imagery brings to the fore sets of vivid experiences that contain active reflections and themes about an individual's priorities and present life challenges. Journal writing can often reveal concerns and perspectives about life that have been unavailable to simple introspection. By defining the process of narrative as more than just the verbal creation of stories, we can identify how each of these internal experiences is shaped by the central narrative themes in our lives.

Narrative enactments can be seen in the patterns of behavior, of relating, and of decision making that steer the course of an individual's life.[128] Why call this "narrative" and not just "learned behavior?" Recognizing the central role of *themes* in bringing some sense of continuity to a person's life directions is helpful in understanding why the person does what he does—and how to help him change that behavior if necessary. Our nonconscious mental models may be revealed as narrative themes. The central, coherence-creating, narrative process has a unifying quality that links otherwise disparate aspects of memory within the individual. Enactments, then, are the behavioral manifestations of this core narrative process that links past, present, and future. Awareness of the role of early life experiences in shaping both *what* is processed and *how* information about the mind itself is handled can help us to negotiate our way through the complexities of the mind and social relationships.

Narratives reveal how representations from one system can clearly intertwine with another. Thus the mental models of implicit memory help organize the themes of how the details of explicit autobiographical memory are expressed within a life story. Though we can never see mental models directly, their manifestation in narratives allows us to get a view of at least the shadow they cast on the output of other systems of the mind.

THE REMEMBERED
AND THE REMEMBERING SELF

Each of us has innumerable anecdotes which can serve to illustrate particular sentiments or sets of events from our pasts. The notion of a single narrative for a human life is too limited, as memory and the nature of our selves are forever changing. As our present state of mind reflects the social context in which our narrative is being told, we weave together a tapestry of selected recollections and imagined details to create a story driven by past events as well as by the need to engage our listeners. Thus the expectations of the audience play a major role in the tone of storytelling. This social nature of narrative means that the remembering self is perpetually in a process of creating itself within new social contexts.[129] Indeed, as we continue to change as individuals through time, our narratives will also evolve as a reflection of the dynamic nature of life and human relationships.

Edward Reed states that "perception is to self as memory is to selves,"[130] emphasizing the important point that in any given moment we perceive and interpret experience from a new view. As we accumulate lived moments across time, we are capable of recalling not as one self but as the many types of selves that have existed in the past. Narrative recollection, then, is the opportunity for those varied states to be created anew in the present.

To extend this argument a bit further, we actually perceive in the present in various dimensions. The "self" at any given moment in time is filled with a myriad of layers of mental representations, only some of which are selected as a part of conscious experience. Thus the remembered self is multilayered. As time passes and we shift across various states, we can indeed recall various ways of being from the past. As our state in the present may also vary from one moment to the next, the state-dependent quality of retrieval suggests that we will also narrate our lives from the standpoints of multiple selves.

With all of this flexibility and change in response to the environment and to internal factors, what makes for any kind of continuity in the narrative process? Though states of mind, social context, and selective recollection certainly influence narrative telling, specific and consistent patterns in the structure of the narrative process do appear to emerge within an individual. One feature that may lend longitudinal continuity to the narrative process is the important role of mental models in shaping the themes of stories. These pervasive elements of implicit memory help create the "between-the-lines" messages of the stories we tell and the lives we live. Another element is the structure of the individual's narrating process itself. As we shall see in the next chapter, early attachment experiences are associated with specific patterns of how people narrate their lives.

REFLECTIONS: SELF AND OTHER ACROSS TIME

From the beginning of life, the brain responds to experience with the establishment of connections among neurons. Those pathways activated simultaneously become associated with one another and are more likely to be activated together again in the future. As noted earlier in this chapter, this is Hebb's axiom. Before the development of the hippocampus in the medial temporal lobe, the brain is only able to have implicit memory. This diverse form of memory is thought to include behavioral, emotional, perceptual, and possibly somato-sensory memory. When implicit memory is reactivated in the future ("retrieved"), it does *not* have a sense of self, time, or of something being recalled. It merely creates the mental experience of behavior, emotion, or perception. The condensation of such experiences are generalized in the creation of schemata or mental models, which are fundamental to implicit memory.

During the second year of life, the hippocampus matures enough for a second form of memory to become available. Explicit memory requires focal attention for encoding and leads to the long-term and then permanent accessibility of elements of first factual and later autobiographical memory. The encoding of explicit memory, which is dependent upon the hippocampus, yields a form of retrieval that involves the sense of recollection—and, if autobiographical, of the self at some time in the past. A process called "cortical consolida-tion" appears to be essential for items in long-term explicit storage to be placed in permanent memory within the associational regions of the neocortex, where they become independent of the hippocam-pus for retrieval.

The autobiographical narrative process is directly influenced by both implicit and explicit memory. Autonoetic consciousness is the experience in which we are able to perform "mental time travel," creating representations of the self in the past, present, and future. As the child develops into the third year of life, the orbitofrontal cor-tex becomes capable of mediating episodic memory or autonoesis. In a fundamental manner, the narrative process allows individuals to shape the flow of information about the self and others.

When we attend a funeral and are surrounded by others who have also known and shared the life of someone we love who has now passed away, we can feel the deceased's "spirit" within us. And, indeed, the patterns of activation of those trillions of neuronal con-nections within each of us at the memorial service may have similari-ties because of our parallel experiences with the deceased. As survi-vors, we attempt to deal with the loss by creating a sense of coherence with the loved one within the narratives we construct of our lives together. At such a memorial service, stories often will be told to "capture the life and the essence" of the person who has just died. This sharing of stories reflects the central importance of narra-tives in creating coherence in human life and connecting our minds to each other. Stories are passed from generation to generation and help keep the human soul alive.

The psyches of those who have been an intimate part of our development live on within us in both the details and the structure of the ongoing story of our lives. Altering our life paths may require examination of these influences on our core narrative structures and themes. Through an elaborative form of contingent communication—the connection between two individuals' mental states, and their joint attention to each other's life stories—interpersonal relationships of many forms may facilitate turning points in individuals' lives, reflected in the changing architecture of their narrative processes. Enabling people to achieve a fuller coherence within their own minds and in their connections to others may help them meet the challenge of living, in which the self is continually emerging in ever-enriching and complex ways. In the next chapter, we will explore the research findings highlighting the features of human relationships that facilitate the development of emotional resilience and a coherent narrative process.

CHAPTER 3

⁂

Attachment

THE ATTACHMENT SYSTEM

"Attachment" is an inborn system in the brain that evolves in ways that influence and organize motivational, emotional, and memory processes with respect to significant caregiving figures.[1] The attachment system motivates an infant to seek proximity to parents (and other primary caregivers) and to establish communication with them. At the most basic evolutionary level, this behavioral system improves the chances of the infant's survival. At the level of the mind, attachment establishes an interpersonal relationship that helps the immature brain use the mature functions of the parent's brain to organize its own processes.[2] The emotional transactions of secure attachment involve a parent's emotionally sensitive responses to a child's signals,[3] which can serve to amplify the child's positive emotional states and to modulate negative states. In particular, the aid parents can give in reducing uncomfortable emotions, such as fear, anxiety, or sadness, enables children to be soothed and gives them a haven of safety when they are upset.[4] Repeated experiences become encoded in implicit memory as expectations and then as mental models or schemata of attachment, which serve to help the child feel an internal sense of what John Bowlby called a "secure base" in the world.[5]

Studies of attachment have revealed that the patterning or organization of attachment relationships during infancy is associated with characteristic processes of emotional regulation, social relatedness, access to autobiographical memory, and the development of self-reflection and narrative.[6] In 1995, Mary Main summarized the following principles:[7]

1. The earliest attachments are usually formed by the age of seven months.
2. Nearly all infants become attached.
3. Attachments are formed to only a few persons.
4. These "selective attachments" appear to be derived from social interactions with the attachment figures.
5. They lead to specific organizational changes in an infant's behavior and brain function.

Qualitative terms describing the nature of the attachment are utilized: Attachments are seen as "secure" or "insecure," with a variety of descriptions within these two broad categories.

The attachment system serves multiple functions. For an infant, activation of the attachment system involves the seeking of proximity.[8] Proximity seeking allows an infant to be protected from harm, starvation, unfavorable temperature changes, disasters, attacks from others, and separation from the group. For these reasons, the attachment system is highly responsive to indications of danger. The internal experience of an activated attachment system is thus often associated with the sensation of anxiety or fear and can be initiated by frightening experiences of various kinds, as well as by a threat of separation from the attachment figure.[9]

Attachment relationships thus serve a vital function in providing the infant with protection from dangers of many kinds. These relationships are crucial in organizing not only ongoing experience, but the neuronal growth of the developing brain. In other words, these salient emotional relationships have a direct affect on the development of the domains of mental functioning that serve as our conceptual anchor points: memory, narrative, emotion, representations, and states of mind. In this way, attachment relationships may serve to create the central foundation from which the mind develops. Insecure attachment may serve as a significant risk factor in the development of psychopathology.[10] Secure attachment, in contrast, appears to confer a form of emotional resilience.[11]

Although attachment behavior is seen primarily in children, adults continue to manifest attachment throughout the lifespan.[12] Especially under times of stress, an adult will monitor the whereabouts of a few selected "attachment figures" and seek them out as sources of comfort, advice, and strength. For adults, such attachment figures may be mentors, close friends, or romantic partners.

HUMAN COMMUNICATION
AND STATES OF MIND

A thirty-year-old woman sits quietly in the chair in her therapist's office. She looks puzzled as her therapist repeats his question: "How was your visit with your mother last weekend?" She bites her lip, looks away, and gazes down toward the floor, saying nothing. She reaches up and covers her eyes with her arm. Her breathing becomes more rapid and shallow. She taps her foot nervously on the floor. Silence. The therapist's heart begins to accelerate. He finds himself looking down at the floor and notices his own foot tapping. The therapist's own state of mind is revealed in nonverbal signals: facial expression, eye gaze, bodily motion, tone of voice, and the timing of verbal signals (whether fast, slow, in response to other comments, or the like). His voice is low in volume, and he slowly says, "Oh . . . it was a hard weekend." His head feels as if it is about to burst. "HORRIBLE!" the woman suddenly exclaims. The pressure in the therapist's head dissipates with a sense of relief. The muscles in his own face begin to relax from their drawn, tightened state as hers also relax. The patient's body becomes less tense. "Horrible . . . , " she moans, now with tears in her eyes.

As this therapist and patient illustrate, engaging in direct communication is more than just understanding or even perceiving the signals—both verbal and nonverbal—sent between two people. For "full" emotional communication, one person needs to allow his state of mind to be influenced by that of the other.[13] In this example, the therapist's sensitivity to the patient's array of signals allows his own state to become aligned with that of the patient. The sense that his head is "about to burst," followed by the release of pressure, shows how the patient's shifts from bewilderment to rage to sadness is experienced by the therapist. This shift in his own state may be a part of the internal process that makes him aware of the often subtle and rapid nonverbal signals sent in this direct form of emotional communication. The alignment of the therapist's state allows him to have an experience as close as possible to what the patient's subjective world is like at that moment. Sensitivity to signals allows for the therapist's internal response in his own state, which permits an awareness of his perceptions of the patient's experience. In addition to yielding important experiential information for the therapist, such an alignment permits a nonverbal form of communication to the patient that she is being "understood" in the deepest sense. Her state directly influences his; she is "feeling felt" by another person. This attunement of states forms the nonverbal basis of collaborative, contingent communication.[14] The capacity to achieve this attuned form of communication, sometimes called "affect attunement,"[15] is dependent on an individual's sensitivity to signals. Parental sensitivity to signals is the essence of secure attachments[16] and can inform us about how two people's "being" with each other permits emotional communication and a sense of connection to be established at any age. In these transactions, the brain of one person and that of another are influencing each other in a form of "co-regulation."[17]

This chapter examines the developmental evidence from attachment research demonstrating the importance of this co-regulating contingent communication and the attunement of states of mind in secure attachment relationships. This is the fundamental way in which the brain activity of one person directly influences the activity of the other. Collaborative communication allows minds to "connect" with each other. During childhood, such human connections allow for the creation of brain connections that are vital for the development of a child's capacity for self-regulation.[18] Studies reveal that such relationship experiences are grounded in *patterns of communication*. We will review how the infant's mind develops within these emotional relationships, in order to understand the research-based views of what forms of interpersonal experience facilitate the development of psychological resilience and emotional well-being.

One essential message is that the developing mind uses the states of an attachment figure in order to help organize the functioning of its own states. The momentary alignment of states is dependent upon parental sensitivity to the child's signals and allows the mind of the child both to regulate itself in the moment and to develop regulatory capacities that can be utilized in the future.[19] The sensitivity to signals and attunement between child and parent, or between patient and therapist, involves the intermittent alignment of states of mind. As two individuals' states are brought into alignment, a form of what we can call "mental state resonance" can occur, in which each person's state both influences and is influenced by that of the other. There are moments in which people also need to be alone and not in alignment; an attuned other knows when to "back off" and stop the alignment process. Intimate relationships involve this circular dance of attuned communication, in which there are alternating moments of engaged alignment and distanced autonomy. At the root of such attunement is the capacity to read the signals (often nonverbal) that indicate the need for engagement or disengagement.[20]

As we shall see, states of mind involve various aspects of brain activity. The flow of energy and of information are both fundamental components of a state of mind. In this way, *attuned communication involves the resonance of energy and information.* For the nonverbal infant, this intimate, collaborative communication is without words. This need for nonverbal attunement persists throughout life. Within adult relationships of all sorts, words can come to dominate the form of information being shared, and this can lead to a different form of representational resonance. Such a verbal exchange may feel quite empty if it is devoid of the more primary aspects of each person's internal states.[21] Infant attachment studies remind us of the crucial importance of nonverbal communication in all forms of human relationships.

ASSESSING ATTACHMENT

Attachment Theory

When children develop secure attachments to parents, these allow them to go out into the world to explore and develop relationships with others.[22] Initially, children seek proximity to their attachment figures which gives them a sense of security. Being near parents can help provide a soothing safe haven, especially when children are upset. As they grow, children internalize their relationships with attachment figures; this gives them the ability to develop a schema or mental model of security called a "secure base." It is postulated that children can use a form of remembering called "evocative" memory by the age of eighteen months to bring an image of an attachment figure forward in their minds, which helps to comfort them.[23] Children carry those to whom they are attached inside of them, in the form of multisensory images (faces, voices, smell, taste, touch), a mental representation of the relationship with them, and the sense that they can be with them if this is needed.

An "internal working model of attachment" is a form of mental model or schema.[24] As described in Chapter 2, the formation of mental models is a fundamental way in which implicit memory allows the mind to create generalizations and summaries of past experiences. These models are then used to bias present cognition for more rapid analysis of an ongoing perception, and also to help the mind

anticipate what events are likely to happen next. In this way, forming mental models is the essential manner in which the brain learns
from the past and then directly influences the present and shapes
future actions.

Attachment studies examine the active nature of both children's
and parents' mental models of attachment relationships. How can
such learned, implicit models be assessed? Models exert their effects
on an array of observable phenomena, including overt behavior,
interpersonal communication, emotional regulation, autobiographical memory, and narrative processes. For example, these models
directly influence how a parent interacts with a child. Parental expectations, perceptions, and behavior interact with the inborn temperamental features of the child in determining what the exact nature of
the parent–child transaction will be like. Attachment research has
shown that parents' expectations and patterns of relating are profoundly influenced by their own attachment history and attitudes in
the present, as revealed in what Main has termed their "state of
mind with respect to attachment."[25]

In the middle of the twentieth century, a British psychoanalyst
and psychiatrist, John Bowlby, turned to animal behavior studies to
enrich the traditional analytic views of child development.[26] Bowlby
wrote about attachment, separation, and loss in ways that powerfully influenced such practices as the establishment of primary caregivers in orphanages and in pediatric hospital wards. His idea was
simple and powerful: The nature of an infant's attachment to the
parent (or other primary caregiver) will become internalized as a
working model of attachment. If this model represents security, the
baby will be able to explore the world and to separate and mature in
a healthy way. If the attachment relationship is problematic, the
internal working model of attachment will not give the infant a sense
of a secure base, and the development of normal behaviors (such as
play, exploration, and social interactions) will be impaired. Of
course, if circumstances change, a securely attached infant or young
child can become insecurely attached, and an insecure attachment
can become secure.

Infant Attachment Research: The Strange Situation

Mary Ainsworth, a professor of developmental psychology at the
University of Virginia, collaborated with Bowlby at the Tavistock

Clinic in the 1950s.[27] As a psychologist, she was interested in developing a research measure that would be a quantifiable instrument capable of assessing the security of attachment. Her idea was this: to study mother–infant interactions over the first year of life, and then to do something that would enable observers to access and classify the proposed internalized working model of attachment. Her Baltimore study[28] did just that and has been replicated hundreds of times since then by other researchers throughout the world. In this study, after a year of observations in the home, each mother–infant pair or dyad was brought to a laboratory setting. At various times in the twenty-minute procedure, the infant stayed with the mother, with the mother and a stranger, with only the stranger, and then alone for up to three minutes. The idea was (and still is) that separating a one-year-old from her attachment figure within a strange environment and at times with a stranger should activate the infant's attachment system. One should then be able to study the infant's responses at separation and at reunion. The most useful assessments came at the reunion episode of this paradigm.

What Ainsworth found in her initial landmark study was that infants' behavior at reunion fell into specific patterns of responding.[29] Each of these patterns corresponded in a statistically significant way to the independently performed home observation ratings for the year prior to the laboratory assessment. This lab measure is called the Ainsworth or Infant Strange Situation.[30] The initial study classified three distinct attachment patterns. Now we also use a fourth, developed by Mary Main and Judith Solomon,[31] which helps further define the nature of some infants' behavior.

At the time of reunion, the infant's response to the mother's return is coded for the way he seeks proximity to the mother, the ease with which he can be soothed, and the rapidity of his return to play. The idea is that an infant who has developed an internal working model of a secure attachment will be able to use the parent to soothe himself quickly and return to his childhood task of exploration and play. If the infant has an insecure attachment model, then the return of the parent will not facilitate such an emotional regulatory function or allow the child to use the parent to return to playing.

The Strange Situation classifications (see Table 2, right side) at one year of age have been associated with numerous findings as children grow into adolescence, such as emotional maturity, peer relationships, and academic performance.[32] These correlations suggest that patterns of relating between parent and child have significant

TABLE 2. AAI Classifications and Corresponding Patterns of Infant Strange Situation Behavior

Adult state of mind with respect to attachment	Infant Strange Situation behavior
Secure/autonomous (F)	Secure (B)
Coherent, collaborative discourse. Valuing of attachment, but seems objective regarding any particular event/relationship. Description and evaluation of attachment-related experiences is consistent, whether experiences are favorable or unfavorable. Discourse does not notably violate any of Grice's maxims.	Explores room and toys with interest in preseparation episodes. Shows signs of missing parent during separation, often crying by the second separation. Obvious preference for parent over stranger. Greets parent actively, usually initiating physical contact. Usually some contact maintaining by second reunion, but then settles and returns to play.
Dismissing (Ds)	Avoidant (A)
Not coherent. Dismissing of attachment-related experiences and relationships. Normalizing ("excellent, very normal mother"), with generalized representations of history unsupported or actively contradicted by episodes recounted, thus violating Grice's maxim of quality. Transcripts also tend to be excessively brief, violating the maxim of quantity.	Fails to cry on separation from parent. Actively avoids and ignores parent on reunion (i.e., by moving away, turning away, or leaning out of arms when picked up). Little or no proximity or contact seeking, no distress, and no anger. Response to parent appears unemotional. Focuses on toys or environment throughout procedure.
Preoccupied (E)	Resistant or ambivalent (C)
Not coherent. Preoccupied with or by past attachment relationships/experiences, speaker appears angry, passive, or fearful. Sentences often long, grammatically entangled, or filled with vague usages ("dadadada," "and that"), thus violating Grice's maxims of manner and relevance. Transcripts often excessively long, violating the maxim of quantity.	May be wary or distressed even prior to separation, with little exploration. Preoccupied with parent throughout procedure, may seem angry or passive. Fails to settle and take comfort in parent on reunion, and usually continues to focus on parent and cry. Fails to return to exploration after reunion.
Unresolved/disorganized (U/d)	Disorganized/disoriented (D)
During discussions of loss or abuse, individual shows striking lapse in the monitoring of reasoning or discourse. For example, individual may briefly indicate a belief that a dead person is still alive in the physical sense, or that this person was killed by a childhood thought. Individual may lapse into prolonged silence or eulogistic speech. The speaker will ordinarily otherwise fit Ds, E, or F categories.	The infant displays disorganized and/or disoriented behaviors in the parent's presence, suggesting a temporary collapse of behavioral strategies. For example, the infant may freeze with a trance-like expression, hands in air; may rise at parent's entrance, then fall prone and huddled on the floor; or may cling while crying hard and leaning away with gaze averted. Infant will ordinarily otherwise fit A, B, or C categories.

Note. From Hesse (1999). Copyright 1999 by the Guilford Press. Reprinted by permission. Descriptions of the adult attachment classification system are summarized from Main, Kaplan, and Cassidy (1985) and from Main and Goldwyn (1984, 1998). Descriptions of infant A, B, and C categories are summarized from Ainsworth, Blehar, Waters, and Wall (1978), and the description of the infant D category is summarized from Main and Solomon (1990).

influences later in life. Since most of these children have continued to have the same parents, these correlations by themselves only support, but do not prove, some views that the first year of life is a critical period of development.[33] Parents and other caregivers continue to influence us throughout childhood. Bowlby's term "internal working model of attachment" was coined in order to emphasize the manipulable working nature of the attachment system.[34] Patterns established early in life have a major impact on functioning, but the individual's experiences continue to influence the internal model of attachment. This suggests that new relationship experiences have the potential to move individuals toward a more secure state of mind with respect to attachment. Intervention studies support the idea that a relationship-based treatment focus can enable proper development to occur.[35]

It may at first seem artificial to reduce complex behavior into segmented, distinct categories. But research must often try to cluster subjects into groups in order to find statistically meaningful patterns. These groupings are general patterns, and a given individual or relationship may reveal elements of several classifications. Nevertheless, this way of thinking scientifically about organizational forms can inform us greatly about global patterns of behavior. Longitudinal attachment studies, which follow parents and infants as they grow throughout the lifespan, require such classifications and have yielded some fascinating and powerful findings useful in understanding the nature of human experience.[36] As we review the specific attachment categories, keep in mind that a given individual may experience a number of elements from each classification. The manner in which an individual has come to integrate a coherent model across numerous experiences may in fact be at the heart of how attachment experiences shape the integrating functions that create a coherent mind.[37]

A Brief Overview of Infant Attachment Classifications

Parents who are emotionally available, perceptive, and responsive to their infants' needs and mental states—that is, those who are sensitive to their children's signals—have infants who are most often "securely" attached. These children seek proximity and quickly return to play in the Strange Situation. The Strange Situation activates the attachment system; this leads a child to engage in proximity-seeking behavior, which is then terminated after contact with the figure to whom the child has a secure attachment.[38] In low-risk, nonclinical populations, security of attachment to mothers is found in about fifty-five to sixty-five percent of infants.[39]

Parents who are emotionally unavailable, imperceptive, rejecting, and unresponsive are associated with "avoidantly" attached infants. These babies seem to ignore the return of their parents in the Strange Situation. Their attentional and representational state is a "deactivating" one, which leads to an external behavior that minimizes proximity seeking.[40] In low-risk samples, twenty to thirty percent of infants are found to be avoidantly attached to their mothers.

Those parents who are inconsistently available, perceptive, and responsive, and who tend to intrude their own states of mind onto those of their children, tend to have children who have "resistant" or "ambivalent" attachments. These infants seem anxious, are not easily soothed, and do not readily return to play in the Strange Situation at the time of reunion. In this case, there is an "overactivation" of the attachment system, in which a child's attentional/representational state leads to external proximity-seeking behavior that is *not* terminated by contact with the parent. In other words, the relationship with the parent is not able to turn the attachment behavior "off" after reunion, and the child remains with an overactivating or maximizing strategy toward attachment filled with a sense of anxiety.[41] In nonclinical, low-risk populations, five to fifteen percent of infants display this type of attachment to their mothers.

Finally, parents who show frightened, frightening, or disoriented communications during the first year of life tend to have infants who Main and Solomon identified as "disorganized/disoriented" in their attachments.[42] During the Strange Situation, such an infant appears disorganized and disoriented during the return of the parent: for example, some have been observed turning in circles, approaching and then avoiding the parent, or entering a trance-like state of "freezing" or stillness.[43] Dyads falling into this attachment category are also given a best-fitting alternative primary classification of one of the prior three organized forms of attachment; for this reason, the sum of all of the percentages reported here is over one hundred. In nonclinical populations, disorganized attachments are found in twenty to forty percent of infants studied. In parentally maltreated infants, disorganized attachment is found in as many as eighty percent.[44]

For each of these classification categories of the Strange Situation, attachment theory suggests that the pattern of communication between parent and child has shaped the way the child's attachment system has adapted to the experiences with the attachment figure. In this way, the genetically preprogrammed, inborn attachment system has been shaped by experience. This adaptation produces characteristic organizational changes in the way the child's mind develops. This can be seen as a fundamental way in which the mind and patterns of communication of the adult directly shape the organization of the developing child's brain.

In particular, these patterns of brain function—these states of mind—become activated within the context of a specific relationship. One child can have distinct attachment strategies for each parent. In this manner, we can propose that the interpersonal relationship directly shapes the neurobiological state of the infant's brain within interactions with each caregiver. These states create an attentional and representational set of activations that are thought to minimize distress, regulate behavior, and help the child organize the self.[45] The activation of a particular state in the presence of a particular caregiver is an adaptive process. As we'll see below, both secure attachment and the "organized forms" of insecure attachment (avoidant and ambivalent) reveal effective modes of adaptation. In contrast, Main and Hesse have proposed that the nonorganized form of attachment (disorganized/disoriented) reveals that the infant has been presented with an unsolvable problem or "paradoxical injunction"[46] in which the parent, being the source of fear and disorientation, makes an organized, effective adaptive state impossible to achieve.[47]

Adult Attachment: Moving to the Level of Mental Representations

By pursuing the question of why parents act in such distinctly different patterns with their children, Mary Main—a graduate student working with Mary Ainsworth just following her original attachment studies in Baltimore, and presently a professor at the University of California at Berkeley—was able to move the field of attachment beyond the study of infant behavior and into the representational level of analysis.[48] Main, with her students Carol George and Nancy Kaplan, asked the parents in her attachment studies about their recollections of their own childhood experiences.[49] What they found was that a parent's pattern of narrating the "story" of her early family life within the semistructured setting of an adult interview could be correlated with the Strange Situation classification of that parent's child. In this manner, Main began what is now a powerfully rewarding set of investigations by creating a research instrument called the

Adult Attachment Interview (AAI).[50] Studies using the AAI are being carried out throughout the world.[51]

The AAI is a narrative assessment of an adult's "state of mind with respect to attachment," which reflects a particular organizational pattern or engrained state of mind of that individual at the time of the interview.[52] The method of analysis of assessing an adult's state of mind with respect to attachment was developed by Mary Main and Ruth Goldwyn (then a visiting and graduate student from London) in the early 1980s. Its robust correlation with that adult's relationship with his offspring suggests that such a stance is in fact quite tenacious in the person's life.[53] Furthermore, attempts to correlate the AAI with features of an adult's personality have not revealed any significant associations.[54] This demonstrates that some of the measures of personality found in behavioral genetics to have a large degree of heritability are not associated with AAI findings; it therefore supports the notion that the AAI is measuring some feature of the adult derived primarily from the individual's experiences.[55] Recent results from carefully performed longitudinal studies using Main and Goldwyn's analysis of the AAI in fact have now found that secure versus insecure childhood attachment status as observed in Ainsworth's Strange Situation can often predict later adult attachment findings.[56] Though all indications point to a primary role of experiential factors (including childhood attachment and more recent relationship experiences in certain AAI results as discussed), Main has noted that the possible contributions of genetic factors will need to be further examined in future studies that utilize standard behavioral genetics approaches, such as twin and adoption studies.[57]

The strength of the AAI's correlations with the Strange Situation results has been reinforced by a number of findings suggesting that it is measuring some feature of the subject that is robust, persists across time, and is independent of other variables. These psychometric properties of this instrument[58] include that the AAI is stable with repeated assessments across a one-month to four-year period[59]; unrelated to most measures of intelligence[60]; and unrelated to both long- and short-term memory, social desirability, or interviewer style.[61] The AAI is even more predictive of the Strange Situation results than it is predictive of direct research observations of parenting behavior available at the present time. van IJzendoorn has termed this a "transmission gap"[62]—a finding that has yet to be fully understood. However, it reinforces the notion that the AAI is assessing some fundamental mental process of the parent. All of these findings suggest that understanding the processes underlying the AAI, including memory, social communication, and some integrating process creating coherence of mind, will enable us to explore more fully the interpersonal nature of the development of the mind.

The AAI is a semistructured autobiographical narrative in which an adult, or sometimes a teenager (usually a parent or parent-to-be), is asked a series of questions about her own childhood.[63] These questions include versions of the following: What were growing up and the person's early relationship with each parent like? What was the experience of being separated, upset, threatened, or fearful? Was there an experience of loss, and, if so, what was the impact on the individual and the whole family? How did the person's relationship with her parents change over time? How have all of these things shaped the development into adulthood of the individual's personality and parenting approach?

The AAI narrative is a subjective account of the recollections of the individual. It does not claim to be an exact accounting of what occurred in the past. The method of interview analysis developed by Main and Goldwyn begins with an examination of the elements of the recalled and inferred experiences with parents, and each of the speaker's parents is ultimately scored for the extent to which the rater concludes that he or she was loving, rejecting, involving/role-reversing, neglecting when present, and pressuring to achieve.[64] However, the most critical aspects of the process of interview analysis rest upon the speaker's ways of presenting and evaluating his history. It is here that the AAI offers a unique perspective on the relationships among attachment, memory, and narrative.

The AAI narrative is classified through an extensive review of the interview transcript; the rater examines elements of the described experiences from the past, as well as the pattern of communication between the interviewer and the subject.[65] In the discourse, and indeed in our daily conversations, how we talk with people reflects our internal processes and our response to the social situation of a conversation with another person. The analysis leads to ratings of what is called the current "state of mind with respect to attachment." Domains of this state of mind include the overall coherence of the transcript, idealization of parent, insistence on lack of recall, involved/involving (preoccupying) anger, passivity or vagueness of discourse, fear of loss, dismissing derogation, metacognitive monitoring, and overall coherence of mind. In some individuals there is some disorganization or disorientation in reasoning or discourse when focusing on the topic of loss (of a family member by death) or abuse; this is assessed by scales for unresolved loss and/or trauma.[66]

The final classification, ascertained after several in-depth readings of the transcript, is based on examination of the numerically determined profiles across the domains of mental states with respect to attachment, together with directions for classifying the speaker's current state of mind (determined by the discourse analysis). This interview has a tremendous capacity to bring out subtle aspects of autobiographical narratives. Subjects are often amazed at how this forty-five- to ninety-minute interview with a stranger can bring out such personally meaningful and often previously unrealized aspects of their early histories. As a parallel to the Strange Situation, the AAI also places a subject in an unusual setting in which "the unconscious is surprised" by the discussion of such intimate attachment issues, early memories, and reflections on how these experiences have shaped the adult's development and parenting behavior.[67]

As Erik Hesse has suggested, the AAI requires that the subject perform the dual tasks of collaborative communication and searching for memories.[68] The search for memories of one's own childhood and the challenge of maintaining normal discourse—including respecting Grice's four maxims of discourse, pertaining to quality, quantity, relation, and manner—can lead to characteristic violations, which are seen as types of incoherences in the narrative process.[69] These maxims form a core feature of the AAI assessment: "1) Quality—be truthful, and, have evidence for what you say; 2) quantity—be succinct, yet complete; 3) relation—be relevant or perspicacious, presenting what has to be said so that it is plainly understood; and 4) manner—be clear and orderly."[70] According to Main and Goldwyn, optimal discourse can be succinctly described as "truthful and collaborative," and they conceptualize violations of Grice's maxims as having to do with (internal) consistency (quality) versus collaboration with the interviewer or interview process (quantity, relation, and manner).[71] Assessment of the AAI examines how a subject's state of mind at the time of the interview facilitates or impedes the ability to carry out a truthful/collaborative discourse while simultaneously conducting autobiographical reflections.

The ways in which the narrative reflects such a process is encoded in the scale assessing the overall coherence of the transcript. With the addition of the other elements that examine features of the narrative process, an overall "coherence-of-mind" rating is achieved, which assesses the global state of mind with respect to attachment. It is important to note that generally this adult stance represents an overarching state of mind toward attachment—not the attachment to each of the adult's parents. In contrast to a child's Strange Situation classification, an adult receives a single "state-of-mind" classification, not a relationship-specific category. Hesse has described an emerging "cannot classify" category—revealed in about five to ten percent of low-risk samples—which may reveal those individuals who are unable to attain such a unifying overall stance toward attachment.[72] As we'll explore in detail in the last chapter of this book, the capacity to integrate various elements of mental functioning, including autobiographical memory and social communication, can be viewed as a fundamental integrating process with which the mind creates coherence across its various states and mental processes.

The AAI results in an interviewee's being assigned a classification (see Table 2, left side, for a listing of these classifications) that tends to correspond to the quality of her infant's attachment to her in sixty-five to eighty-five percent of cases.[73] These percentages are actually statistically quite meaningful, even though there is no one hundred percent predictability.[74] In fact, of all available measures—including intellectual functioning, personality assessments, and socioeconomic factors—the AAI is the most robust predictor of how infants become attached to their parents.[75]

The AAI has been administered to parents at various ages of a child: five years after the Strange Situation, which is performed when the infant is one year of age; at the same time as the Strange Situation; and during pregnancy, with the Strange Situation performed when the infant reaches the first birthday.[76] In each of these contexts, the AAI has a robust association with the specific classification of the infant–parent attachment. This means that the AAI findings are strong, seem to be stable across time, and have predictive power even before an infant is born. The parent's narrative processes are not merely some reaction to the infant's temperamental characteristics or a function of the parent–child relationship. Recent studies are now becoming available in which children who have received Strange Situation classifications as infants are being administered the AAI in late adolescence. In the majority of these studies, the anticipated findings are now being realized, in that the Strange Situation results generally predict, about two decades later, the AAI classifications for the now grown children.[77] Some deviations from these predictions seem to be related to adverse life events, such as trauma and loss during the later years of childhood and adolescence.[78]

An infant's attachment is specific to each parent and corresponds with each parent's AAI classification in a largely independent manner.[79] This parent specificity also suggests that the adult–infant correlations are not merely determined by genetic or other features of the child alone, but are a function of the history of parent–child interactions. Having differing attachment statuses dependent on the state of mind with respect to attachment of each parent (or other caregiver) is an important factor in understanding the development of these attachment patterns. Also, the four prebirth research studies support the idea that the AAI is measuring some variable of a parent, not just some reaction of the parent to a feature of the child's inborn characteristics, such as temperament.[80] Overall, these findings support the view of childhood attachment as relationship-based.[81]

Temperament may play some role in eliciting particular reactions from parents, but it is not the major variable in determining attachment behavior within the child–parent relationship.[82] The temperament and genetically determined features of the parent certainly play a role in overt behavior. Some studies of parenting behavior suggest a strong genetic influence on particular patterns of emotional availability, for example.[83] As noted earlier, future studies of infant attachment and of the AAI will need to specifically examine the genetic contribution to these different patterns of attachment. Studies of identical twins raised apart and of adoptive children, not available to date, will be helpful in exploring the role of genetic factors in attachment. At this point, the findings from attachment studies support the notion of child attachment as the result of a relationship, not of a feature of the child alone.

If a child has a different attachment pattern with different caregivers, how does this affect the child's future adult attachment status? The most dominant experiences—for example, those with a primary caregiver—may be those that tend to exert the most influence on the adult's narrative and attachment status.[84] Research correlations between Strange Situation status with later AAI classification are based on the infant's primary attachment relationship, most often with the mother. One notion is that different attachment models may be activated in the future, depending on the social situation.[85]

Certain child–parent pairs may evoke specific patterns of relating from the parent, which may lead to different attachment classifications for different offspring of the same parent. These variations may explain why the AAI does not have one hundred percent predictability to the Strange Situation.[86] It also raises the important issue of how the AAI may change with life experiences, such as the establishment of new forms of emotional relationships in parenting, romance, friendship, or psychotherapy.[87] In this way, relationships may evoke different patterns of relating in each of us. The states of mind we experience, including the mental models activated in response to communication patterns with others, can in turn shape the manner in which we establish new relationships. We can find ourselves with a very different experience of the self and the self with others within different relationship contexts.

These social-context-dependent changes reflect the capacity of the mind to adapt to new situations. However, attachment research and clinical experience suggest the existence of some tenacious process that maintains similar characteristics of the individual over time. Some of these traits can be seen as elements of implicit memory: mental models of the self and others, behavioral response patterns, and emotional reactions. As an individual reflects on the self across time, these characteristic traits can be seen within the autobiographical narrative process within the AAI. Main's term "state of mind with respect to attachment," refers to an engrained, temporally stable, self-organizing mental state.[88] This is not a transient, randomly activated state; rather, from repeated experiences with caregivers, it has become a characteristic self-defining state—or "trait"—of that individual. We will explore the notion of self-defining states of mind later in the book.

We will now review in more detail the findings from attachment research with both children and adults, in order to explore these topics more fully. A complete review of this fascinating and important area of research is beyond the scope of this chapter, but such surveys are available in a number of helpful references.[89] Attachment research provides us with a set of rigorously collected data about human communication and mental coherence, which, as noted earlier, can teach us important principles about how the mind develops within interpersonal relationships. In the detailed discussions that follow, we will explore the implications of this important work for understanding developmental processes, as well as the functioning of the human mind.

ATTACHMENT, MIND, AND PSYCHOPATHOLOGY

Experiences throughout life shape the functioning of the mind. Those that occur in the early years may set the stage for continued transactions with the world, which then reinforce those mental functions.

Longitudinal research on attachment suggests that certain early relationship experiences promote emotional well-being, social competence, cognitive functioning, and resilience in the face of adversity.[90] However, because development is a process, older children, adolescents, and adults may be able to continue to grow and change despite suboptimal early life experiences.

Insecure attachment is not equivalent to mental disorder, but rather creates a risk of psychological and social dysfunction.[91] For example, social competence in those with avoidant attachments is severely compromised. Avoidantly attached children have been found to be controlling and disliked by their peers.[92] Disorganized/disoriented attachments are sometimes associated with dissociative symptomatology, which, if such individuals are exposed to overwhelming experiences later in life, may make them prone to developing posttraumatic stress disorder.[93] Persons in this group also have deficits in attention and the regulation of emotion and behavioral impulses.[94] Intervention studies that offer young children the opportunity to develop secure attachments with their caregivers have yielded positive outcomes in terms of the development of emotional, social, and cognitive competence.[95]

For example, if an infant does not receive predictable, warm, and emotionally available communication from caregivers, he may adapt by avoiding dependence on others in the future.[96] If his caregiver's behavior does not undergo a favorable change, or if other secure attachments do not predominate, this adaptation may make him withdraw from others' attempts to establish close, warm relationships with him. At five, ten, or twenty years of age, such an individual may be experienced by others as "aloof." Some might interpret such a trait as constitutional rather than as adaptive to the past environment. Of note is that recent studies of rats have found that maternal deprivation is associated with social behavioral problems, which are ameliorated by serotonin medications.[97] These findings support the notion that early attachment experiences directly affect the development of the brain.[98] The fact that the behavioral problems return after cessation of these medications also supports the view that these brain changes are engrained within the neural pathways regulating basic functions, such as behavior, emotional regulation, and social relations.[99] Furthermore, such findings remind us that an individual's favorable response to a medication does not deem the dysfunction as "due to genetics, not experience." Early experience shapes the structure and function of the brain. This reveals the fundamental way in which gene expression is determined by experience.[100]

As Brodsky and Lombroso have noted, "The fact is that neither genetics nor environmental theories have led to a fundamental understanding of the etiologies of the vast majority of psychiatric disorders. If we have learned anything from recent studies, it is that a delicate interplay exists between nature and nurture." In addressing the consistent finding that even in studies of inherited disorders with identical twins the concordance is rarely complete, they go on to state, "These results suggest that although genetic factors may provide [the] underlying diathesis or vulnerability for a disorder, environmental factors play a critical role in the ultimate expression of symptoms."[101] Environmental factors play a crucial role in the establishment of synaptic connections after birth.[102] For the infant and young child, attachment relationships are the major environmental factors that shape the development of the brain during its period of maximal growth. Therefore, caregivers are the architects of the way in which experience influences the unfolding of genetically preprogrammed but experience-dependent brain development. Genetic potential is expressed within the setting of social experiences, which directly influence how neurons connect to one another. Human connections create neuronal connections.

One example of risk for emotional disturbances is seen in the experience of children who experience trauma at an early age.[103] Allan Schore addresses a relevant aspect of the neurobiology of this situation: "Although the critical period overproduction of synapses is genetically driven, the pruning and maintenance of synaptic connections [are] environmentally driven. This clearly implies that the developmental overpruning of a corticolimbic system that contains a genetically encoded underproduction of synapses represents a scenario for high risk conditions."[104] "Developmental overpruning" refers to a toxic effect of overwhelming stress on the young brain: The release of stress hormones leads to excessive death of neurons in the crucial pathways involving the neocortex and limbic system—the areas responsible for emotional regulation.[105] Children who may have a "genetically encoded underproduction of synapses" may be at especially high risk if exposed to overwhelming stress. In this way, we can see how experience and genetics interact in the development of risk for future disorder. Such risk is ultimately expressed within the neural connections of the brain.

An individual's personality is created from the continual interaction of genetically determined constitutional features and experiential exchanges with the environment, especially the social environment.[106] Vulnerability to dysfunction emerges from this interaction—not from genes and experience in isolation from each other. If the capacity of the mind to adapt remains into adulthood, then the emotional relationships we have throughout life may be seen as the medium in which further development can be fostered. These attachment relationships and other forms of close, emotionally involving interpersonal connections may serve to allow synaptic connections to continue to be altered, even into adulthood.

But how "plastic" is the brain? How open is the brain to further development beyond the early years of life? Which circuits remain capable of establishing new connections, and which are relatively "fixed" after certain early periods of development? These are open questions in neuroscience.[107] For some individuals who have experienced suboptimal attachment experiences, the brain may remain open to further growth and development. For others, early life histories of absence of any attachment experience (as in severe neglect) or the experience of overwhelming trauma (as in physical, sexual, or emotional abuse) may markedly alter the neurobiological structure of the brain in ways that are difficult if not impossible to repair.[108] The questions that need to be asked are these: How can such experiences be prevented? And, if they have already occurred, how can lasting improvement in these individuals possibly be achieved? A major theme of attachment research and effective treatment studies is that intervention via the medium of the attachment relationship is the most productive approach to creating lasting and meaningful results. Attachment research suggests a direction for how relationships can foster healthy brain function and growth: through contingent, collaborative communication that involves sensitivity to signals, reflection on the importance of mental states, and the nonverbal attunement of states of mind.[109]

Research at present into the relationship of attachment to psychopathology suggests a number of findings.[110] A meta-analysis of AAI studies conducted by van IJzendoorn and Bakermans-Kranenburg indicates that insecure attachment appears to be associated with a higher incidence of psychiatric disturbance, including anxiety and mood disorders. A study conducted by Carlo Schuengel and his colleagues suggests that the presence of an unresolved loss in a parent who has a primary insecure state of mind with respect to attachment leads to a less optimal outcome for children than does the presence of unresolved loss in a parent who has a primary secure status.[111] Adult security of attachment therefore appears to convey a form of resilience—at least for offspring—even in the face of trauma or loss.

This finding is consistent with the general conclusions that attachment provides a framework for adaptation to life experiences: Security conveys resilience, whereas insecurity conveys risk. van IJzendoorn's meta-analysis indicated that in psychiatric populations, insecurity in the AAI is far more prevalent and security ("secure/autonomous" status; see below) is far less prevalent than in the general population.[112] By itself, then, adult or child attachment classification is *not* synonymous with pathology, but should be viewed as an organizational component of the mind that provides flexibility and adaptability with security—or, in contrast, rigidity, uncertainty, or disorganization and disorientation with insecurity.

The essential issue here is how the pattern of communication with attachment figures has allowed the mind to maintain proximity to attachment figures and establish self-organizing processes.[113] In this manner, Main suggests that the "maintenance of a 'minimizing' (avoidant) or 'maximizing' (resistant) behavioral strategy is therefore likely eventually not only to become dependent on the control or manipulation of attention but also to necessitate overriding or altering aspects of memory, emotion, and awareness of surrounding conditions."[114] The finding that attachment history is correlated with a wide variety of mental processes central to the regulation of emotion and behavior may be understood by the examination of neurobiological studies that implicate the same attachment experience-dependent (orbitofrontal) region in integrating these functions.[115] In this way, the link between insecurity of attachment and risk for psychopathology may be found within the brain regions that are both dependent upon patterns of communication early in life for proper development, and responsible for the regulation and integration of various processes (including attention, memory, perception, and emotion). Dysregulation of this central integrating process will undermine successful self-organization, which may produce various forms of disturbances in emotional regulation and lead to mental suffering.

SECURE ATTACHMENTS

In the Strange Situation, securely attached one-year-old infants (classified as "B") seek proximity after separation, are quickly soothed, and return rapidly to play. In Ainsworth and her colleagues' home observations of secure parent–child dyads during the first year of life, the parents were sensitive to the children's signals—emotionally available, perceptive, and effective at meeting the children's needs.[116] One could say that these parents were "tuned in" to the infants' emotional state of mind.[117] Peter Fonagy and colleagues have described this ability as a product of the adults' "reflective function," in which parents are able to reflect (using words) on the role of states of mind in influencing feelings, perceptions, intentions, beliefs, and behaviors.[118] For this reason, reflective function has been proposed to be at the heart of many secure attachments, especially when the parent has had a difficult early life. The nonverbal component of this reflective ability can be seen in the capacity for affect attunement as seen in these dyads, in which the emotional expression of each member of a pair is contingent with that of the other.[119] Attunement involves the alignment of states of mind in moments of engagement, during which affect is communicated with facial expression, vocalizations, body gestures, and eye contact. This attunement does not occur for every interaction.[120] Rather, it is frequently present during intense moments of communication between infant and caregiver.[121]

Healthy attunement therefore involves the parent's sensitivity to the child's signals and the collaborative, contingent communication that evokes what has been described earlier as a "resonance" between two people's states of mind: the mutual influence of each person's state on that of the other. Such attunement involves disengagement at moments when alignment is not called for and reengagement when both individuals are receptive to state-to-state connection. The states being aligned are indeed psychobiological states of brain activity.[122] Each individual becomes involved in a mutual co-regulation of resonating states.[123]

In emotional relationships of many sorts—including romance, close friendships, psychotherapy, and student–teacher relationships—there may be aspects of attachment present in which there are the basic elements of seeking proximity, using the other as a safe haven to help soothe oneself when upset, and internalizing the other person as a mental image providing a sense of a secure base.[124] These later forms of attachment can be established in the same manner that allows a secure attachment to develop in childhood. For the first two, "symmetrical" forms of relationship—friendship and romance—each member of the dyad demonstrates consistent, predictable, sensitive, perceptive, and effective communication. In therapist–patient and teacher–student relationships—which like parent–child relationships, are "asymmetric"—the sensitivity to signals is the primary responsibility of the former individual, who serves as the sole "attachment figure" providing a safe haven and secure base for the other. The capacity of an individual to reflect upon the mental state of another person may be an essential ingredient in many forms of close, emotionally engaging relationships. This reflection on mental states is more than a conceptual ability; it permits the two individuals' minds to enter a form of resonance in which each is able to "feel felt" by the other. This intense and intimate form of connection is manifested both in words and in the nonverbal aspects of communication: facial expressions, eye contact, tone of voice, bodily movement, and timing of responses. This type of communication is what reveals attunement of states of mind.

The verbal component of communication can encompass many issues. Communication that is about the content of the other person's mind—such as "memory talk" or the elaborative style of discourse that focuses on the perceptions, memory, and imagination of another, as discussed in Chapter 2—enhances the mental processes of memory and self-reflection.[125] Intimate elaborative dialogues also focus on the other essential features of mental states: thoughts, feelings, intentions, beliefs, and perceptions. At the most basic level, therefore, secure attachments in both childhood and adulthood are established by two individuals' sharing a nonverbal focus on the energy flow (emotional states) and a verbal focus on the information-processing aspects (representational processes of memory and narrative) of mental life. The matter of the mind matters for secure attachments.

ADULT SECURE/AUTONOMOUS STATE OF MIND WITH RESPECT TO ATTACHMENT: FREEDOM TO REFLECT

Securely attached children tend to have parents who have an AAI classification of "secure/autonomous" present state of mind with respect to attachment (coded as "F"; think of "free").[126] A parent of a securely attached child stated,

> "My mother was a very caring person, and I remember feeling very close. My mother used to ask me what happened during the day after I came home from school. I remember one day when I was very upset. She was a very busy person. I came in the room, and I remember her putting her books down, and she

went with me to my room so that we could talk in private. I
don't remember exactly what she said, but I do remember how
good she made me feel."

This portion of this adult's AAI narrative reveals a balanced perspective that is not overly idealizing. There is an ease of access to general
autobiographical knowledge (e.g., the person's mother was caring
and she felt close to her), and specific autobiographical details are
provided to support these terms. This narrative segment reveals that
there is general knowledge of what occurred and evidence for what is
being said. The overall coherence of the narrative is very high and
satisfies Grice's maxims of discourse. As Hesse has noted, such narratives reveal that an adult has the capacity to engage in collaborative and coherent discourse while simultaneously examining memories of attachment-related experiences.[127] Another aspect frequently
found in these adults is the ability to reflect on mental processes
within these narrative accounts.[128] Such a reflective function, in
which the mind is able to represent other minds, reveals that the
adult has what Fonagy and colleagues suggest a "mentalizing"
capacity.[129] This may be essential for a child's states of mind to be
perceived and responded to by a parent.

Even though some narratives may contain descriptions of less-
than-ideal parenting experiences, a coherence of mind is reflected in
the flow of the narrative discourse; this coherence reveals an ease in
talking objectively about the past and an ability to see parents as
influential in the adult's development. The parent quoted above had
this to say about her father:

"My father was very troubled by his being unemployed. For several years, I think that he was depressed. He wasn't very fun to
be around. He'd go out looking for work, and when he didn't
find any, he would yell at us. When I was young, I think that it
was very upsetting to me. I didn't feel close to him. As I got
much older, my mother helped me understand how painful his
situation was for him, and for me. I had to deal with my anger
with him before we could have the relationship we developed
after my teen years. I think that my drive today is in part due to
how difficult that period was for all of us."

These reflections on her relationships reveal an ability to balance positive and negative aspects of her experiences and to reflect on how they
may have affected her during youth and then into adulthood.

Adults with a secure/autonomous state of mind may have a flu-idity in their narratives, self-reflection, and access to memory. They may have a range of mental models of attachment relationships, which allows them to be flexible in their perceptions and plan of action. As Main has described, their attentional/representational state does not require a minimizing or maximizing strategy in addressing attachment-related issues.[130] Informal observations suggest that they can also be seen as having the ability both to enjoy and to modulate high levels of emotional intensity, and to experience rewarding emo-tional connections with others.

The narratives of secure/autonomous parents reveal that their internal working models of attachment are secure, that they ack-nowledge the importance of attachment relationships, and that they are free to live in the present. If their internal working models of attachment are secure, there is little "leftover business" that inter-feres with their narratives or, presumably, with their parenting approach to their children. There is a sense that secure/autonomous parents have life stories that allow them to live fully in the present, unimpaired by troubles from the past, denial in the present, or attachment-related worries about the future. The minds of such indi-viduals can be described as having an organized and unimpaired flow of energy and information. We can propose that the coherence of narrative seen in this group of individuals may reflect a well-functioning ability to integrate aspects of the self over time—a sub-ject we will explore in greater detail in Chapter 9.

An informal subset of secure/autonomous adults consists of those with an "earned" secure/autonomous status.[131] These are indi-viduals whose described experiences of childhood would have been likely to produce some form of insecure attachment (avoidant, ambivalent, or disorganized). However, the coherence of their tran-scripts reveals a fluidity in their narratives and a flexibility in their reflective capacity, such that their present state of mind with respect to attachment is rated as secure/autonomous. These individuals often appear, from impressions of the information contained within their AAI narratives, to have had a significant emotional relationship with a close friend, romantic partner, or therapist, which has allowed them to develop out of an insecure status and into a secure/autono-mous AAI status.[132] In studies comparing "earned" secure/autono-mous, "continuous" secure/autonomous, and insecure parents, sev-eral findings emerge. One is that the attachment of children to parents in the "earned" and "continuous" secure/autonomous categories appears to be indistinguishable.[133] When parent–child interactions were assessed, even under conditions of significant stress, these two groups were indistinguishable from each other. "Earned" secure/autonomous parents, however, reported more depressive symptomatology than the "continuous" secure/autonomous group, and as much as or more than the insecure group. Whether this finding is revealing the continuing effects of a history of suboptimal parenting, or whether these depressive states of mind are affecting the narrative process within the AAI to yield a more pessimistic set of recollections, has yet to be clarified.

In terms of our discussion of the flow of energy and information, these findings with the "earned" secure/autonomous adults may reflect a flow of knowledge about the self across time. Implicit elements from early life experiences are quickly activated in intense emotional relationships, such as those with children and spouses. If this "earned" category truly represents the emotional development of an individual from an insecure to a secure/autonomous state of mind with respect to attachment, then the narrative coherence within the AAI may reflect some important integrative process that enables parents to break the transgenerational passage of insecure attachment patterns.[134] Further studies of this population may be helpful in understanding the factors and mechanisms the mind can use to achieve a coherent integration of mind in the face of suboptimal attachment history.

AVOIDANT ATTACHMENTS

In the Strange Situation, avoidantly attached ("A") one-year-old infants demonstrate no overt response to the return of their parents, who are likely to have a "dismissing" stance toward attachment (see below).[135] They continue to play and behave as if the parents didn't leave or return. Studies have revealed, however, a significant response by their nervous systems, as measured by heart rate changes.[136] Externally, to an observer, they appear avoidant of the parents' return.

Ainsworth and colleagues found that during the first year of life, these pairs were characterized by emotional distance and by neglectful and rejecting behavior on the part of the parents.[137] These parents appeared to be emotionally unavailable, relatively insensitive to their children's state of mind, imperceptive of their children's needs for help, and not effective at meeting those needs once perceived. Later studies would show that such parents demonstrated low degrees of affect attunement; language expression independent of facial emotions; and difficulty in relating to their children at the children's level of development in various situations, such as problem-solving tasks.[138]

The view of such a child's internal working model of attachment is that the parent has never been useful at meeting his emotional needs and is not attuned to his state of mind; therefore, behaviorally, it serves no purpose to seek the parent upon reunion. Connecting or emotionally joining in an avoidantly attached pair is limited, keeping parent and child relatively isolated compared to a securely attached dyad. In this manner, the organized adaptive strategy is to have an attentional/representational state that minimizes proximity seeking, reduces expectations, and shapes other attachment-related behaviors and mental processes accordingly.[139]

In an avoidantly attached dyad, the parent is significantly lacking in the ability to conceptualize the mind of the child.[140] This lack may be evident in the inability of the parent, and then of the child, to reflect on the mental states of others or of the self. Some individuals may have a sense of disconnection of which they may be quite unaware. This sense of distance from others, and from the self, may dominate their experiences. It may also be apparent in how they describe their awareness of their own emotions. Informal observations suggest that they tend to engage in dry, logical, analytic thinking that lacks a sensory or intuitive component. As we'll see below in the discussion of adults classified as dismissing with the AAI, there is also a characteristic lack of richness and depth in the autobiographical narrative and self-reflections.[141]

As described at the beginning of this chapter, and as Bowlby proposed many years ago,[142] like other ground-living primate infants, human infants have an inborn, genetically determined motivational system that drives them to become attached to their caregivers. Although infants become attached to their caregivers whether or not those caregivers are sensitive and responsive, attachment thrives especially on predictable, sensitive, attuned communication in which a parent shows an interest in and aligns states of mind with those of a child. Shared states allow for the amplification of positive emotional states and the reduction of negative states in secure attachments. If primary caregivers do not offer these elements of secure attachment, then the child must adapt to suboptimal interactions. In avoidantly attached children, such experiences seem to shape expectations and produce an organized adaptation involving a behavioral response that minimizes frustration: The children act as if the parents never left and show no outward signs of needing the parents. At the same time, the physiological studies of avoidantly attached children and their dismissing parents clearly demonstrate that the internal value placed on attachment has remained intact and intense, however.[143] The behavioral adaptation in infants, and the cognitive adaptations in older children and adults (paucity of autobiographical memory and narrative, beliefs in the unimportance of relationships in development and in life), are in contrast to the continued internal and nonconscious importance placed on attachment.

ADULT DISMISSING STATE OF MIND WITH RESPECT TO ATTACHMENT: MEMORIES FROM AN EMOTIONAL DESERT

"My parents were very helpful to me growing up. They gave me excellent experiences with classes in school and outside of the regular curriculum. I was able to learn a foreign language and to play two instruments proficiently. [In response to a query about her relationship with her parents from early on, she stated:] My parents were very generous people. My father was very, very funny, and he taught me the importance of a good sense of humor. My mother was very neat, and she taught me the benefits of organization. Overall, my family was very good. [When asked for specific memories of her childhood, she stated:] I have very fond memories of my childhood. I don't remember specific experiences, but I do know that we had a very good family life. There were a lot of good times."

This adult repeatedly insisted that she did not recall specific childhood experiences. She also stated, "I believe in hard work and finding your own way in life. I am raising my children to achieve what I was able to: independence and stick-to-it-ness."

This excerpt from an AAI narrative shows the individual's lack of interpersonal connections from her childhood development. Adults with this type of narrative often have the unique feature of insisting that they do not recall their childhoods. Their general descriptors are not supported by specific memories, and hence their transcripts have an incoherence defined by violations to Grice's maxim of quality (consistency) of discourse. Their responses are also generally excessively brief, violating Grice's maxim of quantity. For example, in response to a question about the mother–child *relationship*, they may state, "My mother was good. I cannot remember anything she did to support that word. I just think she was good, that's all." Often the implied sense in the interview is that there was not much emotional connection between parent and child. There are also reported examples of subjects' describing rejecting or neglecting behaviors on the part of the parents to support positive general statements offered about them. Overall, these narratives suggest that the mentalizing processes of the interviewees and their primary attachment figures may have been minimal.[144] The parent–child interaction appears to have had a suboptimal quality and quantity of mutual sharing of reflections on the mental states of others.

The internal working model of attachment in a "dismissing" (coded as "Ds") adult is thought to resemble that of an avoidantly attached child: "My parent is rejecting, and I cannot expect any emotional comfort or connection from this parent, so I will live on my own as an adaptation." This is a mental adaptation, not a conscious, deliberate choice on the part of the young infant. If a parent has shown little attunement to a child's internal state, the child will experience a world that remains emotionally isolated from that of the parent. The child's sense of self also remains fundamentally separate from that of the parent.

The narrative of past experiences quoted above has an underlying theme: "Life was good. I learned important things from my parents. I want my children to learn to be independent too." This person's account does not actually address the question about the quality of her relationship with her parents. Her past is summarized positively in terms of the products her parents gave her, not their connection to or communication with her. As noted earlier, another feature of the narrative is the person's insistence on her inability to recall details of her childhood. This amnesia seems to include a period way beyond five years of age (the time when most of us begin to have ease of access to explicit autobiographical memory). Her "blockage" of memory for her childhood experiences includes most of her adolescent years as well. We can view these findings as suggestive of the possibility that autonoetic consciousness may be quite underdeveloped in dismissing individuals, at least for childhood events.

Dismissing adults' insistence that they do not recall their childhood is often robust. Main and Goldwyn are cautious, however, in their interpretation of this insistence on lack of recall, since it could also be that it serves to block discourse. This lack of recall should not be misinterpreted as a blocked memory of some trauma. Attachment studies suggest that this lack of recall is associated with the neglecting, rejecting, and emotionally disconnected pattern of relationships seen in avoidant attachments, rather than with some form of trauma-induced blockage as might be seen with physical or sexual abuse.[145] Studies also suggest that other aspects of personal knowledge, such as which television shows were popular or what major world events occurred at particular times in the subjects' lives are normally present.[146] In other words, noetic consciousness appears to have developed normally in these individuals.

The emotional distance and rejection that dominate avoidant relationships create a kind of low-affect environment. It is particularly interesting that preliminary findings from the prospective, longitudinal Minnesota Parent–Child Project suggest that avoidantly attached children reveal dissociative symptoms throughout childhood, which seem to remit as adulthood approaches.[147] This project is an ongoing study examining adaptation in an "at-risk" sample of over 150 children and their families, who have been followed since the late 1970s (before the births of the children). These children were considered to be at high risk for poor adaptational outcome due to poverty conditions and other factors, such as the youth of the mothers. In general, the findings from this study support the view that interpersonal relationships shape the way the mind develops. Specifically, the relationships that lead to avoidant attachments appear to foster a dis-association among, or disavowal of, elements of mental life.[148] For example, the need for emotional connection is repeatedly met with frustration within the interpersonal matrix of avoidantly attached dyads.

Why would such an emotional climate produce a lack of access to explicit autobiographical details of family life? Are these events encoded, but is access then blocked? Is there some different process of encoding in avoidantly attached children and in adults with dismissing states of mind with respect to attachment? Could it be that the lack of emotion does not allow the relationship experiences to be encoded as "value-laden" memories, which are then more likely to be recalled? Do these families not engage in the sorts of elaborative discussions that would develop the contents of the children's memories and imaginations more fully and enable them to express these more readily? The answers to these questions are open for investigation.

These questions suggest a number of possible routes to the lack of recall and lack of autobiographical narrative richness seen in dismissing and avoidant attachments. If future studies confirm their validity, then they may also point the way to what approaches might be useful to enable reflection to develop in these individuals' lives: emotionally involving, elaborative, and contingent communication with others. As noted briefly earlier, and as we'll explore in the chapters ahead, the region of the brain most central to attachment also appears to be the primary mediator of autonoetic consciousness. This right orbitofrontal region serves the vital integrative function of coordinating social communication, empathic attunement, emotional regulation, registration of bodily state, stimulus appraisal (the establishment of value and meaning of representations), and autonoetic consciousness.[149] These exciting convergent findings suggest a preliminary view of how early emotional relationships shape self-knowledge and the capacity to integrate a coherent state of mind with respect to attachment.

The assessment of AAI narratives examines how specific explicit recollections correspond with generalized autobiographical themes and descriptions. In this way, the rater is able to uncover inconsistencies among the subjects' episodic recall, their semantic knowledge, and the themes of their life stories. Life narratives are not merely accumulations of autobiographical detail, but are driven by both explicit memory and implicit recollections of repeated experiences. We've discussed in Chapter 2 how the themes of life stories may be created by generalizations of the past (such as mental models), as well as by nonconscious wishes for, and fantasies of, what could have been a more desired past. This reconstructive aspect of memory can have strategically adaptive functions in creating a narrative sense of self that can serve to reduce anxiety about the actually lived past.[150] The "minimizing" strategy of the avoidant or dismissing stance may produce very specific adaptations of the access to and focus of autonoetic consciousness. As we'll see next, the "maximizing" strategy of the ambivalent or preoccupied stance may also produce characteristic patterns of autonoetic consciousness in which there is a blurring of past, present, and future representations during the AAI. Because autonoesis permits mental time travel, it can involve quite distinct dimensions of the experience of recollection during the challenging setting of the AAI.

Autobiographical memory can be conceptualized as being organized into three categories of recollection: general periods, general knowledge, and specific events.[151] We can first think of our past in general periods, such as "when I was in high school." Next, we may have general autobiographical knowledge, such as the view that "I was good at basketball." Finally, we may recall specific events from our past, such as "when I was at that last game in basketball during my junior year in high school." AAI narratives show that dismissing adults appear to lack recall for the details of specific relationship-related events in their lives.

This finding may be understood by viewing Wheeler, Stuss, and Tulving's notion of autonoetic consciousness as distinct from autobiographical memory.[152] In particular, this distinction focuses on autonoesis as the mind's ability to perform mental time travel as described in Chapter 2. Within the focus of autonoetic awareness is the sense of the self in the personally experienced past. Memory for general periods or general knowledge of events in one's past can exist as a part of autobiographical memory, but may be experienced only within noetic consciousness: We may know that a past event occurred, but we do not have a sense of ourselves in the past. This factual knowledge of even personal past events is recalled as a semantic (factual) recollection, rather than as part of the episodic process of mental time travel. In episodic recall, the self as experienced is represented in memory. The finding that differing brain structures support autonoetic versus noetic recollection suggests that those with dismissing states of mind with respect to attachment may in fact be utilizing differing neurological mechanisms in their narrative recounting. Most individuals look to the left when recalling autobiographical memories, a process thought to activate right-hemisphere circuits predominantly.[153] Do those with dismissing states of mind look to the right side during the AAI—suggestive of the activation of the left hemisphere, where semantic recall is thought to be mediated? Main and Hesse are currently examining the answer to this question both with respect to the AAI and with respect to a self-visualization task conducted at Berkeley.[154]

But some of those with dismissing states of mind insist on complete lack of recall for personal events in their lives. Not only do they appear not to recall themselves in the past; they do not seem even to recall the facts of experiences. Beyond mere autonoetic impairments, there appears to be a blockage in recall or impaired encoding of facts about relationship-related experiences. To attempt to understand this insistence on lack of recall, we can look toward the general studies of memory and emotion, which suggest that emotionally charged experiences are more likely to be remembered.[155] The parts of the brain responsible for assigning priorities to incoming engrams, including the amygdala and orbitofrontal cortex, probably mediate this "red-flagging" of experiences as being value-laden, emotionally meaningful and therefore memorable.[156] Emotional experiences are more likely to be remembered in the long term, suggesting that the cortical consolidation process selects these memories above others for entry into permanent storage. This may be the way in which our life stories come to contain emotionally meaningful themes and corresponding supportive details.[157]

Could it be that in avoidantly attached children, the lack of emotional involvement keeps the amygdala, orbitofrontal cortex, and other appraisal centers from labeling relationship-related experiences as worthy of recall? In one study, ten-year-olds who were found to be avoidantly attached to their primary caregivers at one year of age were also found to have a unique and marked paucity of autobiographical narrative detail.[158] They would say things like "I don't know what to say about my life," or "I live at home with my brother; that's about it." Their dismissing parents had this same quality of minimal elaboration of their life stories, especially as these pertained to relationships with other people.

If parents are uninterested in reflecting or unable to reflect upon their children's minds, then we can hypothesize that they may also provide less elaboration via memory talk and co-construction of narrative, both of which appear to be important in making memories accessible. With these diminished mentalizing or reflective functions (thinking about the subjective experience of one's own or another's mind), narrativization, autobiographical memory, and emotional connections with others, it may well be that these individuals' subjective experience of life lacks a certain vitality shared by those in the other attachment groups. Overall, self-awareness and autonoetic consciousness itself may differ as a reflection of these differences in developmental experience.

Avoidant or dismissing attachment can be conceptualized as involving restrictions in the flow of energy and information through the mind. Acquired from emotionally distant communication patterns, this pattern of attachment organizes the mind to reduce access to emotional experience and information in memory. These restrictions impair the mind's ability to develop an integrated sense of the self across time in relationship to others. The view of the self is limited to nonemotional domains, which are seen as quite independent of the influence of interpersonal relationships. Although one can certainly argue that this is just an "adaptation" to prior experience and not an impairment in mental functioning, an organization of the mind that excludes emotion and interpersonal relationships is quite inflexible. If one believes that emotion and relationships play an important role in determining meaning and mental health throughout the lifespan, then such a restrictive approach to living in the world can be seen as an impairment to the healthy functioning of the mind.

AMBIVALENT ATTACHMENTS

The second form of insecure attachment is called "resistant" or "ambivalent" ("C"). I prefer to use the term "ambivalent," because it denotes the mixed and anxious feelings often associated with this form of relationship. During the Strange Situation, ambivalently attached infants return to their parents upon reunion, but are not easily soothed and do not quickly return to play. They cry, show relief, then cry again; they appear difficult to console.

In their home observations during the first year of life, Ainsworth and colleagues found that the parents in these dyads were inconsistently available, sensitive, perceptive, and effective.[159] Such a parent would have moments of intrusiveness that appeared to be emotional invasions into the infant's state of mind. These were generally not hostile in nature; a parent might suddenly grab a happily playing child and shower him with excited hugs and kisses without warning, disrupting the child's focus of attention and state of mind. That is, the parent would try to be connected, but in a way that was not contingent to the child's communication. In ambivalently attached dyads, the parents' emotions and mental states appear to interfere repeatedly with the ability to consistently and accurately perceive those of their infants. As a result, the infants remain uncertain whether their own emotional states and hence needs will be attuned to and satisfied. Sometimes they will, sometimes they won't. As Mary Main has suggested, this leads to an attentional/representational state that "maximizes" a focus on the attachment system.[160] Mental state resonance or alignment does occur in these dyads, but is unpredictably available and is at times dominated by the parents' intrusion of their own states onto those of the children.

Each of us goes through cycles of needing connection with others and needing to be left alone. These natural oscillations between an external focus with communication to others and an internal focus with periods of solitude are part of what sensitive caregivers perceive in the changing states of their children. Knowing when to go toward a child (or adult) in an effort to communicate, versus knowing when to "back off" and give emotional space to another person, is a fundamental part of attunement. In ambivalent attachments, there appears to be a significant inconsistency in the parents' ability to perceive and respect these natural cycles.

How do parents create an ambivalent attachment strategy in their children? Examination of AAI findings (see below) reveals that "preoccupied" parents have significant intrusions within their own narratives of elements of the past that shape their experience in the present. Is there anyone for whom the past *doesn't* shape the present? Of course not; our minds are always automatically comparing past experiences with present perceptions as we anticipate the next moment in time. This comparing process is a natural outcome of the interplay among memory, perception, and consciousness, and defines the mind as an "anticipation machine." However, the states that children evoke in us as parents create challenges beyond merely cognitively comparing forms of representations and matching our expectations. These parental states of mind are in fact responses to the child's behavior, some might argue. But are they contingent? The issue is that with parents with a preoccupied stance toward attachment, their responses to the AAI and to their children's behavior are dominated by their entanglements with their own past. Their responses to the external world are shaped intermittently by their internal mental processes, which are independent of the signals sent by their children.

In this way, an ambivalently attached child experiences inconsistent parental sensitivity and has a degree of distress that is not reliably soothed by the parent. Unlike the avoidantly attached child, who learns to dismiss the mental state of the parent and develops a deactivating strategy, an ambivalent attachment forces the child to be more preoccupied with her own distress[161] and to maximize her attention to the (unpredictable) attachment relationship.

One way of conceptualizing this finding is seen in Aitken and Trevarthen's discussion of intersubjectivity.[162] In this view, attuned communication has an initial phase during the first few months in which there is a direct form of contingent communication between infant and caregiver. This is called "primary intersubjectivity." By about nine months, the infant's increasingly complex representational capacities allow for the development of an internal image of the parent, which Aitken and Trevarthen call a "virtual other." This is "secondary intersubjectivity," in that now the infant (like the parent since the beginning of their relationship) has the filtering process of perceiving the other person and representing those perceptions in the secondary process of a "virtual other" representation. This intermediate step is the normal way in which the mind connects the memory of past experiences with ongoing perceptions. Beyond the first half year of life, we each have a set of "virtual others," which are continually evoked during interactions with other people. If past attachments have been filled with uncertainty and intrusion, then the virtual other—the internal representation of the attachment figure—may interfere with the ability to clearly perceive others' bids for connection. The individual may (mis)perceive others' behaviors in light of a virtual other that creates caution and uncertainty.

Daniel Stern has described in detail the ways in which such interactions become represented and generalized in the infant's mind.[163] These generalizations form the building blocks of the internal working models. As Main has clarified Bowlby's original meaning, parenting that generates multiple, contradictory models of attachment creates a sense of insecurity.[164] In the Strange Situation, the child is not easily soothed by the return of a parent who, in this particular setting, may be acting in a perfectly attuned and comforting manner. The past, encoded within the child's memory, directly shapes both the implicit mental models and the "evocative memory" that creates the image of the virtual other in the child's mind during interactions. As Main has noted, insecure attachment is generated by multiple "incoherent" models of attachment.[165] We can propose that these processes are state-dependent and can be activated in certain mood states (such as feeling threatened) or within interactions with specific people. The virtual other can be so dominant in an individual's mind that an actual other has little chance of being directly and accurately perceived. Informal observations suggest that for the child of such a person, the sense of being "unseen" or "absent" may fill many interactions and create a sense of a "false self." The result is that this attachment history shapes the child's perceptions and expectations of the world, others, and the self in the direction of ambivalence.

The ambivalently attached child has learned that his own mental state may be intruded upon by the parent in unpredictable ways. The flow of energy and information within the child will be unpredictably disrupted rather than predictably enhanced by communication with the parent. Nevertheless, the developing child needs to have the attachment figure psychologically accessible in order to feel secure. Ironically, the ambivalently attached child is left with an internal sense of uncertainty, which gives him an even more urgent and continuing need for comfort from external interactions. In this way, the unpredictable and intrusive patterns of communication have established ambivalence in the child's self-regulatory capacities. Combined with the parent's own continuing preoccupations and inconsistent sensitivity to the child's signals, the dance of (mis)attuned communication in such a dyad continues to reinforce the intense, inconsistent, and intrusive nature of the alignment of states of mind.

ADULT PREOCCUPIED STATE OF MIND WITH RESPECT TO ATTACHMENT: INTRUSION OF THE PAST UPON THE PRESENT

"We were a close-knit family. We used to play all the time, have fun, walk around. There were never any times when things became too loud, or sometimes they would. But it was OK. One time we went to Disneyland with my uncle. It was a lot of fun. But last week my parents took my brother's kids there and they didn't even call us. Why they do this, I don't know. It doesn't bother me now, but it does. I mean it did. I think. I wish they would stop favoring him over me; but I'm through caring about it, I'm through with the whole thing. When will it stop?"

The person just quoted was responding to the direct request, "Tell me about your family from your earliest memories." Her account reveals an adult with an AAI classification of "preoccupied" (coded as "E"; think of "entangled") state of mind with respect to attachment.[166] The narrative indicates that the past is emerging into this adult's present. The response to the question about early memories begins to include issues about current relationships that contain overt hostility, fear, and passivity. According to Main and Goldwyn, the linguistic analysis reveals the violation of the discourse maxims of quantity, manner, and relevance:[167] The narrative is not succinct and does not directly address the interviewer's queries. Individuals like this woman have easy access to a flood of memories of their childhood, which begin to blend with the reality (directly stated or not) that their past childhood experiences with their parents still actively and profoundly influence their lives in the present.

Preoccupied adults' contradictory models of attachment include concerns that their attachment figures may or may not be able to meet their needs. There is simultaneously a powerful wish for closeness and at times a disabling fear of losing it. This preoccupied state is filled with emotional turmoil centering around attachment-related issues. Mental models of relationships will bias present perceptions and expectations, as we have seen, in such a way that these persons may create their own worst nightmare of uncertainty in their relationships with others, including their own children. The inconsistent emotional availability and intrusiveness of these adults can be seen as resulting from their preoccupation with previous attachments. Using Aitken and Trevarthen's model of the virtual other, I would propose that one way of conceptualizing this preoccupation is that the virtual other of an adult's attachment figure is so dominant that it distorts the parent's ability to perceive the child directly. In this way, the child may be repeatedly seen through the filter of the parent's preoccupations with the dominant virtual other, and thus may be at risk of developing a sense of inauthenticity within the parent–child relationship. As noted above, such a process may encourage the development of a sense of a "false self" in the child. In this manner, both parent and child become filled with representations of the self and of the other that interfere with contingent, collaborative communication. Their inner worlds may each be dominated by intrusive emotional concerns ("Am I loved enough? Will I be abandoned?"), which will be activated within a variety of relationships.

A parent's emotional turmoil and preoccupations with the past and with his own mental state can create repeated patterns of inconsistent attunements with his child. Preoccupations with the past dominating the parenting pattern may also repeatedly lead to an adult's relating to a child as if the child were a mirror of himself at an earlier age. In this way, entanglements with his own childhood intrude on the way he relates to his child. This may be especially true in one particular subcategory of this adult classification, "preoccupied/overwhelmed by trauma," in which the AAI reveals frequent references to past traumatic experiences.[168] Though these repeated references are not disoriented, they do reveal that the adult continues to have the trauma intrude upon his narrative discourse.

In ambivalently attached children and their preoccupied parents, mental models of the self with others are full of leaky boundaries between past and present. The adults' experience becomes influenced by activations of models of insecure attachment from their own childhoods. As perception and emotional meaning are established through the filter of this uncertainty, a self-fulfilling prophecy is created: New relationships are again experienced as inconsistent and unreliable. Emotional joining or connecting is a longed-for but inconsistently achieved goal in the minds of ambivalently attached individuals.

A parent's preoccupation with her own past—for example, how she felt abandoned by her mother or how her father was disappointed in her—can continually intrude itself onto her present perceptions. Being with a child can produce the most intense entanglements with these images and ideas from the past within the parent's mind. The parent enters an old state of mind and can become filled with sensations of fear, rejection, disappointment, or anger, which color her experiences with her own child. The parent often remains unaware of how disabling this preoccupation with the past is to her functioning as an effective parent in the present.

In memory terms, such parents are being "primed" to recall their childhood experiences in two fundamental ways. Priming is a normal part of memory, in which elements become more likely to be retrieved following certain contextual cues.[169] For preoccupied parents, the context of being with children who may share some of the features of their own childhoods (for example, shyness or being rejected by the mother) creates a context in which the parents begin to relive their own childhood struggles. Marital difficulties can also evoke emotional states that tend to reinstate old memories. For example, a father may feel a sense of rejection because of his wife's possibly distant, emotionless pattern of relating, which then creates a mental state within him that resembles the rejected, frustrated state of mind of his youth. His wife's interest in a child may also evoke a sense of rejection resembling the feeling of the birth of a sibling in the father's own childhood history.

"State-dependent" memory is a term referring to the way in which events encoded in particular mental states will be more likely to be recalled if a person is in a similar state in the future.[170] This normal feature of memory is prominent throughout life and is particularly relevant to how being a parent can induce states resembling those of one's youth. This happens in everyone, regardless of attachment history. But how these memories are experienced may vary considerably with attachment history. For example, preoccupied parents may be flooded with emotional and behavioral responses within implicit memory. They may begin to remember, both explicitly and implicitly, particular aspects of memories from their own childhoods as they raise their children through the various stages of development. Explicit recollections may return in the form of facts about child-rearing or other autobiographical events, or general knowledge from the past. Implicit recall may take the form of many components of "personality," including learned behavioral responses, emotional reactions, mental models, attitudes and beliefs, perceptual images, and possibly internal bodily sensations. The activation of implicit memory by itself does not involve a sense of recollection. When situations activate implicit memories without their explicit counterparts, parents merely act, feel, perceive, or sense in the here-and-now. These implicit recollections are not usually subject to a process of self-reflection, as in "Why am I doing this or feeling this way?" Individuals may sense these experiences as just defining who they are.

There is a direct connection between how past experiences have shaped implicit memory and how they are reactivated in the setting of being with a child. If parents do not recognize this link, then they are at risk of enacting, without conscious awareness, learned behaviors and emotional responses that will dominate their actions and create their children's attachment experiences. If these implicit memories are of healthy forms of relating, then the outcome will be a secure attachment. If instead the parents had less than optimal experiences, without self-reflective work they may be at risk of passing on either imitated patterns or adaptations to these relationships, which will keep their children from experiencing a dependable emotional closeness (which secure attachments require).

Preoccupied attachment can be described as reflecting an impairment in the flow of information and energy in attachment-related contexts. The intrusion of information (memory) from the past into present situations impairs an adult's ability to have contingent, collaborative communication with a child. We can propose here that one mechanism by which this intrusion of memory influences social communication is within the integrating circuits of the orbitofrontal region, described earlier. As autonoetic consciousness mediates the mind's ability to travel through time—to experience the self in the past, present, and future—then the settings of the AAI, emotional relationships, or ongoing parenting experiences may evoke attachment-related contexts that activate the orbitofrontal cortex's retrieval of autonoetic representations. For the preoccupied state of mind, autonoetic awareness then evokes a range of intense mental representations that slip easily into this state of roving among past, present, and future preoccupations. This may be how the characteristic AAI pattern is created.

The orbitofrontal region also specifically mediates the perception of emotional signals and social cognition. The dual tasks of the AAI[171] (as described by Hesse)—to carry out collaborative and coherent discourse while searching for memory—may be particularly challenging to the orbitofrontal region in insecure states of mind with respect to attachment. For the preoccupied state, such a challenge may lead to a flood of episodic representations, which can be postulated to impair the emotional perception and social cognition functions of this same region. Furthermore, within the context of parenting, such flooding may also impair the capacity of the orbitofrontal region to mediate sensitivity to the child's signals, to achieve attuned communication, and to regulate emotional states within the parent—the processes that ordinarily allow a child to achieve consistent and predictable social referencing. In an ambivalently attached dyad, these processes, in which the child looks to the parent's often nonverbal responses to "know how to feel,"[172] are inconsistently useful in helping the child learn to regulate her own internal states. These transactions may be at the core of the inconsistency and intrusiveness of the ambivalently attached child's experience with the preoccupied parent.

In such a dyad, the energy arousal often associated with the flooding of intense emotional states onto interpersonal interactions can be seen as an impairment in the flow of energy both within the mind of the parent and in its interactions with other minds. The intrusion of mental representations from the past will also influence the direct perception and representation of the child's signals. Patterns of the flow of energy and information from past experiences intrude onto the natural collaborative flow of the preoccupied state of mind interacting in the present with other minds.

DISORGANIZED/DISORIENTED ATTACHMENTS

After reunion following separations, a one-and-a-half-year-old girl would seek her father's attention and get on his lap, but continued to cry and did not return readily to play. This behavior was quite distinct from her secure attachment to her mother, in which she sought proximity and then was easily soothed and then returned to exploration in the room. Unfortunately, the Strange Situation for this young girl and her father revealed more than these elements of an ambivalent attachment. When he returned to the room, she first got up from playing and moved toward the wall, away from him; then she seemed to walk toward him, but with her gaze focused in the opposite direction from where she was walking. Main and Solomon classified this type of approach–avoidance during the Strange Situation with a parent as disorganized/disoriented ("D"), with a primary or best-fitting alternative classification of ambivalently attached.[173]

During the reunion in the Strange Situation, an infant with a disorganized/disoriented attachment ("D") frequently exhibits chaotic and/or disoriented behavior.[174] Examples of this may include first going toward the mother or father and then backing away. In more severe cases, children may go in circles, fall down, enter trance-like states of "freezing," or avert their gaze and rock back and forth. In the first year of life, these dyads are characterized by unusual forms of communication from the caregiver. This communication has the quality of a "paradoxical injunction."[175] "Come here and go away" is a mild version of this conflictual communication. These communications present a child with an unsolvable and problematic situation. Main and Hesse have proposed that these dyadic interactions involving parental frightened, disoriented, or frightening behaviors toward the infant are inherently disorganizing.[176] They are disruptive to an organized strategy because the infant cannot make sense of the internally generated and confusing parental responses. Furthermore, the child cannot use the parent to become soothed or oriented, because the parent is in fact the source of the fear or disorientation. There is no organized adaptation available for the child. The internal state of mind is thought to lack internal coherence, because the attachment system is such that the caregiver is intended to confer safety to the child. Hesse has pointed out that disorganized attachment is seen in many situations that do not involve abuse in which parents exhibit frightened, dissociated, or disoriented behavior.[177]

At another extreme, however, are children who experience physical, sexual, or emotional abuse who also develop disorganized/disoriented attachments. In one clinical study of these high-risk, parentally maltreated infants, disorganized attachment was found in about eighty percent; in another study, in the context of home intervention, the incidence was fifty-five percent.[178] In this setting, a child experiences fear or terror of the attachment figure, not just loss of the ability in the moment to use the attachment figure as an orienting and soothing haven of safety. When this parent returns, the infant experiences a bind in which the feeling of fear cannot be modulated by the very source of that fear. Without the option to fight or flee, stuck between approach and avoidance,[179] the infant can only "freeze" into a trance-like stillness, which may be the beginnings of a tendency toward clinical dissociation—the phenomena in which consciousness, states of mind, and information processing become fragmented.[180] The parental behavior of either abuse (frightening) or sudden shifts into mental states independent of the child's signals (frightened or disoriented) are thought to be the mediators of disorganized/disoriented attachment.[181]

Children with disorganized/disoriented attachment have been found to have the most difficulty later in life with emotional, social, and cognitive impairments.[182] These children also have the highest likelihood of having clinical difficulties in the future,[183] including affect regulation problems, social difficulties, attentional problems, and (as suggested just above) dissociative symptomatology. Unlike the other forms of insecure attachment, which are "organized" approaches to the pattern of parental communication, this form of insecure attachment appears to involve significant problems in the development of a coherent mind. The sudden shifts in these children's states of mind yield incoherence in their cognitive, emotional, and behavioral functioning. Their social interactions become impaired. Studies have found that these children may become hostile and aggressive with their peers. They tend to develop a controlling style of interaction that makes social relationships difficult. These peer interactions in the school-age child often occur when the child is having continuing difficulties in the home environment that engender unsolvable paradoxes or overwhelming feelings without solution. Disorganized attachment has been associated with serious family dysfunction, such as impaired ability to negotiate conflicts, chronic and severe maternal depression, child maltreatment, and parental controlling, helpless, and coercive behaviors.[184] As the children develop and continue to have such experiences, the recursive aspect of mental development suggests that they will reinforce the very incoherence that is creating their difficulties. Disorienting relationships create internal disorganization that in turn impairs future interactions with others, which disorganize the development of the mind still further.

In these dyadic situations, the child has the double trauma of experiencing terrifying events and the loss of a trusted attachment figure. Terrifying experiences that have occurred early in life, during the normal period of infantile amnesia (before explicit episodic memory is available), will be processed in only an implicit manner. If such experiences occur later in life, then the family denial and lack of memory talk can impair explicit recall after the traumatic event, which in turn may impair the consolidation process and prevent experiences from becoming a part of permanent explicit autobiographical (narrative) memory.[185] Instead, these events may remain in an unresolved, unconsolidated form. In this state, they may be more likely to influence implicit recollections automatically, creating elements of emotional, behavioral, perceptual, and perhaps somatic reactions without conscious awareness of their origins.[186] The ability of the mind to integrate these aspects of memory is severely impaired in unresolved trauma and in disorganized/disoriented attachments, leading to dissociative tendencies and incoherence of mind.

ADULT UNRESOLVED/DISORGANIZED STATE OF MIND WITH RESPECT TO ATTACHMENT: INCOHERENT LIFE STORIES AND ABRUPT SHIFTS IN STATES OF MIND

In Main and Goldwyn's adult attachment studies, episodes of marked disorganization and disorientation in reasoning or discourse during attempted discussions of loss or abuse in the AAI lead to assignment of the transcript to unresolved/disorganized status. As Main and Hesse first discovered, unresolved parents tend to have infants whose Strange Situation behavior is disorganized.[187] A meta-analysis conducted by van IJzendoorn has shown that across a full set of existing studies, a child with a disorganized attachment (D) indeed often has a parent with an AAI classification of "unresolved" trauma or grief/disorganized (coded as "U/d").[188] As with the child classification, the adult is also given a primary, best-fitting alternative adult classification (F, Ds, or E; see Table 2, left side).

An example of disorientation or disorganization during an interview includes an individual's referring to a deceased person as if she was still alive (loss) or becoming confused and disoriented when discussing fearful experiences with a parent (trauma).[189] Examples of narrative findings *not* classified as unresolved would be a person's crying during the interview or stating that the subject matter is too painful and he does not wish to discuss the topic. These latter two examples reveal that the emotional pain of the loss or trauma can still be active and available to the person's conscious mind, but the person is not showing signs of discourse disorientation or disorganization. In this view, unresolved trauma or loss is defined as being reflected in a disruption in the representational processes necessary for coherent discourse.[190] We can propose that the mind's ability to integrate various aspects of representations within memory into a coherent whole is impaired in unresolved states. The orbitofrontal cortex can be hypothesized to be playing a central role in such impairments in integration.[191] Abrupt shifts in state of mind, intrusive "dissociated" elements of implicit and explicit memory, transient blockages in the capacity to carry out collaborative social communication, and difficulty maintaining a fluid flow in consciousness across these processes may be at the root of unresolved states of mind as assessed in the AAI.[192]

If one examines the incidence of loss or of trauma *alone* (and not the indicators of its lack of resolution), there is little statistical correlation with the disorganized attachment status of offspring or with any other developmental feature.[193] It appears that the AAI is uniquely eliciting this usually unstudied feature of unresolved loss, and that it is unresolved loss, not loss itself, which leads to disorganized infant response patterns. Lack of resolution of traumatic events or loss from the past directly affects emotional experience.[194] Hesse and Main have emphasized the role of unintegrated fear in the lapses in reasoning or discourse observed in the speaker.[195] Unresolved trauma or grief creates pain and suffering in both these individuals and their children; for this reason, helping people resolve trauma and grief is of vital importance for present and future generations. Failure to identify lack of resolution can permit dysfunction to continue across the generations within the devastating effects of disorganized attachment. Again, these children have a marked inability to regulate emotional responses and the flow of states of mind establishing a tendency toward dissociation, disruptive behaviors, impairments in attention and cognition, and compromised coping capacities, as well as a vulnerability toward posttraumatic stress disorder.[196]

It is clear that there may in fact be many individuals who do have unresolved grief or trauma, but whose AAI narratives may not reveal this as disorganization in discourse. It is assumed that the percentages of subjects placed in the unresolved category may actually represent underestimates of the prevalence of lack of resolution. In spite of this unavoidable procedural limitation, the unresolved category has a robust correlation with the group of infants with disorganized/disoriented attachments.[197]

One father revealed a marked disorientation during discussions about his own father's alcoholism. This incoherence in his narrative suggests unresolved trauma. When asked about times when he may have felt threatened by his parents, he stated:

> "I know I didn't like my mother's depression, but I don't think I felt threatened by it. She would be OK sometimes, other times not. I think I was mostly disappointed and sad. About my father, well, that is a different sort of thing. I try not to think about it much. He is always unpredictable, though I think he can control himself, though sometimes he can't, and I couldn't figure out when he would, so I don't, I mean I couldn't, know how to deal with him . . . [twenty-second pause]. There were things that would happen . . . [seventeen-second pause]. And they weren't very fun, I mean they were scary. Yes, I feel frightened. He is very big, and very threatening. Yes."

Note the use of the present tense to describe the past—a sign of disorientation. The incomplete sentences and prolonged pauses in speech are other signals of cognitive disorganization. During this part of the interview, something was happening in this father's mind that was incompletely processed and was impairing his usual ability to tell a coherent story while searching for memories.[198]

Disorganizedly attached children and their parents with unresolved trauma or grief each have the potential to activate incoherent, conflictual, or unstable mental models. Abrupt shifts in states of mind can occur within these individuals, leading to a disorganized form of behavior externally and to the experience of a dissociation in consciousness internally. AAI narratives such as the one above reveal breaks in the normal flow of communication—both in the extended pauses without explanation and in the incoherent content of discourse. Unresolved traumatic experiences or unresolved grief over loss of a loved one can be revealed through this disorganization in narrative flow.

A young infant, attempting to make sense of the world, is particularly vulnerable to a parent who has abrupt shifts in his own state of mind. These state shifts are primarily functions of the internal processes of unresolved trauma or grief, rather than directly contingent and hence predictable responses to the child's own behavior. The child's capacity to anticipate the parent's behavior is severely impaired, and expectations, mediated via mental models, cannot be created in an organized manner. As the two individuals interact, the child's state attempts to align with the shifting sands of the parent's rapid changes. With these noncontingent shifts, the child's mind may be unable to develop smooth transitions and will continue to have abrupt and at times chaotic shifts in state, which are ordinarily seen primarily during the first year of life. States of mind begin to have significantly smoother transitions by the second year unless mitigating factors, such as frightening or conflictual parental responses, prevent this developmental milestone.[199] Furthermore, the child may begin to take on a disorganized state as a learned, engrained, repeated pattern of neuronal activations. The child learns to recreate the parent's incoherent behavior by attuning to the chaotic shifts in parental state.

Parental lack of resolution may explain the findings that, as Hesse and Main have hypothesized[200] and as several researchers have recently demonstrated,[201] these parents may behave with fear or fear-inducing actions that are conflictual and confusing.[202] Their children cannot incorporate an organized approach to this behavior. Parental lack of resolution of trauma or loss involving an attachment figure can produce future disorganization in these parents' minds as well as their actions. The conditions that elicit such shifts may include questions about the topic (as in the AAI), or relationship contexts that resemble those of the adults when they were children with their own attachment figures. Examples of the latter include many crucial moments in parenting, such as setting limits, tuning in to a child's distress, responding to a child's testing of limits, and negotiating bedtime and other separations. Hesse and van IJzendoorn have found that in a nonclinical sample of young adults, individuals whose parents had experienced the loss of a child or another loved one within two years of their own birth tended to have higher rates of "absorption," one element of dissociative reactions.[203] Loss in a caregiver around the time of raising an infant may be less likely to have been resolved at that time, and these findings support the view that such lack of resolution may contribute to the development of disorganized attachment and the tendency to dissociate.

Parental confusion, internal conflict, intrusive emotional memories, rapid shifts in state of mind, overt trance states in response to stress, and difficulty with their own and their children's affect regulation are some of the fear-inducing and confusing parental elements that may directly produce disorganized/disoriented attachment in the children. For example, with the father whose AAI was described above, abrupt shifts into dramatically different states of mind would often occur when he initially felt rejected, either by his wife or by his daughter. He described the experience as if something would then happen that would activate a "crazy feeling"—as if "something was about to pop." He would sense a pressure in his head and a trembling in his arms. He would feel that he was going out of his mind, ready to explode, "receding from the world," and drawing away from people as if in a tunnel. At this moment he could no longer stop the process. He knew that his face looked enraged and tightly drawn, and that the muscles in his body were stiff. Sometimes he would hit his daughter. Sometimes he would squeeze her arm. Other times he would just yell at her, at the top of his lungs, filled with a rage he could not control.

The father tried to deny his repeated and sudden shifts into a frightening rageful state. He felt so ashamed of these outbursts that he did not engage in any repair process with his daughter during or after such terrifying interactions. These repeated discontinuities without repair in their communication produced a mental model in her of a confusing and unreliable relationship with her father. Her implicit memories of these frightening experiences might emerge as she grew older and be revealed as sudden shifts in her own state of mind, behavioral responses toward others, bursts of rage, or images of her enraged father. She might have the general sense that whenever she needed something, others might become irritated and betray her.

Such parental behaviors as these reflect parents' unresolved traumatic experiences from their own childhoods. How does this occur?

Traumatic experiences often involve a threat to the physical or psychological integrity of the victim.[204] If the traumatizing individual is someone in a position of trust, such as a parent, relative, friend, or teacher, then the sense of betrayal can play an important role in the meaning of the experience(s). As a child, the father described above was repeatedly subjected to the alcoholic outbursts of a drunk and angry father. His withdrawn mother was unavailable to protect him, and he was vulnerable to his father's unpredictable whims. The son learned that these sudden shifts in his father could be anticipated from the amount of alcohol the father had consumed. He would keep a vigilant eye on how much his father drank each night. If it was too much, his father would pass out. If it were just a little, he would get berated. If it were "just the right amount," he would be at risk of being chased and beaten.

When this man grew up and had a daughter, and the daughter would insist on things being done her way (as children often do), he found it difficult to be flexible. Her irritation with him (also a normal childhood response) was felt by him as a rejection, and set off the patterns of abrupt shifts in his state of mind and the enraged reactions that established the disorganized pattern of attachment. What happened after that was a sign of an unresolved traumatic experience, which we can hypothesize involved the father's present experience with the intrusive elements of his past. The perception of his daughter's irritation with him induced a shift in his mental state. In memory terms, his present perception of her irritation was represented in his mind as a perceptual representation, or engram. This engram became linked with other representations connected with the perception of an irritated face. We can conceptualize these as part of the virtual other from his own childhood. For the father, these linkages included the emotional representation of feeling rejected and the associated implicit memories from past experiences: behavioral impulses to flee, perceptual images of his enraged father or depressed mother, and bodily sensations of tension and perhaps pain. These linkages were made quickly and out of his awareness. He did not feel that he was recalling anything. As implicit memories, they were experienced in the here-and-now, as part of his present reality. These implicit processes created his subjective world and organized his internal experiences.

In those crucial moments in which his perception of his daughter's response initiated a cascade of implicit memory activations, he would become flooded with an emotional response that rapidly shifted his state of mind.[205] This sudden shift could be a sign of a discontinuous experience of the flow of consciousness—in other words, dissociation. At times, such a shift might appear as the entrance into a frozen, trance-like state of mind. At other times, this shift might reveal the sudden onset of explosive rage. The father described the sensation of feeling that he was going out of his mind, that he was about to explode. In this situation, he was overwhelmed with implicit memories and suddenly shifted into a childhood mental state filled with that old and all too familiar sense of rejection, fear, anger, and despair. His sense of impotence and disconnection was experienced as shame. His subsequent perception of his daughter's irritation as anger at him induced a feeling of humiliation within himself. Before he could pull himself out of this avalanche, he would become enraged. In this altered, dissociated state, he would behave in a way terrifying to his daughter, which he would never ordinarily choose to do. He was, literally, out of control.

This father's repeated entry into these states of mind as a child had allowed these states to become engrained in his neural networks. These were dreaded states, filled with shame and humiliation—painful, despairing, imprisoning and terrifying. States of mind that are repeatedly activated can become traits of an individual.[206] The unresolved nature of this man's traumatic experiences placed him at risk of uncontrolled entry into these dreaded states. This disorganization in his internal experience was now directly shaping his interactions with his daughter, who in turn was beginning to experience the disorganization of her own internal world. Therapeutic work with this family would require an understanding of these rapid shifts in states and their connection to patterns of relationships from the past. If we can help those with unresolved trauma heal, then we can alter the cycle of intergenerational transmission of relationship disturbances—a cycle that produces and perpetuates devastating emotional suffering.

RUPTURE AND REPAIR

Repeated and expectable patterns of interpersonal connection between a child and an attachment figure are necessary for proper development. There are always times of disconnection, which can be followed by repair and reconnection. In each of the forms of insecure attachment, there is a problem with connection and repair. In the avoidantly attached dyad, connections are consistently infrequent and unsoothing; there is no repair. In the ambivalently attached dyad, connections are unpredictable and at times overwhelming and emotionally intrusive. There is inconsistent respect for the cycling of needs for interaction versus solitude. Repair in these situations may be overstimulating, such as an intrusive parent's wanting to reestablish a connection and not letting the infant avert his gaze as a means of regulating his level of arousal/distress. Parents who persist at trying to make direct contact or alignment when attunement actually calls for them to back away from such efforts will overwhelm their children and teach them that there is no reliable comfort in connection with the parents.

In a dyad with disorganized/disoriented attachment, interactions can be a source of overwhelming terror and despair, going well beyond misattunement or missed opportunity for connection or repair. In this case, the child is left in an overaroused state of distress without any comfort from the caregiver, who is in fact the source of distress. Disorganized attachment develops from repeated experiences in which the caregiver appears frightened or frightening to the child. As Lyons-Ruth and Jacobwitz have recently observed,[207] repair in such a dyad after these interactions does not occur. Often following such frightening encounters, the parent may be so disoriented or in denial that the child is not given the opportunity to experience repair. The child remains frozen, in a state of disconnection, and with the overwhelming feelings of terror that have created such a large and frightening distance between child and parent.

REFLECTIONS: ATTACHMENT AND MENTAL HEALTH

It is amazing that such a complex process as interpersonal communication and parent–child relationships can actually be understood in a fairly simple manner: Attachment at its core is based on parental sensitivity and responsivity to the child's signals, which allow for collaborative parent–child communication. Contingent communication gives rise to secure attachment and is characterized by a collaborative give-and-take of signals between the members of the pair. Contingent communication relies on the alignment of internal experiences, or states of mind, between child and caregiver. This mutually sharing, mutually influencing set of interactions—this emotional attunement or mental state resonance—is the essence of healthy, secure attachment.

Suboptimal attachments arise with repeated patterns of non-contingent communication. A parent's communication and own internal states may be oblivious to the child's, as in avoidant attachment. In contrast, an ambivalently attached child experiences the parent's communication as inconsistently contingent; at times it is intrusive, and yet at other times there is an alignment of their internal states. If the parent is a source of disorientation or terror, the child will develop a disorganized/disoriented attachment. In such a dyad, not only is communication noncontingent, but the messages sent by the parent create an internal state of chaos and overwhelming fear of the parent within the child.

These characteristics of the relationship with a child are features that emerge in specific relation to each parent. Furthermore, a parent's "state of mind with respect to attachment" is the most powerful predictor of how the parent–child relationship will evolve. The narrative process of the AAI reveals characteristic ways in which parents' coherent or incoherent states of mind are associated with their secure or insecure attachment to their children, respectively. The AAI finding of an "earned" secure/autonomous status is an important point for our understanding of coherent functioning. In some cases, therapeutic and personal relationships appear to be able to move individuals from an incoherent to a more integrated functioning of the mind. The fact that these adults are capable of sensitive, attuned caregiving of their children, even under stress, suggests that this "earned" status is more than just being able to "talk the talk"; they can also "walk the walk" of being emotionally connected with their own children, despite not having such experiences in their own childhoods. We may serve a vital role for this and future generations in enabling each other to achieve the more reflective, integrated functioning that facilitates secure attachments.

We can also propose that a transforming attuned relationship would involve the following fundamental elements: contingent, collaborative communication; psychobiological state attunement; mutually shared interactions that involve the amplification of positive affective states and the reduction of negative ones; reflection on mental states; and the ensuing development of mental models of security that enable emotional modulation and positive expectancies for future interactions.

In those adults whose early life probably included a predominance of emotional neglect and rejection, a dismissing stance toward attachment may be found. These adults often have relationships with their children marked by avoidant attachments. Communication appears to have little sensitivity to signals or emotional attunement. The inner world of such adults seems to function with independence as its banner—living free from the entanglements of interpersonal intimacy, and perhaps from the emotional signals from their own bodies. Their narratives reflect this isolation, characterized by the specific finding of insisting that they do not recall their childhood experiences. Life is lived without a sense that the past or others contribute to the evolving nature of the self.

In those adults who probably experienced inconsistently available caregiving and intrusive emotional communication, there is a preoccupied stance toward attachment filled with anxiety, uncertainty, and ambivalence. The children of these adults experience these preoccupied states as often impairing their parents' ability to perceive their needs consistently. Mental models of others may create a sense of caution about impending loss or intrusion from others. The result for the inner experience of these adults is to be perpetually overwhelmed by doubts and fears about relying upon others. Their AAI narratives are marked by intrusions of these past states upon their ability to focus clearly on the present. These narrative intrusions are reflections of the shifting emotional states that impair their ability to have consistent contingent communication with their own children. In this way, what they may have learned from inconsistent and intrusive experiences is laid down directly within their pattern of relating to others and within their own narrative process.

Finally, we have discussed how parental lack of resolution of trauma or loss has been demonstrated by attachment research to be a major factor associated with the most disturbed child form of attachment, disorganization/disoriented. Examining the nature of memory processes makes it possible to begin to address this basic question: What does lack of resolution truly mean for the functioning of the human mind? Answering this question is of pressing concern, given the impairment that these adults and their offspring may come to experience. These parents appear to enter rapid shifts into states of mind that are terrifying to their children. In studies of posttraumatic stress disorder, those individuals who utilize dissociative mechanisms (entering into altered states of mind) during and after a trauma appear to be those most likely to suffer later disability.[208] Understanding how unresolved trauma or loss relates to the dis-association of various processes from one another, including explicit from implicit memory, is essential to gain insight into what later may become terrifying parental behaviors.

The individuals at greatest risk of developing significant psychiatric disturbances are those with disorganized/disoriented attachments and unresolved trauma or grief. From our conceptualization of the developing mind and mental health, these attachments involve the most profound disturbances in how the self is able to organize the information and modulate the energy of emotional states. At a most basic level, these individuals appear to have the most seriously impaired capacity to integrate coherence within the mind. They are not able to create a sense of unity and continuity of the self across the past, present, and future, or in the relationship of the self with others. This impairment reveals itself in the emotional instability, social dysfunction, poor response to stress, and cognitive disorganization and disorientation that characterize both children and adults in this attachment grouping. As we've discussed, children with disorganized attachment tend to become controlling in their behaviors with others and may be hostile and aggressive with their peers. Disorganized attachment in children and unresolved/disoriented attachment in adults has been proposed by a number of authors to predispose these individuals to violent behavior.[209] Finding ways as a society to identify these high-risk individuals and help them to heal their unresolved trauma and repair the devastating effects of such chaotic attachment histories may enable us to help them develop more coherent internal function and more socially adaptive and rewarding interpersonal relationships.

The inability to integrate a sense of self and of the self with others across time may be due to the disorganization in a more fundamental self-organizational process. Studies of early trauma and neglect reveal that neural structure and function within the brain can be severely affected and lead to long-lasting and extensive effects on the brain's capacity to adapt to stress.[210] As we explore the nature of relationships, emotion, and representational processes in the next chapters, we will lay the groundwork for a more in-depth discussion of how the mind regulates its own functioning. It is clear that certain early experiences create a fundamental impairment in self-organization. At one extreme are dismissing or avoidant attachments, which reveal excessively restrictive processes. At the other are preoccupied or ambivalent attachments, which have intrusions of past elements onto the present. In unresolved or disorganized attachments, there is a primary difficulty in organizing the self, which leads both to internal flooding and to disruptions in interpersonal relationships.

CHAPTER 4

Emotion

APPROACHING EMOTION

Defining Emotion

Attachment relationships differ in the ways in which states of mind and emotional communication are shared between parent and child. We have seen how a "state of mind" can be defined as the clustering of a profile of activation within the brain's neural network. These states organize brain functioning and thus the experience of mind. A child uses a parent's state of mind to help organize her own mental processes. The alignment of states of mind permits the child to regulate her own state by direct connection with that of her parent. For example, in the process of "social referencing," the child looks to the facial expressions and other nonverbal aspects of the parent's signals to determine how she should feel and respond in an ambiguous situation.[1] Social referencing reveals the fundamental way in which nonverbal communication is the medium in which states are aligned. What do these nonverbal signals actually represent?

The study of emotion suggests that nonverbal behavior is a primary mode in which emotion is communicated.[2] Facial expression, eye gaze, tone of voice, bodily motion, and the timing of response are each fundamental to emotional messages. But what exactly is "emotion"? We can know when others are upset and "emotional," but what does this really mean? This chapter attempts to define emotion and to explore its central role in human relationships and the developing mind.

A much-emphasized universal finding has been that certain types of affective expression seem to be both expressed and recognized in all cultures throughout the world; however, professionals often have quite different notions about what these affective expressions actually represent.[3] There is a wide range of ideas about how to define emotional processes. The definitions that follow incorporate both research and clinical concepts in an effort to outline some fundamental aspects of emotion. The specific purposes of providing these definitions are (1) to attempt to clarify the basic functions of emotions, and (2) to characterize which features of emotions are shared among different individuals and which may be quite distinct.

There is quite a bit of controversy among scientists from various disciplines about what emotions actually are.[4] For example, some physiological and cognitive psychologists view emotions as existing within the individual, whereas more interpersonally oriented social psychologists and cultural anthropologists view emotions as being created between people.[5] Even within the field of neuroscience, there is a heated debate about the nature of emotion in the brain.[6] For example, it was generally accepted for many decades that emotions emanate from the part of the brain called the limbic system. Various authors defined this system as the "primitive" or "old reptilian" brain, and described it as including such structures as the amygdala, orbitofrontal cortex, and anterior cingulate. Research paradigms attempted to delineate the boundaries and specific functions of this frequently cited system, but often failed to identify its functional limits.[7] The essential point here is that emotion is *not* limited to some specifically designed circuits of the brain that were once thought to be the center of emotion. Instead, these same "limbic" regions appear to have wide-ranging effects on most aspects of brain functioning and mental processes.[8] The limbic system is specialized to carry out the appraisal of meaning or value of stimuli. It is also a center for the mental module or information-processing system which carries out social cognition, including face recognition, affiliation, and "theory of mind" (the view that another person has a subjective experience of mind). Some authors use these findings to argue for the socially constructed nature of emotion.[9] These findings also support the idea that emotion is found throughout the entire brain.[10]

Within cognitive psychology, debate exists over the importance of the "discrete" or "basic" emotions: what they are and how important they are in helping us understand emotional experience. Some authors argue that there is little "basic" about these discrete emotions,[11] while others suggest that studying the manifestations of these universally expressed states is crucial to understanding the role of emotions in both cognitive processing and interpersonal relationships.[12] Within the field of developmental psychology and psychopathology, emotion and emotion regulation are seen as woven from the same cloth.[13] In this manner, emotions both are regulated and perform regulatory functions. One might surmise from these viewpoints that emotions are everywhere in the processes of the mind. For instance, Kenneth Dodge states that "all information processing is emotional, in that emotion is the energy that drives, organizes, amplifies, and attenuates cognitive activity and in turn is the experience and expression of this activity."[14] This view describes both the ubiquitous nature of emotion and the way in which the common distinction made between thought and feeling, cognition and emotion, is artificial and potentially harmful to our understanding of mental processes.

Despite these controversial points, most theories of emotion share some common themes. One is that emotion involves complex layer of processes that are in constant interaction with the environment. At a minimum, these interactions involve cognitive processes (such as appraisal or evaluation of meaning) and physical changes (such as endocrine, autonomic, and cardiovascular changes), which may reveal some repeated patterns over time. As Alan Sroufe has described, emotions involve "a subjective reaction to a salient event, characterized by physiological, experiential and overt behavioral change."[15] A similar view suggests that emotion can be seen as involving neurobiological, experiential, and expressive components.[16]

For our purposes, it will be helpful to approach a unifying definition of emotions with an open mind. Our everyday ideas about emotions will undoubtedly influence how we approach these definitions, but looking at what is known in science about how the brain functions may help to open our minds to some new and helpful perspectives. Let us assume that the familiar end products of emotion—what we usually consider in everyday thinking as the common feelings of anger, fear, sadness, or joy—are actually *not* central to the initial experience of emotion. Let us also assume that emotions do not necessarily exist at all as we may usually think of them: as some kind of packets of something that can be experienced, identified, and expressed, as implied in the statement "Just get your feelings out." Instead, let's consider that *emotions represent dynamic processes created within the socially influenced, value-appraising processes of the brain.* Finally, as we examine what emotion might be in the individual, let us recall what we have learned about attachment relationships and the alignment of states of mind. This requires that we continue the challenging task of thinking about the individual mind within the context of human relationships, rather than in isolation from social meaning.

Initial Orientation, Appraisal, and Arousal

In the brain, a signal of heightened activity can be called an "initial orienting response." This expression refers to how the brain and other systems of the body enter a state of heightened alertness with an internal message of "something important is happening here and now." This initial orienting response activates a cognitive alerting mechanism of "Pay attention now!" that does not require conscious awareness and does not initially have a positive or negative tone.[17] Very rapidly (within microseconds), the brain processes the representations of the body and the external world generated with this initial orienting process. As this occurs, processes that can be called "elaborative appraisal and arousal" begin and direct the flow of energy through the system. Elaborative appraisal and arousal serve to modulate the state of mind by directing the flow of activation of certain circuits and the deactivation of others. In this way, initial orientation sets off a cascade of subsequent elaborative appraisal–arousal circuits, which serve to differentiate the unfolding states of mind within the individual.[18]

Elaborative appraisals assess whether a stimulus is "good" or "bad" and determine whether the organism should move toward or away from the stimulus. The evolutionary benefit of having core processes that rapidly assess the value of events in the world helps us to understand why the appraisal and arousal processes are so central to the functioning of the brain.[19] As the circuits are activated in response to this "good–bad" evaluation, the mind has a further elaboration of the flow of energy through its various mental processes involved in approach or withdrawal.[20] *Emotional processing prepares the brain and the rest of the body for action.* Elaborative appraisal and arousal extend the initial orienting process of "Pay attention!" to "Act!" within a short period of time. The appraisal process evaluates the informational meaning of stimuli; the arousal process directs the flow of energy through the system.

Appraisal involves a complex web of evaluative mechanisms, in which both external and internal factors play active roles. The specific nature of appraisal incorporates past experience of the stimulus, including emotional and representational elements of memory; present context of the internal emotional state and external social environment; elements of the stimulus, such as intensity and familiarity; and expectations for the future.

Alan Sroufe has described the central role of "discrepancy" of the stimulus from internal expectations in the generation of emotional engagement with the environmental surround.[21] In Sroufe's terms, the emotional arousal generated in response to such a discordance between internal set and external features is called "tension." Emotion and its regulation are examined within a "tension modulation hypothesis": Such tension is not in need of reduction, but is managed within an individual's interaction with the environment, especially with significant others in the social world. Emotional forms of arousal are distinguished from other forms of arousal— such as those arising from exercise or drinking caffeinated beverages—in that they reflect a subjective sense of meaning, which is evaluated in response to engaging with experience (internal or external). The framework offered here is consonant with this view of emotional tension, and I use the general term "arousal" with this emotional engagement frame in mind.

Primary Emotions

The term "primary" emotions can be used to describe the textures of the shifts in brain state that are the results of both initial orientation and elaborative appraisal–arousal processes. This concept is distinct from that of "basic" or "discrete" emotions, sometimes also called "categorical," which refers to differentiated emotional states. The use of the term "primary" is suggested here to emphasize the initial, core, and ubiquitous quality of these essential emotional features. As in "primary" colors, the term also implies that various combinations of primary emotional elements may constitute a wide range of textures within the spectrum of emotional experience.

These primary emotional sensations of the mind's state are without words and can exist without consciousness. They reflect the nonverbal sensation of shifts in the flow of activation and deactivation— the flow of energy and evaluations of information—through the system's changing states. Primary emotions directly reflect the *changes* in states of mind. These changes may be subtle or intense; they may be fleeting or persistent; they may continue as gentle sensations, like waves lapping on a shore, or they may evolve into larger, global changes, like a storm pounding on the beach. Primary emotions are dynamic processes of change; again, they are not packets of something, but rather are fluctuations in the energy and informational flow of the mind. As such, the idea of primary emotions is congruent with Ross Thompson's notion of "emotion dynamics," which involve the timing/immediacy, magnitude, and specificity of emotional response.[22]

When an event has meaning for an individual, because it is discrepant from prior experiences or because other evaluative processes label it with significance, the brain is alerted to focus attention: "This is important! Pay attention!" At this point, the orientation serves as a kind of jolt to the system. The primary emotional experience is one of increased energy and alertness. Second, the brain must further appraise the meaning of the stimulus and of the aroused state itself. At this moment, primary emotions are now being experienced as developing "hedonic tone" or "valence." For example, the elaborative appraisal and arousal processes may create a sensation such as "This important thing is bad. Watch out! There is danger here," and the flow of energy through the system becomes channeled toward a cautious, hypervigilant stance. At this point, the rush of energy has now been directed to a fearful, unpleasant state reflected in a high primary emotional intensity with a sense of danger. In contrast, elaborative appraisal and arousal may assess the initial orientation as good, something to seek more of; this creates a primary emotional state of eager anticipation. In this way, appraisal and arousal create a state of mind that is predisposing the individual to act in a certain fashion. At the most basic level, valence can be labeled as good and involve approach, or can be labeled as bad and involve withdrawal.[23]

Primary emotions themselves, in addition to the stimulus itself, can be appraised by the value systems of the brain. This evaluation of primary emotions reflects the basic flow of emotions from initial orientation to elaborated appraisal–arousal processes. In this manner, the mind begins to assess the value of its own evaluative and activation processes. The recursive nature of such a continuing "appraisal of appraisals" is actually quite common in the complex system of the mind (we shall return to this characteristic in Chapter 6). This also raises the issue of how both temperament and learning directly affect core emotional responsiveness.[24] Some individuals may react to their own intense arousal with a negative appraisal and a tendency to withdraw both behaviorally and cognitively from the further elaboration of their own emotional states, as in the case of shy individuals.[25] Others may have learned that certain intense emotional states are not tolerated by others.[26] Such lack of attunement to intense states may lead to the sense that they are "out-of-control" states, and thus "bad" and to be avoided. Such individuals learn to avoid emotional intensity. In contrast, Jerome Kagan has demonstrated that parents who support and encourage shy children to explore novel situations actually enhance the children's capacity to tolerate new experiences.[27] In either of these examples, the appraisal of states of arousal is influenced by interpersonal experience and leads to further elaboration of appraisal–arousal circuits, which directly influence the unfolding primary emotional states.

Differentiation and Categorical Emotions

Following the first two steps of initial orientation and elaborative appraisal–arousal, a third phase that can occur in the experiencing of emotions is the "differentiation" or channeling of activation pathways. The more highly categorized activations represent the differentiation of primary emotional states. Sometimes we may feel "neutral," being unable to identify any particular verbalizable feelings. At other times, however our primary emotional states—the flow and change of energy through our emerging states of mind—become further differentiated into more well-defined states.

The differentiation of primary emotional states into specific classifications of emotions, such as fear, brings us to the more familiar notion of "categorical emotions."[28] "Categorical," "basic," or "discrete" are terms commonly used for those classifications of sensations that have been found universally throughout human cultures, such as sadness, anger, fear, surprise, or joy.[29] These internal emotional states are often communicated through facial expressions, and each culture seems to have words to describe their unique manifestations.[30] They also appear to have unique physiological profiles in which they manifest themselves. *Categorical emotions can be thought of as differentiated states of mind that have evolved into specific, engrained patterns of activation.* The cross-cultural similarities in the manifestation of categorical emotions suggests that the human brain and body have characteristic, inborn, physiologically mediated pathways for the elaboration of these states of mind.

The brain has a physical reality to its construction through which internal states are expressed via our genetically and experientially created bodies. Throughout the world, human beings share common pathways to the expression of categorical emotions. In every culture, we can identify these characteristic expressions of "basic" emotions[31]—for example, as sadness, anger, or fear. In sadness, the face will show the typical findings of turned-down lips and squinted eyes, together with slower bodily motions. Anger will involve dilated pupils, widened orbital area, raised eyebrows, furrowed brow, and pursed lips. Fear reveals the combination of raised eyebrows, flattened brow, and open mouth. Though we can categorize emotions within an individual and across cultures,[32] this does not mean that one person's categorical emotion, such as sadness or fear, is identical to that of another individual.

Affect and Mood

The way an internal emotional state is externally revealed is called "affective expression" or simply "affect." Affect appears within nonverbal signals, including tone of voice, facial expression, and bodily motion. These external expressions can be defined as "vitality affects" or as "categorical affects,"[33] revealing the primary or the differentiated nature of the emotional states, respectively. For many researchers, affect is essentially a social signal.[34] The purpose of the expression of emotion is considered to be social communication, as supported by the general finding that individuals reveal more affective displays in social settings than they do when alone.

It is interesting how often people consider the categorical emotions the only emotional processes they can try to know, or attempt to communicate to others. Examining the three phases of emotional response—states of initial orientation, elaborative appraisal and arousal, and then categorical emotions—yields a new way of thinking about how to respond to the question "How are you feeling?" The term "feeling" can be used to describe the conscious awareness of either an emotion or an affect.

We can feel (categorically) "sad" or "mad" or "happy." We may come to be aware of this by how we sense our minds or our bodies, or by what we detect on our faces. We may, as children so often do, be aware of just feeling "bad" or "good," or just "normal" (neutral), reflecting our initial appraisals without further differentiation into categorical emotions. Often we may also be aware of only feeling less differentiated primary emotional states, such as surges of energy, a sense of deflation, images of one sort or another, diffuse fogginess, or nervous agitation. These flows in our states of mind—the changes in activations within our brains—are defined here as our primary emotions, and can be seen externally as what have been termed vitality affects. Primary emotions are a frequent part of our basic "feelings."

Parents attune to the subtle changes in a baby's state of arousal, not merely the categorical affect that the infant may or may not be expressing.[35] In fact, this expression of internal state through vitality affects is the primary mode of communication between an infant and a caregiver during the early years of life. These affective expressions reveal the profile or energy level of the state of mind at a particular moment. The profile contains within it a picture of how the individual's internal state is being expressed in a changing state of activation of the face, motion in the body, and tone and intensity of the voice. Vitality affects reveal aspects of the primary nature of emotion—the changes in the system's state of arousal.

Individuals may attune to vitality affects across sensory modalities. For example, a facial expression of joy can be mirrored in the response of another person's tone of voice, with the rising and falling of intensity of the sounds reflecting those of the muscles of the face. It may be that primary emotional experience reveals both how we know ourselves and how we connect to one another. In parent–child relationships in which the parent is depressed, vitality affects may reveal a "depressed" state, with low energy and a global negative hedonic tone. Research also suggests that depression is associated with a decreased capacity to perceive the emotional expressions of others.[36] The impaired ability to perceive facial expressions has been correlated with alterations in the activity of the parts of the brain responsible for such perceptual capacities.[37] Studies of dyads with a depressed parent reveal significant effects on the emotional development of the child.[38] The experience of expressing one's emotional state and having others perceive and respond to those signals appears to be of vital importance in the development of the brain. Such sharing of primary emotions does not merely allow the child to feel "good"; it allows the child to develop normally.

Primary emotions are expressed in a unique manner in the moment, just as an individual's state of mind at a particular time is a one-of-a-kind state. The flow of states moves forward in time and never repeats itself. This flow of states is unique. Vitality affects are the external expressions of primary emotions. In contrast, the external expressions of categorical emotions may reflect the very specific routes through which the physical body is able to reveal certain aspects of these differentiated internal states. The mechanisms facilitating this movement toward these different forms of categorical emotions, such as the differentiation of sadness, anger, or fear from one another, are not fully understood at this time. The view proposed here is that the process from primary to categorical emotions is influenced directly by the unique components of neural processes that form a state of mind. In other words, the mental state active at a given time may shape the elaboration of arousal and meaning from primary to categorical emotions. More often, however, our changing states of activation within the mind, our primary emotions, may ebb and flow without necessarily becoming intense, entering consciousness, or becoming further differentiated into categorical emotional states.

The term "mood" refers to the general tone of emotions across time. Mood can be thought of as a bias of the system toward certain categorical emotions. Mood shapes the interpretation of perceptual processing and gives a "slant" to thinking, self-reflection, and recollections. For example, a person who is in a "down" mood may find himself interpreting things as evidence of his failures, think of the future in dismal terms, reflect upon himself as a "loser," and have increased recollections of the numerous times he has made mistakes in his life. The influence of mood upon all of these cognitive functions reveals how general emotional tone reinforces itself in a feedback loop that keeps one's mood spiraling in the same direction. This may explain the tenacious nature of emotional disturbances such as depression or chronic anxiety, in which a given mood becomes a relatively fixed and disabling state. In certain individuals, the ability to maintain a flexible flow of primary emotional states may be quite impaired and reflect difficulty in their ability to modulate their emotions.

THE CONVERGENCE OF SOCIAL PROCESSING AND EMOTION

By clarifying the distinction between primary emotions and the more familiar idea of categorical emotions, we can become more sensitive to the early stages of meaning-making interactions with others. As we'll see in the pages to follow, emotion in general is a complex series of processes and is of central importance in the mind. It involves the dual nature of the essence of mind: the flow of energy and the processing of information. Emotion also reflects the essential way in which the mind emerges from the interface between neuro-physiological processes and interpersonal relationships: It serves as a set of integrating processes linking various systems in a dynamic flow across domains and through time. Within the brain itself, emotion links various systems together to form a state of mind. Emotion also serves as set of processes connecting one mind to another within interpersonal relationships.

The appraisal centers of the brain are located within the limbic system. A brief review of the anatomy involved will help us to visualize how these processes converge.[39] These centers involve such areas as the amygdala, anterior cingulate, and orbitofrontal cortex. External stimuli enter the brain via the sensory systems, such as vision, hearing, and touch. The representations generated from these perceptual processes are then filtered through the thalamus and passed on to the amygdala, where they are appraised and given initial value: "Pay attention? Is this good or bad?" The amygdala is able to directly affect these basic evaluative and perceptual processes. It also sends these representations on for further evaluation by the anterior cingulate and orbitofrontal cortex.[40] Like the amygdala, these centers are processing information about the social environment: the facial expression, direction of eye gaze, and other aspects of others' nonverbal behavior that reveal their state of mind.[41] *Information about the social context directly affects the appraisal process.* These areas of the limbic system also register the state of the body and directly affect its states of activation.[42] Information from these areas is passed on to the hippocampus for "cognitive mapping" and, in some cases, transfer into explicit memory. The orbitofrontal cortex also plays a major role in coordinating these appraisal and arousal processes with the more complex representations of "higher thinking" and social cognition.[43]

This brief review of the limbic system's neurophysiological coordination of input and brain/body response highlights the general statements made throughout this book about the mind: Neural processes and social relationships both contribute to the creation of mental life. The limbic system functions as the center of processing of social information, autobiographical consciousness, the evaluation of meaning, the activation of arousal, and the coordination of bodily response and higher cognitive processing. These processes are not limited to the limbic region, however; rather, they emerge as a convergence of information processing and energy flow that directly influences a wide array of both basic and more complex processes of the brain.

NONCONSCIOUS AND CONSCIOUS EMOTION

Emotions are primarily nonconscious mental processes. In their essence, they create a state of readiness for action, for "motion," disposing us to behave in particular ways within the environment. Emotional reactions create this disposition by determining the brain's activation of a wide array of circuits leading to changes in the state of arousal within the mind/brain and other areas of the body. The amygdala is a cluster of neurons that serves as a receiving and sending station between input from the outer world and emotional response. As a coordinating center within the brain, the amygdala, along with related areas such as the orbitofrontal cortex and anterior cingulate, plays a crucial role in coordinating perceptions with memory and behavior. These regions are especially sensitive to social interactions. They nonconsciously assign significance to stimuli; their actions influence a wide array of mental processes without the involvement of conscious awareness. These circuits are widely connected to other regions that directly influence the functioning of the entire brain as a whole system.

In fact, the limbic system also registers the state of the body and directly influences the body's state of activation via regulation of the autonomic nervous system.[44] In this manner, the limbic system serves as a source of social processing, stimulus appraisal, and brain/body ("emotional") arousal; these may originate within particular limbic regions, but there are no clear boundaries to their effects.[45] Once again, emotion is not merely a function restricted to the areas defined as central to the limbic system; emotion directly influences the functions of the entire brain and body, from physiological regulation to abstract reasoning.[46]

The amygdala has been studied more than any other appraisal center and has been found to play a crucial part in the fight-or-flight response. Classic studies have examined its role especially with regard to fear states.[47] Let's look at the amygdala as an example of the elaborative feedback mechanism of the appraisal process that occurs without the requirement of consciousness. Studies of the amygdala have examined how the initiation of an appraisal leads to subsequent perceptual biases that reinforce the nature of the initial appraisal. The flow of activation of the brain's circuits begins a process of further assembly of various activations, which then ready the individual organism for a particular response. The amygdala receives and sends signals directly from and to the visual system, reacting to visual stimuli without the involvement of consciousness. The amygdala responds to the initial visual representation—say, of a dog—by sending signals back to the same and even earlier layers of the visual processing system, and then by producing initial orientation of the attentional and perceptual apparatus of the brain: "Watch carefully; this is important!" If the amygdala also registers the visual input as dangerous, it can establish elaborative appraisal–arousal processes that create a state of fear in the brain and then feed back to the visual system. First receiving from and then sending signals to the visual centers, the amygdala can rapidly bias the perceptual apparatus toward interpreting the stimuli as dangerous. All of this occurs within seconds and does not depend on conscious awareness.

Nonconsciously, the brain is wired, at least with regard to the fear response, to create a "self-fulfilling prophecy." If the amygdala is excessively sensitive and fires off a "Danger!" signal, it will automatically alter ongoing perceptions to appear to the individual as threatening. This may be a basis for phobias and other anxiety disorders. For example, if a child encounters a dog that growls and lunges at her, she may have a response of fear. At this time, the amygdala directly activates arousal centers (located in the brainstem and forebrain) that create a general state of increased excitability through the release of substances such as noradrenaline in the brain and adrenaline in the body. The whole child becomes hyperalert and ready to deal with the "danger." If particular mental representations are active at the time of this arousal, then they will become associated in memory with a feeling of danger. This association occurs via Hebb's axiom (neurons that fire together wire together; see Chapter 2). Now a learned feedback loop has been established in which a dog can be a source of amygdala activation firing in the future. The brain learns to anticipate a bodily response of hypervigilance to the animal, and a constellation of fear and avoidance behaviors to dogs can then unfold. Such early experiences of fear may become indelible subcortical emotional memories, which may have lasting effects.[48]

How does this rapid, automatic process become conscious? Consciousness is a controversial subject that has long intrigued philosophers and more recently neuroscientists.[49] Though there is no universally accepted explanation for the experience of consciousness, either in the sense of awareness or in the qualitative sensation of subjective experiencing, there are some substantiated views that are quite helpful in understanding aspects of the mind. One such view of the internal experience of conscious awareness is the view of consciousness as involving a system in the brain responsible for working memory, the "chalkboard of the mind." In this perspective, perceptual representations from external stimuli or internally generated images from imagination or memory are functionally connected within an area of the brain called the lateral prefrontal cortex. It is in this region that attention is modulated, so that an "attentional spotlight" can be focused on particular representational profiles in the brain.[50] Working memory is able to handle only a limited amount of units of information, usually in a serial fashion. Neural activation profiles can be linked to the activity of the lateral prefrontal cortex and give the internal sensation of being within an attentional focus of consciousness. The lateral prefrontal cortex is located to the outer side of the front part of the brain, just to the side of the orbitofrontal cortex; it is thought to act by linking items together within conscious awareness, where they can be focally attended to and manipulated.[51]

What exactly it means for neural activation profiles to become "linked" is a central concern for scientists of the brain and mind. How do simultaneously activated processes bind together to form a continuity of experience? One approach to trying to answer this binding question comes from studies of the waves of electrical activity sweeping across the brain on a regular basis. A forty-cycle-per-second ("forty-hertz" or "40-Hz") pattern has been noted, in which the brain becomes active from back to front.[52] This activity occurs in both halves of the brain and has been identified as a "thalamo-cortical" sweep, going from the deeper areas such as the thalamus up toward the higher cortical regions. One view is that representational processes (the neural net profiles activated at a particular moment in time) that are "on" at the time of the sweep are bound together as one seemingly continuous flow of conscious experience. This view allows us to see how the phenomenon of consciousness creates a sense of continuity out of what is really a set of quite discontinuous representational processes, such as sights, sounds, thoughts, bodily states, and self-reflections.[53] This "40-Hz" view also gives us insight into how the lateral prefrontal cortex may become "linked" to a particular set of representations—those that are active during the sweep. The attentional focus of working memory can select from those representations the limited number it may be able to handle at any one time. Because of the nature of the sweeping, each hemisphere can function quite independently of the other. There are probably left-hemisphere and right-hemisphere forms of consciousness that are quite distinct from each other, based on the unique nature of the representational processes of each hemisphere. This will be explored briefly below and in depth in the next chapter.

A related view[54] is that when distributed neural assemblies become active in a rapid and strong manner such that they can achieve a certain degree of functional clustering, a temporarily stable state of complexity is achieved. When these assemblies achieve a certain level of integration, they can become "linked" to the thalamocortical system and their mental processes become a part of consciousness. This view is also compatible with the notion of some core thalamocortical 40-Hz sweeping process and the linkage with the activity of the lateral prefrontal regions. As we shall discuss in more detail in later chapters, these models of consciousness will be useful in helping to understand a number of aspects of mental life.

One view of how emotions become conscious is when their effects are connected to the activity of the attentional mechanisms of the lateral prefrontal cortex.[55] For example, when we say that we have a "gut feeling" about something, we may be referring, literally, to a somatic representation in our brains of our "gut response"—the body's response—to a stimulus.[56] This feedback loop of bodily response leading to emotional reaction has been a perspective long held by researchers with much scientific validation.[57] What is crucial to note, however, is that our brains frequently receive this bodily information without the involvement of conscious awareness. The binding of consciousness may be an "epiphenomenon" in many situations—something that is not essential for other neural reactions subsequently to occur. We may frequently have nonconscious "gut reactions" that profoundly influence our decision-making processes without our awareness of their impact.

We can also become aware of a sense that something feels "meaningful." In this case, we have caught a conscious glimpse of emotion as a value system for the appraisal of the significance of stimuli. Some aspect of the effects of emotional processing has become bound in consciousness. Another example of emotion's becoming a part of our conscious experience is when we feel ourselves becoming lost in a "sea of emotion." Our minds are capable of being bombarded by a flood of stimuli from emotional processes, which fill us with an overwhelming feeling. These sensations may reflect primary emotions (such as internal shifts in states of arousal) or categorical emotions (such as anger, fear, sadness, excitement, or joy). Emotions are what create meaning in our lives, however, whether we are aware of them or not.

Some people have very little awareness of their emotional reactions to things. For one man, for example, it was easy to be conscious of his thoughts about interactions with others, but he had a difficult time letting his wife know verbally "how he felt" beyond simple statements of "good," or "bad," or "I don't know." We could say that for some reason, the representations of his emotional state—things like his bodily response or shifts in his mental state—did not get linked to his lateral prefrontal attentional processes. We cannot say whether they in fact were present or not in his mind. In a sense, this person was emotionally blind. Unfortunately, this blindness to emotions included his unawareness of his wife's states as well as his own.

This illustrates the importance of recognizing that emotional processes are primarily nonconscious. Some people, and certainly this man's wife, would be prone to say that he "has no feelings." As we've seen in Chapter 3, avoidant attachment fosters an emotional disconnection of the child from the parent. There is some suggestion that this disconnection may also be prominent in this man's lack of conscious access to his own nonverbal experience of primary emotions. The lack of connection between consciousness and the arousal–appraisal system does not mean that there is a lack of emotion, however. Instead, we can state that there is a lack of binding of emotion to consciousness. Consciousness may be necessary for an intentional alteration in behavior patterns beyond "reflexive" responses. Without the involvement of consciousness and the capacity to perceive others' and one's own emotions, there may be an inability to plan actively for the future, to alter engrained patterns of behavior, or to engage in emotionally meaningful connections with others.

EMOTION AS A VALUE SYSTEM
FOR THE APPRAISAL OF MEANING

The functioning of the brain as a complex system of neuronal circuits requires it to have some way of determining which firings are useful, neutral, or harmful. Without such an appraisal mechanism, stimuli from the outside world and internally generated states and representations would all be equally welcome. Such an organism would not be able to organize its behavior, to accomplish tasks that allowed it to survive, or to pass on its traits.[58] The brain must have a way of establishing value in order to organize its functions. Value disposes us to behave in particular ways. At the most basic level, the first phase of this process, initial orientation, lets the organism "know" whether to pay attention to something that is important. The second phase, consisting of elaborative appraisal and arousal, gives the individual the value of whether the stimulus is good or bad. Good things should be sought; bad things should be avoided. *Value systems in the brain function by way of increasing states of arousal.* Evaluative circuits serve as a neuromodulatory system with extensive innervation throughout the brain that can lead to hyperexcitability and increased neuronal plasticity. Chemically, this makes the neurons hypersensitive and more readily activated. By initiating attentional mechanisms, arousal enhances the focus of attention on a particular stimulus. In this way, attention is often considered the process that directs the flow of information processing. For perceptual processing, this means, for example, that a person will pay more attention to an object. For memory, arousal leads to enhanced encoding via increased neuronal plasticity and the creation of new synaptic connections and therefore increased likelihood of future retrieval.[59]

As the activations within the brain change, energy flows through the system. Changes in the state of the system are changes in this flow of energy. Many factors in addition to appraisal influence what determines how the system's state changes over time. These determining factors include present input from the external world or from other components of the body, as well as constraints established from prior experience (such as Hebbian connections) and present appraisals. Moreover, there are many forms of arousal, which involve different circuitry. Initial orientation may then activate specific elements of attention. This initial stage "energizes" attentional and perceptual circuits, which then lead to further, elaborated appraisals. This elaboration can produce different forms of subsequent arousal, depending on the nature of the appraisal. At the most basic level, stimuli appraised as "good" will arouse elements of cognitive and behavioral approach. Stimuli appraised as "bad" will arouse withdrawal patterns of neural circuitry activation. When we think of the concept of "arousal," we need to keep in mind that it is a general notion referring to a wide range of specific activation patterns.

It is interesting to note that some of these approach/avoidance distinctions may in fact be hard-wired into the brain. For example, recent studies suggest that the ability to process others' facial expression of emotions, an ability thought to exist in the anterior cingulate, the orbitofrontal cortex, and the amygdala, may have distinct characteristics in different regions. Preliminary findings suggest that the amygdala appears to contain face-recognition cells that exist solely to respond to expressions of fear and anger—not positive emotions or even other negative ones, such as disgust.[60] The limbic regions use input of others' emotions to regulate a person's internal state and external responses directly. As Main and Hesse have proposed, disorganized attachment is commonly associated with parents who show frightening or frightened behaviors.[61] Perhaps these findings reflect the role of parental anger and fear in repeatedly activating specific face-recognition cells within the amygdala as well as generating the characteristic fight–flight response mediated by this limbic region. Could such a specific and ingrained set of limbic states be at the core of the disorganized behaviors (and dissociation) exhibited by these children? As we've discussed in Chapter 3, as they grow older, such children tend to develop controlling, hostile, and aggressive behavior with their peers.[62] These behaviors can be proposed as elements of an excessively sensitized amygdala's fight response. Low levels of stress may be able to activate these reflexive responses and may trigger the rapid perceptual–amygdala feedback loop, which reinforces the sensation of threat. In general, the communication of different types of emotions in children's home environments and the unique neurobiological effects of these emotions may be important in determining the children's patterns of response over time.

Some aspects of a value system are inborn, and some are acquired through experience. Some constitutional aspects of a value system include the motivational systems of attachment and novelty seeking. Within the brain are clusters of cells that are designed to fire in response to eye contact and facial expressions.[63] These clusters of social responders are located within the value centers of the brain, such as the amygdala and the orbitofrontal cortex. For example, *seeking proximity to a caregiver and attaining face-to-face communication with eye gaze contact is hard-wired into the brain from birth.* It is not learned. Similarly, infants are "natural explorers," seeking out new stimuli within their increasingly sophisticated ability to search the environment. Discussions of the genetic determinants of emotional behavior offer helpful insights into the way in which our value systems organize our behavior to increase the chance of survival. Evolutionary theory suggests that those organisms with genetically encoded specificity to their appraisal, such as fearing a snake or becoming aroused by a suitable mate, will have a significantly increased likelihood of passing on their genetic information to future generations.[64] Genes clearly play a large role in the value system of the brain.

Action, learning, and development can be viewed as interrelated sets of phenomena throughout life.[65] For infants, interactions with the environment are driven by the emergence of the increasingly complex capacities of their brains to represent the world around them. The inborn aspects of the value system are in place from the beginning of life, but the system is also shaped by learning from experience. For example, a child will naturally make eye contact with a parent as a "good" interaction. However, if such eye contact results in her being overwhelmed and intruded upon by the actions of the parent, then such interactions may become associated with a negative value. The child learns that eye contact should be avoided. The brain can learn to modify its response to the evaluative system's initial criteria of what is good or bad, based on past interactions with others. If past eye contact leads to a flood of disorganizing activations, the avoidance of such experiences in the future will help keep the self organized.

The appraisal of stimuli and the creation of meaning are central functions of the mind that occur with the arousal process of emotion. Incoming stimuli are appraised for their value, and the representations of these stimuli are then linked with a sense of "goodness" or "badness." As the child develops, the increasingly complex representational system becomes capable of more subtle evaluative sensations. These variations on the "good or bad" theme are what lead to the wide variety of emotions we are capable of feeling. We are unique individuals precisely because both our value systems and our interactional histories are one-of-a-kind combinations. As the intertwined nature of value system responses and environmental encounters unfolds, each of us continually emerges and defines ourselves.

RESPONSE FLEXIBILITY, RELATIONSHIPS, AND EMOTION

Central to this process of creating meaning and emotion is the orbitofrontal cortex.[66] As noted in Chapter 1, this area of the brain sits at the interface between "lower" regions involved in taking input from the body and the senses, and the "higher" parts involved in integrating information and creating complex thoughts and plans. This integrating region is involved in stimulus appraisal (the meaning, value, or emotional valence given to a stimulus),[67] affect regulation (the capacity of the brain to modulate its psychophysiological state),[68] social cognition (the complex process by which one individual is able to have "mindsight" or the ability to perceive the mental state of another),[69] and autonoetic consciousness (the ability to perform mental time travel).[70] It is this region that is postulated to be one of the core areas of deficit in the major disorder of social cognition, autism.[71] Other cognitive processes involving the appraisal–arousal structures, such as the orbitofrontal cortex, the anterior cingulate, and the amygdala, include emotional memory (especially fear),[72] empathy (feeling what another feels),[73] and categorical emotions.[74]

The orbitofrontal cortex has also been demonstrated as central in mediating a process we can call "response flexibility." As Nobre and colleagues have demonstrated in visual stimulus experiments, this region appears to mediate the "switching or reversing of stimulus-response associations" and is at the "interface between automatic default-mode operations of the CNS [central nervous system] and neural processes that allow for flexible adaptations to shifting contexts and perspectives."[75] In other words, the orbitofrontal region is active in taking changing of unexpected internal and external conditions and creating new and flexible behavioral and cognitive responses instead of automatic reflexive ones.[76]

We can propose that this response-flexibility process may become integrated with the other functions subsumed by the orbitofrontal cortex, as described above, as well as other related regions, such as the lateral prefrontal cortex and its mediation of working memory. As Mesulam has stated, "The prefrontal cortex plays a critical role in these attentional and emotional modulations and allows neural responses to reflect the significance rather than the surface properties of sensory events."[77] The prefrontal mediation of response flexibility may thus entail a coordinated process incorporating sensory, perceptual, and appraisal mechanisms and enabling new and personally meaningful responses to be enacted. We can propose that such an integrating function may allow an individual, for example, to approach life decisions, relationships, and perhaps narrative responses with self-reflection and with a sense of perspective on past, present, and future considerations. In this manner, the capacity for response flexibility may become functionally linked with other prefrontally mediated domains that we have discussed, such as autonoetic consciousness, social cognition, emotionally attuned communication, and working memory. The outcome of such well-developed and integrated functioning can be proposed to play a central role in the individual's ongoing development, subjective experiences, and interpersonal relationships.

Response flexibility enables the mind to assess incoming stimuli or emotional states and then to modify external behaviors as well as internal reactions. Such an ability can be proposed as an important component of collaborative, contingent communication. The capacity for response flexibility may also be revealed in the coherence of the discourse process of the AAI. As suggested by Main,[78] coherent narratives require the flexible focusing of attention on attachment-related issues. The inability to exhibit response flexibility can thus be proposed to contribute to incoherent narratives of the insecure adult attachment findings. Such an impairment may also be revealed in the collapse in the maintenance of a narrative strategy seen in the "cannot classify" adult category described by Hesse.[79] Thus, response flexibility can be proposed to be a contributing link between parent–child attachment and adult narratives. In situations where this function fails to develop or its integration with other processes is impaired, especially with those mediated by the prefrontal regions, we can predict that tenacious, global effects may be exerted within the individual's internal and interpersonal experiences across time. As with other mental processes, response flexibility is likely to be state-dependent: Internal and interpersonal contexts can promote or inhibit the integrative mechanisms on which they are created. In this manner, response flexibility can be seen as an integrative capacity that is achieved under certain conditions, rather than a fixed developmental accomplishment. For these reasons, an individual may exhibit this adaptive flexibility in certain situations and not in others. As we'll discuss in the final three chapters, the ways in which emotional states flexibly integrate and organize widely distributed internal and interpersonal processes—the manner in which the flow of energy and information is adaptively modulated—can be seen as having a direct effect on self-regulation, relationships, and development across the lifespan. Future studies will be helpful in clarifying the nature of response flexibility, its mediation by the orbitofrontal region, its potentially experience-dependent development, and its possible relationship to incoherent narratives and patterns of parent–child communication.

How are response flexibility and other integrative processes influenced by the emotional communication inherent in many interpersonal relationships? Looking toward neurobiological structure and function may shed some light on this question. The orbitofrontal cortex sits at a crucial neuroanatomic position at the uppermost part of the limbic system—the center of our basic appraisals, thought to be the origin of our widely distributed emotional experiences. As discussed earlier in this chapter, a controversy exists as to what the limitations of the limbic region actually are: Its boundaries as a major center for influencing the functioning of the brain cannot be clearly delineated, and in this way the entire brain can be considered "emotional."[80] As we can see, the social/emotional/meaning-making processes of the limbic system help coordinate a wide range of mental functions. The result of the adaptive integration of these functions may be the proposed process of response flexibility.

The orbitofrontal cortex receives direct input from the sensory cortex, which is responsible for perception; the somatosensory cortex and brainstem, which register somatic sensation; the autonomic nervous system, which controls bodily functions; the dorsolateral prefrontal cortex, involved in attentional processes; the medial temporal lobe, involved in explicit memory; and the associational cortex, involved in abstract forms of thought. Allan Schore has described how the development of the orbitofrontal cortex is thought to depend on stimulation from the emotional connections of the attachment figure in the form of eye contact, face-to-face communication, and affective attunement.[81] The orbitofrontal cortex, like the amygdala, has specific cells particularly responsive to facial expression and eye gaze direction.[82] These fundamental aspects of social signals specifically activate these regions of the brain. The orbitofrontal cortex is also crucial in coordinating bodily states and the widely distributed and linked representations that are fundamental to reasoning processes, motivation, and the creation of emotional meaning.[83]

Emotion is a fundamental part of attachment relationships in the early years and throughout the lifespan. The earliest forms of communication are about primary emotional states. This sharing of basic appraisal and arousal processes establishes the fundamental way in which one person becomes connected to another within emotional relationships. We can also propose that the reciprocal collaboration within such contingent communication facilitates the development of a parallel, prefrontally mediated process, response flexibility, that enables the individual to respond to changing internal and interpersonal contexts in an adaptive, "internally collaborative" manner.

Such internal collaboration may be seen as a way in which widely distributed neural processes come to be recruited into a flexible state of mind, one that is adaptive to a range of internal as well as external factors. In this way, we can see how intimate, reciprocal human communication may directly activate the neural circuitry responsible for giving meaning, integrating the capacity for flexible responses, and shaping the subjective experience of living an emotionally vibrant life.

EMOTION AND SOMATIC RESPONSE

The signals from the body also directly shape our emotions. Our awareness of bodily state changes—such as tension in our muscles, shifts in our facial expressions, or signals from our heart or intestines—lets us know how we feel, though bodily feedback occurs even without awareness. Perceptions of the environment certainly occur in the brain, but the subsequent reactions of the body may follow very soon after and become the "data" informing us about what those perceptions mean to us. In this way, our appraisal mechanisms may depend upon bodily reactions to determine the direction of subsequent elaboration. States of mind are created within the psychobiological states of the brain and other parts of the body.[84]

For example, contracting the muscles of the face in a characteristically negative (frown) or positive (smile) manner produces a respective bias in interpreting data.[85] If we sense our own faces smiling, we are more likely to enter a positive state of mind and to view our experience from that stance. Studies even demonstrate that contracting the muscles of the left side of the face (presumably requiring activation of the right hemisphere) is associated with negative bias, whereas contracting those of the right side of the face (presumably requiring left-brain activation) leads to positive appraisals.[86] Somatosensory data from the face are registered in the brain and directly influence the state of activation, so that information processing is shaped by the effects of this information.

The neurologist Antonio Damasio has postulated that the change in bodily state is perceived and represented in the brain as what he calls a "somatic marker."[87] Two forms of bodily response are especially relevant. Muscle changes in our limbs and faces are highly sensitive components of emotional reactions, and these send input directly to the brain and are represented in an area called the somatosensory cortex. Of note is that the portion of the somato-sensory cortex in the *right* hemisphere has more integrated represen-tations than that in the *left* hemisphere, suggesting a more direct role of the right brain in the processing of somatic markers. As we'll see, the brain's asymmetry plays an important role in understanding emotion and the mind. The other form of bodily response is in changes in the viscera, such as the stomach, intestines, heart, and lungs. Visceral changes are registered in the orbitofrontal cortex and related areas, also especially in the right hemisphere. Interestingly, these regions of the brain monitor as well as regulate these visceral reactions.[88]

Experience establishes learned associations between external stimuli and these bodily responses. In this view, our knowledge of how we feel is based in large part upon the nature of these somatic markers. As we develop, Damasio postulates further, we acquire the capacity to have an "as-if" loop, in which an internal stimulus (such as a thought, image, or memory) can activate an "as-if" somatic marker.[89] Our brains create a representation of bodily changes that is independent of the present-day response. A thought can be associated with an emotional response containing a somatic marker that has been generated internally. This is a representation of a shift in bodily state created by our brains from imagination and past experiences. Memories of emotional experiences evoke as-if somatic markers, which can feel as real as direct bodily responses and can deeply enliven the associated imagery of the recollection. In some cases we will also have the actual bodily changes, such as increased heart rate, sweating, and dilated pupils when we are recalling a past frightening event.

For example, if an adult was bitten by a cat as a child, the state of fear and arousal at the time will be registered in the brain as a so-matic marker of fear associated with the image and idea of a cat. In the future, seeing a cat may activate a similar bodily state of fear, instantiating a somatic marker similar to the time of the initial cat bite and activating a set of associational memory processes linked to the time of the original bite. An "as-if" somatic marker reveals how the process of imagination or memory can elicit a sensory response, which then initiates a cascade of fear-related associations that may be quite debilitating. This may be one way in which unresolved posttraumatic conditions continue to perpetuate frightening reactions from long ago; such individuals feel as if they are being traumatized over and over again.

INDIVIDUAL DIFFERENCES
IN EMOTIONAL EXPERIENCE

Some couples experience a kind of "compatibility" that both members of a pair may have felt when they first met: They resembled each other in certain favored ways of being, in certain needs for play and relaxation, or in preferred times for work. In some pairs where there is a discordant match in the partners' attachment histories, the disparity between their individual appraisal systems may lead to difficulty in their pattern of communicating despite this compatibility. For example, a husband with a dismissing state of mind with respect to attachment had experiences with his mother that appeared not to have reinforced the positive effects of emotional intimacy. His relationship with her seemed not to have offered him encounters in which eye gaze and face-to-face contact were associated with a sense of soothing. Recall that studies of avoidantly attached pairs reveal that the body continues to register distress during separation (for children) and in discussion of attachment issues (in adults). This finding suggests that the original value system, which assigned a "good" meaning to affective connections between people, has probably remained intact even after repeatedly disappointing and rejecting experiences. What has been learned is the person's development of behavioral and complex cognitive responses, such as memory and narrative, that serve to minimize conscious access to this persistent distress. The brain has learned to adapt itself to the learned experience by minimizing the manifestations of such distress on other aspects of mental functions.

In this couple, the wife's experience of her husband was that in a quiet way he seemed to enjoy her presence. To her, his lack of focus on her emotional states provided a sense of first safety and then frustration. She seemed to have had an ambivalent attachment with her own mother and a disorganized one with her father; she now had an unresolved adult attachment status, with a best-fitting alternative classification of preoccupied. On some nonverbal level, she felt that her husband liked being "close" to her, though he would never state this directly. She was probably sensing something real—an intact but frightened emotional system in her husband, which did indeed continue to value attachment. Both on the surface of his behavior and in his conscious experience, however, he denied the importance of such connections. In fact, the husband seemed to pride himself on his autonomy, often stating that the sign of healthy development is to "not need anyone, just want them." His wife did not feel needed. She often didn't even feel wanted.

With many couples, the very characteristics that each partner initially found attractive in the other become the same qualities that create intolerable frustration and drive them to a therapist for help. In this couple, the wife was attracted at first to the husband's "autonomy and independence." She felt safe and unthreatened by his emotional distance. The husband liked his wife's "sensitivity and ability to express her emotions." She offered him something he had never had. As time went on, however, she began to feel so isolated that his autonomy made her infuriated. He began to sense her emotional response as attacks on his personality. This couple became stuck in an emotional rut.

In this case example, the wife's capacity to experience emotion was quite different from that of her husband. She was able to notice changes in her body's sensations, such as a tightening in her muscles, a queasy feeling in her stomach, and a trembling in her hands. She might feel her face beginning to smile, or notice tears on her cheeks. Each of these bodily messages let her know some aspect of her emotional state: anger, fear, sadness, joy. The ability to sense this somatic feedback is the kind of self-awareness that has led numerous researchers to postulate that *the body's response lets us know how we feel.*

Somatic markers—actual or "as-if"—can be generated without consciousness. These representations can influence perceptual bias, memory processes, and rational decision making without our awareness. In this couple, the wife often could sense when she was having an intense "emotional experience" by the way her body felt. For her husband, life was not so full of these sensations. He would make decisions, perceive the world, and recall things (or not) without a sense that any kind of biasing was occurring. But we cannot say that he was any less influenced by his hidden value system than his wife, whose emotions were more readily accessible to her conscious experience.

Working memory is able to contain a number of processes and manipulate them within conscious awareness. These processes include present perceptual representations, items from long-term memory, and states of the body. To minimize distress and maximize function, the brain of this dismissingly attached husband might have had the challenge of focusing his conscious attention away from attachment-related experiences. This diverting of attention might have concerned external events, such as the behavioral response of acting as if his mother didn't return (as seen in the infant separation studies), as well as internal events, such as the minimization of the importance of parental relationships (as revealed in the AAI; see Chapter 3). A distressed response is most readily seen in the body's state of increased sweating, heart rate, respiration, and muscle tension. Each of these may become activated in attachment situations with avoidantly attached children and dismissing adults. To avoid impairment of functioning, the representation of these responses must be kept away from working memory. To accomplish such a task means creating a pattern of neural interactions in which somatic markers are not linked to the working memory processes of the lateral prefrontal cortex.

Given the location of these processes, we can hypothesize how this husband might have been affected by such an adaptation. The cortical representations of somatic muscle responses are most highly integrated in the right hemisphere of the brain. Visceral responses are monitored by the orbitofrontal cortex and the closely associated anterior cingulate, also primarily on the right side. The lateral prefrontal cortex is centered just to the side of the orbitofrontal cortex, with which it receives and sends direct connections. Reduction in input to the right lateral prefrontal cortex would be quite helpful to avoid receiving the representations of the right-sided somatosensory and orbitofrontal cortices.

What would this mean for this man and others with a similar attachment history of distant emotional communication from a primary caregiver? Impaired input of the right-sided sources of somatic markers would functionally lead such individuals to be consciously unaware of their bodies' responses. They would therefore not be able to know easily how they feel. Furthermore, if the right lateral prefrontal cortex had more general blockages, we would predict that the other functions of the right hemisphere might also be less accessible to conscious awareness. In this case, the husband had a difficult time seeing the gist or context of things. He also seemed unable to read his wife's state of mind as expressed through her nonverbal signals. Such difficulties are all problems in functions of the right hemisphere. We shall return to the issue of hemispheric specialization in the mind both below and in the next chapter.

A common belief in everyday life is that there appears to be a pattern of differences in emotion, especially the empathic sharing of emotional states, between males and females. Developmental studies have focused on the gender differences in relationships among friends during the school years. In general, these studies find "masculine" and "feminine" styles that most boys and girls, respectively, seem to exhibit.[90] The masculine style has been defined as a form of mutual assertion of one's individual talents and skills. Boys' interest in athletic prowess is one example of such a form of shared assertion. The feminine style has been described as one of mutual empathy; girls' interactions with each other tend to focus on shared expression and resonance with each other's emotional experiences.[91] Clearly, however, many girls have elements of the masculine style, and many boys have elements of the feminine style. Although generalizations of any sort must be carefully examined, it is important to try to understand the genetic, hormonal, developmental, and/or social factors that contribute to such observable gender differences.

EMOTIONAL COMMUNICATION: EMPATHY AND AFFECTIVE EXPRESSION

An important aspect of emotions is their social function. Emotions, both primary and categorical, serve as the vehicles that allow one person to have a sense of the mental state of another. The capacity to feel another person's experience has many labels, such as "empathy," "sympathy," "mirroring," and "attunement." In its essence, the ability of one mind to perceive and then experience elements of another person's mind is a profoundly important dimension of human experience. We are a social species, and having the ability to "mind-read," or having "mindsight," lets us rapidly detect the emotional state of another. Why is this so important? There are several reasons. This form of communication allows us to perceive the intentions, attentional focus, and evaluation of events in others; it therefore allows us to understand social interactions and anticipate the behavior of other people. Our minds are capable of detecting the nonverbal signals of others, which reveal these internal aspects of their states of mind. Young infants begin to differentiate between animate and inanimate objects in the world, attributing intention and emotional responses to the former and not the latter. With the assignment of intention, our minds are able to compare external behaviors with implied internal motivational states.[92] This ability allows us to detect "cheaters" and note when we are being misled. A further evolutionary benefit of mindsight is that our ancestors could rapidly sense when a member of their own social group was detecting danger by the look on her face, her gestures, or her tone of voice. Those social beings capable of such mindsight escaped danger more often, were less often tricked by the destructive motivations of others, and thus were more likely to survive and pass on the capacity for such state-to-state lines of communication.[93]

From a developmental perspective, the most utilitarian of these benefits is that parents can sense the inner needs of their children and therefore maximize the potential of their offspring's survival. Another benefit of empathic attunement is that it creates an attachment bond between parent and child, which provides a source of increasingly complex layers of external and then internal security for the growing child in the increasingly challenging world encountered as he develops. The experience of being understood develops a mental model or inner expectation that needs are important and goals are achievable. Also, the child's system requires the parent's attunement to help organize the child's own mind. Positive emotional states are amplified and negative ones modulated within these attuned communications. As the child grows, these repeated alignments of mental states allow him to develop a self-organizational capacity for autonomous state regulation. Human infants have profoundly underdeveloped brains. Maintaining proximity to their caregivers is essential, both for survival and for allowing their brains to use the mature states of the attachment figure to help them organize their own mental functioning.

The subjective side of these emotional connections is that it allows a sense of belonging to grow within the individual. "Feeling felt" is the subjective experience of mental state attunement. The pleasurable response to such a resonance of minds may be built into our brains as a genetic inheritance of evolutionary history. For us as social animals, our having such a sense encourages group behavior, which has been of great survival value to our species as we evolved. It may also be the reason why large groups are experienced so differently from smaller ones, in which face-to-face eye contact and other aspects of shared nonverbal communication are readily available. Committees of over a dozen people become unwieldy and inefficient (not that some smaller ones do much better!). Feeling felt for some requires even smaller group settings, with one-to-one situations being the ideal for many people.

Empathic emotional connections require some way in which internal states are expressed externally. Primates are the only group of animals with muscle endings on the skin of the face; this gives us the capacity for a huge assortment of facial expressions, which are directly controlled by our nervous systems.[94] Our tremendously rich enervation allows for exquisitely subtle and rapid alterations in facial expression. To match this expressive ability, primates have neuronal groups in the brain that are specialized to respond to faces, and also to particular facial expressions! As we've discussed, these neuronal groups often rest in the value system circuits of our brains, such as in the amygdala and orbitofrontal cortex. We are hard-wired to have meaning and emotion shaped by the perception of eye contact and facial expression.[95] We are also hard-wired to express emotional states through the face.

Complex neural/bodily aspects of emotional processes are not easily translated into words. Nonverbal expressions, including those of the face, tone of voice, and gestures, can transfer information about internal states more fully to the outside world than words can do. Words go only so far. When anyone asks, "How are you feeling?", it is a huge translational challenge to turn such subtle and dynamic neural processes into a verbal statement. Emotion can be seen as an energizing drive toward motion. Seeing what a person does, rather than asking her how she feels, can often be a more direct road into the person's emotional state. Nevertheless, we often feel compelled to ask others how they feel. The social process of "talking about feelings" with each other is much more an interactive event than the mere telling of a linguistic message. Linguistic representations, such as the words "sad" or "angry," are quite limited and distant symbolic packets we send to each other in response to the query, "How are you feeling?" The message is in the medium of how we respond, not in the words alone.[96]

The link between emotion and action is in the appraisal–arousal foundation of these processes. At their core, appraisals define what is good or bad, what should be approached or avoided. Children are often more at ease with the hedonic tone of primary emotional states than with trying to define the categorical emotions they may be experiencing. When children say, "I feel bad," or "I feel good," this may be a very direct statement reflecting this basic aspect of their appraisal system and primary emotional experience.

EMOTION AND THE HEMISPHERES

Affect can be expressed through facial expressions and through modulations in the tone and prosody of the voice. These nonverbal aspects of language communication, in both their expression and perception, appear to be mediated predominantly by the right hemisphere.[97] The body's posture and movement can also blend with the voice and facial expression in sending affective signals that are readily perceived by other people. What is striking is the finding that the registration of the status of the body itself is also much more highly integrated in the right hemisphere than in the left. As we've discussed briefly, even the regulation of the body's autonomic nervous system is primarily mediated by right-brain mechanisms.[98] The right hemisphere therefore appears to play a major role in mediating emotional processes, as well as in permitting the expression of emotional states and the conscious awareness of emotional experience.

For this discussion of emotion, it is important to provide some background information. Appraisal and arousal occur on both sides of the brain, as do other emotional processes. However, the subjective experience and the nature of emotion on either side of the brain may be quite different. Leading theories propose a number of disparate views of emotions and brain asymmetry.[99] One major perspective is that of the valence hypothesis, which suggests that unpleasant emotions are processed on the right side and pleasant ones on the left.[100] Consistent with this suggestion is the view that withdrawal states and processes are located on the right side, whereas approach states and processes are located on the left.[101] Another view is that socially mediated emotions, such as guilt or the enactment of social display rules, are processed in the left hemisphere, whereas more basic, spontaneous emotions are processed in the right hemisphere.[102] Still others argue that raw, intense emotional experience is primarily mediated via the right hemisphere.[103]

From a neuroscientific view of emotion as a socially mediated set of processes affecting all other mental processes, one can look to our basic elements of the mind as composed of the flow of energy and of information within the brain for insights into this dilemma of multiple theories. Primary emotional states are often directly expressed via nonverbal components of communication, including facial expressions and tones of voice. Primary emotional states are directly shaped by bodily response and directly influence bodily responses. These two basic somatic functions of primary emotions have been demonstrated to be mediated and perceived by the right hemisphere of the brain. Furthermore, in studies of patients with blocked communication between the two hemispheres, the left brain appears unable to register the facial expression of others. The right brain both perceives and sends messages through facial expressions and tone of voice.[104] It may therefore be fair to propose that the non-

verbal right hemisphere may be the location for the subjective awareness and expression of primary emotions as we have defined them.
The processing of such emotions, however, is likely to be mediated
by both hemispheres.

Developmental studies suggest that in fact each hemisphere may
mediate quite different processes of engagement with the environment. As noted above, this may mean that approach is mediated by
the left hemisphere and withdrawal by the right. For example,
behaviorally inhibited (shy) children reveal a dominance in right
frontal electrical activity at baseline; more adventurous children demonstrate left frontal activation. Nathan Fox has suggested that such
findings support the notion that characteristic emotional styles may
reflect profiles of frontal activation.[105] Left frontal activation is associated with active approach, positive affect, exploration, and sociability. The absence of left frontal activation leads to an absence of
positive affect and the experience of depression. In contrast, right
frontal activation leads to active withdrawal, negative affect, and
fear/anxiety. Hypoactivation of the right frontal region leads to
disinhibition of approach, with impulsivity and hyperactivity. Such a
view can explain some features of shy and of aggressive children and
the changes in their states as the context may alter their frontal activation profiles.

Further developmental studies suggest that both constitutional/
temperamental and experience/attachment features may directly
shape these patterns of frontal activation.[106] In the case of depressed
mothers, for example, there is a marked decrease in shared positive
affect states, and the infants (and their mothers) are seen as withdrawn. In both parents and children, there is a marked decrease in
left frontal activation. If such depression lasts beyond the first year
of life, the infants may continue to express this pattern of frontal
activity.[107]

SUBJECTIVE EXPERIENCE

Emotion is inherently a subjective experience involving the evaluation of meaning and the interaction with the environment. Experiences evoke within us textured subjective states that create the fabric
of our lives and our relationships with others. Music has been
described as one of the purest expressions of emotions that exists. It
is filled with contours and spacing, varied intensities, and modulations in sound. These could be considered as categorical features,

such as joy or sadness, but perhaps they are more appropriately reflecting profiles of arousal so parallel to vitality affects that we could call primary emotions the "music of the mind." The process of creating and listening to music is a form of emotional experience and affective communication.

Several studies, and my own informal survey of dozens of children, reveal a common preference among unprofessionally trained individuals for the left ear when listening to music.[108] Sound heard with the left ear may induce a more holistic sensation, a floating with the flow of the music, quite distinct from the sensation produced by music heard with the right ear. How can this be? The left auditory nerve goes primarily to the right hemisphere! Though there is some crossover, the auditory stimulation in the right brain appears to evoke a different sensation from that which goes to the left brain from the right ear.

We are filled with representations of all sorts: sensations and images in a context-rich form mediated by the right hemisphere, and linguistic symbols in a linear, logical, detail-oriented mode mediated by the left hemisphere.[109] If this view is true, then our daily conversations are filled with a blending of right-sided and left-sided communication. Some authors argue that emotional attunement is fundamentally right-brain-to-right-brain communication.[110] This view may sound too reductionistic and simple to be either true or useful. But let's take a look at a fundamental notion of attunement: the feeling of another person's experience. Merely to understand another person requires an intellectual grasp of the other's experience. To have the ability to conceptualize the mind of another, as well as to perceive what the other's subjective world might be like, requires special tools enabling the kind of reflective functioning discussed in Chapter 3. The neurological bases of these tools have been established over thousands of years of evolution and are a fundamental part of the social circuitry of the brain so intimately related to emotional experience. These circuits are located primarily in the right hemisphere. To feel another person's experience requires the ability to take in the essential data of how the other person in fact is feeling by way of specific signals generated by this person. These data then directly affect the receiver's state of mind. Would it be such a big surprise to find that the neural processes of one hemisphere are best expressed externally by that hemisphere, and then perceived best by the same hemisphere, but in another person? After all, words generated by the left hemisphere of one person are best perceived and understood by the left hemisphere of the listener. What we are really talking about are the forms of information that the mind is processing. As we'll discuss more fully in the next chapter, the types of mental representations are quite distinct in each hemisphere. Learning about the nature of these differences can give us a better understanding of emotional experience and communication between minds.

Emotions recruit distributed clusters of neuronal groups in the emerging states of mind that organize the systems of the brain.[111] Recruitment can be generally defined here as a process that temporarily links distinct, differentiated elements into a functional whole. In the brain, recruitment involves the binding of the activity of spatially distributed neural circuits at a given moment and across time. Emotion can be proposed to serve this integrative role by way of its involvement of neuromodulatory systems that are themselves widely distributed and have direct effects on neural excitability and activation, neural plasticity and the growth of synaptic connections, and the coordination of a range of processes in the brain. We can suggest that perhaps the most active representations may be the ones that become recruited and then have the potential to enter the spotlight of conscious awareness. Consciousness may in fact be quite distinct on each side of the brain. Some authors have suggested that the right hemisphere is a master at representing social context, whereas the left remains focused on details devoid of contextual meaning.[112] The social context of a situation determines the nature of action of the appraisal systems. Internal context, the history of present and recent representational activity, also directly affects the way the appraisal systems work. The impact of representational processes on each side of the brain may create quite distinct contextual influences on the appraisal process and lead to distinct senses of conscious awareness.

The brain looks to the body's response to "know how it feels." An experiment that illuminated this involved subjects being told to contort their facial muscles in specific patterns. Unbeknownst to them, these configurations represented the various categories of emotions, such as anger, fear, or sadness. When they were presented with a standardized story, their appraisal of meaning was directly influenced by which facial musculature patterns they had activated. If their muscles were held in a sad way, they interpreted the story presented as sad. If their faces were held in a way to show joy, they had a "happy" reaction to the same story. The finding that the right hemisphere has a more integrated representation of the body, including the face, suggests that this form of information will have more impact on the experience of emotion on the right side of the brain.

By our second year of life we have learned the trick of how to show facial affective expressions that are different from our internal emotional states.[113] This form of social deception allows us to act in socially appropriate and sanctioned ways. In a fundamental manner, this behavior creates a division between the private, internal self and the public, external self. Most of us carry out this dual role every day in our private and public lives. If we spend too much of our time attempting to be "socially appropriate" by having a public self, and do not express authentic feelings or thoughts, then we may be vulnerable to developing a "false self" quite distant from our actual primary emotional experience. Of note are findings suggesting that the left hemisphere plays a more significant role in the communication of emotions that conform to social rules.[114]

As noted earlier, words are often quite limited in their ability to convey our internal states. Attunement to one another's nonverbal means of communicating emotional experience is a much more direct and satisfying mechanism for joining with others. However, we must use words and concepts to attempt to understand the nature of emotion if we are to begin to comprehend the human mind. Some might argue that without words, we cannot reflect on the conceptual nature of our own minds. As we've seen in Chapter 3, those parents who have the capacity to reflect on the importance of mental states are more likely to have secure attachments with their children. This reflective function is revealed in both affective attunements and the ability of these individuals to state, in words, the importance of mental states in human experience.[115] In fact, the ability to use "mental state language"—words reflecting mentalizing concepts, such as beliefs, feelings, attitudes, intentions, and thoughts—is associated with parents of children with secure attachments.[116] These ideas can inspire an approach to creating "reflective dialogues" with children in order to help them develop emotionally. In this way, having the capacity for reflecting in one's own mind on the importance of mental life can be revealed in both attuned (nonverbal) and language-based communication. Using both our nonverbal right and verbal left hemispheres, we can find ways to communicate the important subjective emotional experience of ourselves and others.

EMOTION REGULATION

Emotion is indeed a complex set of processes. As we've seen in this chapter, emotion is at the core of internal and interpersonal processes that create our subjective experience of the self. The organization of the self is dependent upon the manner in which emotion is regulated. Research on emotion regulation reveals that emotion as a set of processes is both regulated and regulatory. That is, emotional processes cannot exist without influencing other such processes and being influenced themselves by other such processes. Thus the study of emotion and that of emotion regulation go hand in hand.[117]

Self-regulation—the manner in which the process called the "self" comes to regulate its own processes—consists in part of the regulation of emotion. Sroufe describes the "twin tasks" of emotion in development as the expression of affect and its management. He states, "The ability to maintain flexibly organized behavior in the face of high levels of arousal or tension is a central aspect of stable individual differences in personality organization."[118]

Susan Calkins has described pathways to such differences in emotion regulation as involving both internal and external sources.[119] Internal features include constitutional aspects of neuroregulatory structures (such as neuroendocrine, autonomic, and frontal lobe systems), behavioral traits (such as attentiveness, adaptability, reactivity, soothability, and sociability) and cognitive components (including social referencing, beliefs and expectations, awareness of need for regulation, and ability to apply strategies). External features include interactive caregiving patterns (responsiveness, cooperation, reciprocity, accessibility, support, and acceptance) and explicit training (including modeling, reinforcement, and discipline).

In general, our skills at regulating emotion allow us to achieve a wide range and high intensity of emotional experience while maintaining flexible, adaptive, and organized behavior. The processes of emotion regulation—and dysregulation—can involve any of the basic levels of emotion: physiology, subjective experience, and behavioral change. As we'll discuss in detail in Chapter 7, the regulation of emotion involves the modulation of states of mind. Regulation of the flow of states can involve internal (physiological and cognitive) and interactive (engaging with the social environment) elements. For example, alterations in attentional focus, perceptual bias, or the evaluation of meaning can directly change the course of elaboration of primary emotional states into more differentiated categorical emotions. We can utilize the very processes of emotion to regulate their flow.

Before we can appreciate the details of these complex regulatory processes more fully, we will need to review what is known about how the mind constructs reality with representational processes (Chapter 5) and how states of mind are created within the complex system of the mind (Chapter 6). Then we will be ready to wrestle with the questions of how the brain organizes its own functioning, including how it regulates emotional states within itself and in connection with others, in the creation of the mind.

REFLECTIONS: EMOTION AND THE MIND

An amusing cycle of responses sometimes enters the classroom when a psychotherapy student or teacher asks the question "What is a feeling?" "A feeling," the response sometimes goes, "is an emotion. It is what you feel when you are emotional. Emotions generate feelings." An initial way out of this endless loop of confusion comes from the knowledge of how central these elusive things, these emotional processes, are for human relationships. Emotions are the contents and processes of interpersonal communication early in life, and they create the tone and texture of such communications throughout the lifespan. This view at least brings emotions out of the individual and into the interaction between people. But, still, this leaves us with only a bit more clarity about the challenging task of how to define emotions.

Everyday descriptions of what emotions are may seem to be more appealing than trying to create seemingly restrictive, scientifically derived concepts and definitions. Emotions are what allow us to fall in love. They are the stuff of poetry, art, and music. Emotions fill us with a sense of connection to others. They link families together; they remind us of who is important in our lives. Emotions make life worth living.

For some, the risk of becoming scientific about emotions is that it has the potential to reduce the essential and passionate stuff of subjectivity into some neural-circuitry-based explanation that appears on the surface to be cold and useless. However, ironically, it seems that the application of neural science principles to understanding our feelings can actually expand and enrich the subjective experience of our own emotional minds. Understanding the neuroanatomic reality of the convergence of social interactions, appraisal, and emotional arousal helps us to see how the mind creates and is created by interactions with other minds. We can now move beyond circular definitions and embrace the metaphors of emotion in a deeply impassioned and integrated manner.

At the most basic level, the brain must have value systems that appraise the significance of internal and external stimuli. The centers of these value systems, so often linked to areas that respond to social signals, act by initiating activity or arousal within specific circuits in the brain. This chapter has provided a broad set of specific definitions of emotion that can enable us to understand human experience more fully. At its most basic level, this view sees emotions as the flow of energy, or states of arousal and activation, through the brain and other parts of the body. This process emerges from and directly affects the further processing of information within the mind by way of the appraisal of meaning. Three phases can be identified: First, a stimulus (internal or external) evokes a state of initial orientation, creating a sensation of "Something important is happening; pay attention now!" This focus of attention is automatic and does not need to involve conscious awareness. Next, the value systems of the brain continue to appraise the meaning of that stimulus and of that initial orientation itself by means of elaborated appraisal and arousal processes and the activation of certain circuits. At this point, the sensation may begin to become "This is good" or "This is bad." These first two steps of an emotional response contain activation profiles, such as surges of energy, that can be defined as "primary" emotions. In their essence, primary emotions are the beginning of how the mind creates meaning.

Externally, primary emotions can be seen as vitality affects, expressed by the contours of activation of the body, facial expressions, nonverbal gestures and tone of voice. These vitality affects constitute the primary connection between infant and parent. This finding reveals the exquisite sensitivity of the appraisal centers to social interaction and shows how emotions are initially created within our relationships with others.

A third phase in emotional response is what is more generically thought of as "emotion": the differentiation of initial orientation and elaborated states of arousal and appraisal into categorical emotions. Examples of such emotions found throughout the world in characteristic expressions are sadness, anger, disgust, surprise, joy, fear, and shame. The brain and other body systems appear to have common pathways by which each of these distinct categorical emotional states are physiologically manifested and expressed as categorical affects.

Generated by the value systems of the brain, these emotional activations pervade all mental functions and literally create meaning in life. *In this way, we can say that emotion and meaning are created by the same processes.*

Information processing involves the creation and manipulation of cognitive representations. Attentional mechanisms direct the flow of information processing. Within perception and memory, the appraisal systems of the brain must label representations as significant or value-laden. In this way, the appraisal and arousal processes—the central features of emotion—are interwoven with the representational processes of "thinking." *Creating artificial or didactic boundaries between thought and emotion obscures the experiential and neurobiological reality of their inseparable nature.*

Energy flow is a basic aspect of primary emotions. As states of mind emerge within the individual, the changing activations that create them are often experienced as primary emotions. The regulation of emotion, or the regulation of the flow of information and energy within the brain, creates the self. The capacity to assess the personal significance of events and alter automatic, reflexive responses may be carried out by the prefrontal regions in a process we have called response flexibility. When such an ability becomes integrated with other aspects of emotional and memory processing, the individual may be able to generate a set of internal and interpersonal experiences that enables the self to have a flexible form of regulation. In the next two chapters, we will examine how the mind organizes itself by how it regulates the flow of information and mental states both within itself and with other minds. Emotion and its modulation are in this way a fundamental part of the information processing and energy flow that are central features of the organization of the self.

CHAPTER 5

⚫

Representations

Modes of Processing
and the Construction of Reality

Our experience of reality is constructed by the activity patterns of neuronal groups within the brain. These groups are clustered into functional units capable of representing experiences in different modalities, such as sight or taste, words or sensations, abstract ideas or perceptual images. The ways individuals assemble particular neuronal activations within themselves or in interaction with other people determine the nature of their subjective experience of reality. We can view communication within human relationships in part as the ways in which these mental representations are shared. The patterns of communication within early relationships directly shape the development of the mind.

A frustrated wife looked at her confused husband and said, "You never understand what I am talking about. All you know is what you have learned in books. You couldn't read my face if your life depended on it!" To this challenge, the man responded, "I can tell from what you say that you're probably not happy with me. But, you know, there are two kinds of people in this world: those who are too needy, and those who aren't." The wife got up and left the room.

How do people ever communicate with each other? How does one mind "read" the signals sent by another? How are words and nonverbal modes of communication, such as tone of voice and facial expressions, processed differently by the brain? Why couldn't this husband respond to the emotional content of his wife's message? Insights into the answers to these questions come from the ways in which people's minds construct reality.

In this chapter, we explore these ways by examining how the mind creates representations and processes information. The couple described above clearly had a major problem in how each partner constructed and therefore experienced reality. By examining the different mental modules responsible for representing the world and other people, we can begin to understand the foundations of this couple's profound difficulties. As discussed briefly in Chapter 4, the individual brain is divided into two halves that have distinctly different mental representations and modes of processing. Asymmetry of the brain exists in almost all mammalian species, is present in the human fetus, and is functionally evident in the behavior of the human infant long before complex cognition is available.[1] The developmental origins of bilateral differences in the brain are deeply rooted in our evolutionary and genetic history. The ways in which such asymmetries influence our experiences—both internal and interpersonal—are explored throughout this chapter. The anatomic and functional separation between the two hemispheres permits their processes to be quite independent at times, and it directly shapes the construction of subjective experience. Repeated patterns of neuronal activations help to establish a continuity in the individual's representations of reality across time. How two individuals come to share their individual representational worlds is a fundamental part of "feeling felt" and establishing a sense of interpersonal connection.

This chapter proposes that the *different attachment patterns described in Chapter 3 involve the recruitment of unique patterns of neuronal group activations*. For example, the emotionally distant connection of avoidantly attached children with their dismissing parents can be understood as involving primarily the linear, logical, linguistically based mode of communication of the left hemisphere. Persons in whom the left-brain mode of processing predominates have been shown to be markedly deficient in the ability to read others' nonverbal communications and to sense the emotional expressions of others or of the self. Imagine what being in an interpersonal, emotional relationship with such a person might be like. This may in part have been what the wife in the example above was encountering in her marriage. The experiential reinforcement of particular representational processes can become an engrained pattern in the way an individual comes to experience the world. As we shall see, new forms of experiences within interpersonal relationships may evoke new representational processes. This would be one of the aims of therapy for this couple's mismatch in representational processes.

INFORMATION PROCESSING AND MENTAL REPRESENTATIONS

Within a simple but powerful computational model, the brain has been viewed as a fundamental processor of information. The nature of the brain's processing of information is captured by two fundamental ideas in this model: *A mental symbol (that is, a pattern of neural activation) contains information, and it creates an effect.*[2] Cognitive science has provided a conceptualization of how particular systems within the mind give rise to some fundamental building blocks of internal experience.

Though there is much debate about what the mind is, there is little controversy about the mind's innate ability to process information. The elaborate circuitry of the brain is reflected in the many elegant ways in which it can process information: We can learn, note similarities and differences, make generalizations, categorize, associate, analyze, and create new combinations of information within the intricate firing patterns of our brains. These patterns are not random, but emerge from the arrangements of neural connections that are able to carry out specific kinds of processing. For instance, we have circuits responsible for visual processing and others for the processing of the more abstract representations of ideas.

Within this information processor, we experience desires and beliefs that emanate from the meaning of mental representations. What is the nature of this representational language of the mind? At a very basic level, *the patterns of firing serve as codes or symbols that carry information and cause events to happen in the brain. These events themselves are patterns of neuronal activation, which in turn carry further information.*[3] *The processing of the codes or symbols—the essence of information processing—is based on both the representational and causal properties of the symbols themselves.* This chain reaction of symbols and events cascades into "cognitive processes" such as memory and abstract thought. In other words, the brain creates symbols whose actions are themselves symbolic—they carry information.

How does the brain do this? By altering the activity rates of the firing of neurons, the brain is able to establish a set of signals or codes that serve as symbols as defined above. The term "mental representation" has been used to designate such a mental symbol as created by neuronal firing patterns.[4] Changes in the rate of firing (increases or decreases in the baseline firing rate of a given neuron or clusters of neurons) create a pattern of activation at a given moment. Even a representation is a dynamic process in the brain. Patterns of transformation act upon these representations to further alter their form and action within the brain. Such complex transformational patterns are called "cognitive processes." These processes can make new associations among representations, identify similarities and differences, or extract global themes and principles from patterns of representations over time. In this way, the brain generates new combinations and features of representations, which are further acted upon by specific processes. This is the fundamental framework for the computational mind; it takes place within specific neural pathways in the brain.

Evolutionary pressures have required that the brain become specialized in its problem-solving skills. We inherit the genetically preprogrammed capacity for information processing of a particular sort. The brain cannot process all types of information; a given module of the mind is only able to handle certain kinds of information in specific kinds of ways. For example, one requirement of living in the physical world is to be able to represent specific objects and events. This can be seen in explicit memory, for example, as the encoding of the details of specific autobiographical memories or facts. One evolutionary purpose of explicit memory has been to be able to represent objects in space and time—a capacity that allowed our ancestors to find hidden food or recall where an enemy might be lurking. Our autobiographical memory may reflect this temporal and spatial representational ability of the self in the physical world. At the other extreme, the mind must be able to transform these particular events and facts into more generalized representations, in order to allow learning and adaptation to repeated experiences with the world. This is seen in memory systems as implicit mental models, general autobiographical knowledge (for example, "When I was seventeen I was unhappy"), and semantic concepts or categories of objects. These properties of the specific versus the general can be seen in various aspects of the mind's specialized problem-solving skills. As we come to generalize and abstract features from the originally perceptually based, input-driven representational process, our representational processes become more complex. For example, we can have ideas of "freedom" and "justice," which have their origins in physical reality but contain far more complex and abstract features than spatial and temporal representations permit.

The distinct modules of the mind, from sensory and perceptual processing to abstract reasoning and the conceptualization of other minds, are each designed to solve specific kinds of problems. They do this by creating and handling specific kinds of representations. Interaction among specific modules allows for the transfer of information across modalities, as in the coordination of sight and hearing or in the influence of implicit on explicit memory processing. Artists and poets can extract meaning from sensory experiences, which they then translate back into powerful symbols of more universal concepts within a visual medium or the expressive use of words. In this way, various layers of representational processes, from perceptual images to abstract concepts, can become linked within a single experience. The mind is governed by the ways in which these information-processing modules function and interact with one another. The modules themselves are created by the activity of the brain. Thus the brain's information-processing modules and neural activation features both contribute to our subjective experience of mental function.

FORMS OF REPRESENTATIONS AND SUBJECTIVE EXPERIENCE

The subjective experience of information processing can help to illustrate its relevance for understanding the mind. The information contained within representations can be about many things. For example, Steven Pinker describes a four-part division of representations as follows: visual images containing a two-dimensional pattern or mosaic; phonological representations as a stretch of syllables in a string-like display; grammatical representations carrying the information of nouns and verbs, phrases and clusters, stems, roots, phonemes, and syllables; and "mentalese," the language of conceptual knowledge and the medium in which the gist of an idea is contained.[5] Within this framework, one can see that the mind may include codes for objects, words, and other complex subjects. Other researchers have proposed a three-part division of representations into sensory–perceptual, conceptual (or categorical), and linguistic forms.[6] Whatever perspective one takes, it is clear that the mind has distinct information that it symbolizes, as well as different modes of processing these specific forms of representations. The activation of each of these types, their interaction with each other, and their accessibility to various states can help illuminate some basic aspects of subjective experience. With a wide array of mental processes, individual differences in experience, and a fundamental limitation in how one person can know the subjective experience of another, it may seem an impossible task to define how the mind represents information and therefore constructs reality. We need to be able to have a common language for communicating some of what is known about the basic aspects of the mind's processing of information. For the purposes of this book, then, let us use a basic vocabulary of representational processes as described below.

Sensation and Perception

A "sensory representation" contains information representing sensations, including input from the outside world, from the body, and from the brain itself. External sensory data include sight, hearing, olfaction, taste, and touch. These enter the body through sensory receptors in their respective areas. The signals then travel to the brain, where they are usually processed first in the thalamus at the top of the brainstem and then in their particular sensory areas in the cerebral cortex. Internal sensations include bodily motion and physiological status of the body (such as states of arousal, temperature, and muscle tension). These are registered in the somatosensory cortical areas, which are especially integrated on the right side of the brain. In general, a sensory representation is thought to have a minimal amount of categorization; that is, input is registered in the brain with relatively little "top-down" processing. A blast of sound, a bright light, and a pressure on the skin of the arm are all examples of stimuli that we may sense but be unable to classify into a previously experienced representation, which we can then compare and contrast to prior experiences. We "sense" such stimuli, but we do not (yet) have a category or name for what they are. This is the closest we may come to "the thing itself." Even sensory representations are constructions of our nervous system's ability, via our neurons and sensory receptors, to translate stimuli into the code of distributed neuronal activations within our brains.

A "perceptual" representation is a more complexly processed unit of information than a sensory one. At the level of the sensory cortices, the brain analyzes and compares incoming information with memories from prior experience in order to categorize the sensations into a perception. In contrast to a "basic" sensation, a percept is "symbolized"; it represents a constructed bit of information created from the synthesis of present sensory experience with past memory and generalizations contained within experientially derived mental models. This is the essence of top-down processing.

In the strictest sense, even a sensory representation meets the literal definition of a "symbol"—something that carries information about something other than itself. The sensations we have of putting our hands in cold water are signals generated from the firing of our neurons connected to our temperature receptors in the skin of the hand. This firing pattern is not the "cold" itself; it *stands* for "cold," because it comes from receptors that detect temperature in our skin. This pattern is a basic code directly related to the sensory medium. In an extended definition, however, some scientists refer to a more direct code as a "presymbolic" representation: It is as close to the thing itself as we can get before the mind does a lot of top-down categorizing and manipulating of incoming data based on preconceived ideas and past experiences. I use the term "presymbolic," because it will help remind us of the nature of information processing within the mind, and also because it is often useful to distinguish these forms from those representations that are more easily translated into words.

These presymbolic codes are generated from sensory receptors, take in information from both the outside world and the body itself, and are initially encoded within the deeper structures of the brain. Some might argue that this brain activity is not part of the "mind," often being at a nonconscious level and thought by some to be merely an "automatic" function of the brain. However, these presymbolic representations, these less complex codes, serve a vital function in influencing all other information-processing aspects of the mind.

The flow of processing from sensation to perception is influenced by the state of mind at the time of sensing something. Mental states profoundly influence our construction of reality at this emerging symbolic representational level. The mind constructs perceptual reality from bits of selected information it receives through the senses, in combination with extremely subjective and context-sensitive mental processes, such as mental models and the influence of emotion. Some may ask, "Does the outer world exist in any accurate and direct way in the mind?" A good question! Internal mental experience is not the product of a photographic process. Internal reality is in fact constructed by the brain as it interacts with the environment in the present, in the context of its past experiences and expectancies of the future. At the level of perceptual categorizations, we have reached a land of mental representations quite distant from the layers of the world just inches away from their place inside the skull. This is the reason why each of us experiences a unique way of minding the world.

Conceptual (or Categorical) Representations

In both sensation and perception, we may be aware of sensing or perceiving various things, without the ability to describe them in words. These forms of awareness are sensory and perceptual symbols, which are considered "prelinguistic" representations. Another type of prelinguistic symbol is a "conceptual" representation. It is this form of encoding that carries information about more highly processed entities, such as the gist of an idea, "reading between the lines" of a story, or notions of freedom and justice. These complex conceptual representations are an important part of the information processing of the mind. They are not directly related to the external world and the derived sensory and perceptual representations, but are created by the computations of the mind in its interactions with the world and other people within it. In this sense, sensory–perceptual representations attempt to symbolize the physical world (external or internal); conceptual representations symbolize the mind's creation of ideas and of the mind itself. We can create complex representations of the self, others, and the relationships we have. These conceptual representations are nonverbal. They form the fundamental building blocks of our thoughts, beliefs, and intentions, and aspects of our explicit memories. We will see later in this chapter how this ability to form complex representations allows the mind to create the concept of the minds of other people.

Although the actual word "concept" does not fully capture the range of representations falling under this divisional framework, it is a useful term in contrast to "percept." These conceptual representations appear to have no direct three-dimensional correlates in the external world. How, for example, would the concept of "freedom" or "justice" be simply represented in the world? An artist may be able to portray these concepts in a visual form, but their status in the mind may not be so easily linked to perceptual representations.

Another way of thinking of this is that the mind utilizes a categorical structure in which to classify and organize perceptual representations. (In fact, as described below, some authors use the term "categorical" representations rather than "conceptual.") For example, we can generate a list of mammals that live in the ocean, or fish, or living creatures that swim, or plants that live in water. In each of these categories, there is no single entity in the world that constitutes the category. For instance, there is no such animal as a "mammal"; there are many individual species that fit into the overall classification. These groupings certainly come from patterns observed by the human mind. But in this way, they are abstract creations of the mind, not direct perceptions of actual things in the world.

Linguistic Representations

"Linguistic" representations contain information about sensations, perceptions, concepts, and categories within the socially shared packets called words. Words themselves have physical properties; they can be seen, heard, felt, spoken, and written. But words move beyond the physical world and link the mental representational worlds of separate people. We can throw mental representations out of our minds and into the air or onto the printed page, where they can be detected by a receiver whose mind in turn activates "similar" packets of verbal representations. Human language permits information processing to be shared across individuals. The evolutionary benefit of such an innate ability has been that it has allowed us as social beings to create cultural history and pass on knowledge across generations, across time, and across the huge space that exists between the minds of two people.

Information processing occurs automatically in the mind. The brain's activity occurs in patterns from specific regions that determine the nature of the information being carried. These patterns result in subsequent neural activity, which itself contains information. Most of this process occurs without the participation of conscious awareness and often is not translatable into linguistic representations.

Some people are more aware of certain layers of information than other people are. For example, the capacity to conceptualize the "nature of a relationship" will vary quite a bit. Some individuals may take the phrase and expound for hours on the patterns of their relating with others. Others will hear the phrase and may only be able to respond with "It is good" or "It is bad." These individuals may have the ability to form complex representations of relationships, but these representations may be inaccessible to translation

into words. That is, such persons may be able to form very sophisticated reactions to intricate social interactions, but may be unable to
describe the internal processes which have led to them. Still others
may be quite "concrete" and be unable to make such abstract representations.

Awareness of the body is another example of how people may
differ in their awareness of internal information processing. The
importance of bodily responses in determining emotion and meaning
makes awareness of this form of information vital to grasp. The
ways our functionally distinct modes of representational processing
interact with one another may be keys to understanding the blockages in information processing that are a part of mental dysfunction.
Such impairments in the flow of information can be seen, for example, in the memory disturbances of individuals with posttraumatic
stress disorder. Altering the flow of information processing may be a
fundamental part of psychotherapy for these individuals. Also, being
able to put some of these representations into words may enable the
individuals to reflect on their history and alter the future outcome of
the representations' effects on the self.

CONSCIOUSNESS AND
REPRESENTATIONAL PROCESSES

Gerald Edelman has described a process by which the mind functions
through positive feedback loops that reinforce their own patterns of
firing.[7] This is called "reentry" and is based on the principle that
loops of reciprocal firing—in which one group of neurons activates
another, which then in turn activates the original group—constitute a
major organizing process of the brain. One can visualize this as a
form of interneuronal group "resonance." Reentry stabilizes a
neuronal firing pattern that allows for the subjective experience of
the processing in that moment. At certain times, this stabilizing process permits the activation of consciousness. Edelman has described a
form of "primary consciousness" as occurring when our basic sensory–perceptual processes resonate with our conceptual ones (which
he terms "categorical" processes). This is the "remembered present,"
giving us a sense of awareness and familiarity with something without our being able to name it or to see it from a distanced temporal
perspective involving past and future.

In Edelman's model, there are the three major forms of neuronal

groups as summarized above which function as representational processes; he describes these as "perceptual," "categorical," and "linguistic." Perceptual groups are activated in response to sensations
from the environment or the body. If the mind has experienced these
sensations before and has categorized them with larger informational
meaning, then the neuronal groups for that category will also be activated. For example, if a child has never seen a dog before, the child's
visual sensation of the canine will be experienced without a connected sense of "what it is." If the child has seen pictures of dogs or
actual dogs before, the child will have remembered these and created
a general category, or "schema," for such a sight. In this case, she
will also have neuronal groups activated representing the category or
concept of "dog." The *simultaneous* activation of perceptual (seeing
the dog) and categorical (having a category for "dog") neuronal
groups is thought to produce the internal sensation called primary
consciousness. There is an awareness of the sight as a familiar animal, a "being in the moment" with such a sight, which heightens an
internal conscious sensation. This is the remembered present.

With the development of language, Edelman argues, the neuronal groups responsible for linguistic processing allow a different
form of consciousness to emerge. When the more experienced older
child sees the animal, the perceptual groups activate the categorical
ones, and she has a primary consciousness of the dog. With language, the neuronal groups with the linguistic representation of
"dog" also become active. The simultaneous activation of the categorical and linguistic neuronal groups yields a "higher-order consciousness" in which the child is freed from the prison of the remembered present and is able to reflect both backward and forward in
time. In this view, it is our unique language capacity as humans that
allows us to be both historians and actuaries, reflecting on the past
and consciously planning for the future.

Others, such as Wheeler, Stuss, and Tulving, might argue that
such a form of cross-time representation is a fundamental part of
autonoetic consciousness.[8] We might go on to suggest that such a
form of mental time travel is not dependent upon linguistic representation, but rather on the mind's capacity to represent the self as experienced. For example, the developmental acquisition of autonoetic
consciousness may be more a function of the child's developing self-
awareness and understanding of perceptual processes that permit
experiential awareness than of linguistic abilities alone.[9] In this way,
autonoetic consciousness is a function of an individual's understand-

ing of minds, linking it, as we've discussed in earlier chapters, to the integrating processes of the prefrontal regions, including social cognition, response flexibility, and working memory. As Buckner suggests, however, the specific circuits of the prefrontal area of the brain may carry out quite distinct processes mediating aspects of autonoetic consciousness.[10] What role the left-hemisphere linguistic processing centers may play in the encoding via left orbitofrontal mediation of episodic memory, or in its retrieval via right-hemisphere processes, has yet to be elucidated. In general, the capacity to reflect on the self across time—with or without linguistic representations—may be considered as an extremely evolved, "higher-order" form of consciousness. As we'll see, the development of such a capacity may be intimately influenced by early interpersonal relationships.

Consciousness, as we've discussed in Chapter 4, is a subject of great interest and impassioned debate among academicians ranging from philosophers to neuroscientists. Consciousness has two dimensions: *access* to information, and the *sentience* or subjective quality of an experience. In both of these realms, information processing and mental representations play a central role in determining the nature of our conscious experience. For example, access consciousness can contain within it the awareness of sensation or perceptions, as well as focal attention to aspects of the internal world, including the experience of emotional processing and our beliefs, wishes, and intentions. The sentience of these representations will depend upon the nature of their integration and the information they encode: whether we associate from memory and with conscious awareness the tones of music, the rough surface of a sheet of sandpaper, or reflections upon the various textures and sensations of memories we have of our early days (for example, learning to swim). But this division of consciousness into access and sentience dimensions doesn't fully explain the subjective experiences of consciousness. Some authors argue that perhaps nothing truly can.[11]

Fortunately, this is not an insurmountable problem for our examination of the developing mind. We can in fact gain a deep appreciation of the differences between people in the qualitative ways in which life is experienced. For example, we will discuss soon how those with a history of avoidant attachment seem to have minimal access to the nonverbal signals that reflect primary emotional states. Such an absence is seen in their frequent lack of awareness of other's emotions, and perhaps of their own emotions as well. By examining which representational processes are utilized to perceive such states in others and in the self, we can begin to understand what may be missing or impaired in these individuals. Internal subjective experience may vary, depending upon which systems of representation are activated at a particular time. By definition, subjective experience implies the unique, internal quality of an experience. Understanding how these representational processes are integrated and then bound to the 40-Hz sweeping process and the activity of the lateral prefrontal cortex, discussed in Chapter 4, will enable us to move more deeply into a view of how individuals may differ in the fundamental ways in which they live. In this way, we will utilize this view of information processing to understand some aspects of the qualitative, subjective experience of the mind.

MODES AND MODULES

At the most fundamental level, the activity of the brain's circuitry creates patterns of activation that serve as symbols, which both represent information and cause further mental processes to occur. These processes themselves represent information. This is the information processing of the mind. The difference between the distinct forms of representations lies both in the patterns of firing and in the localization of the neural circuits being activated.

For example, sensory representations are created within the circuits linked directly to the outside world and to the body. Perceptual representations are established as these earlier sensory inputs are processed and transformed into more complex representations. The various layers of the sensory cortex—for example, in visual processing—reveal that they serve as pattern recognition modules capable of firing off with a match between, say, a set of angles and contrasts when one is visualizing a "table." The location of this representation of the table in the visual cortex helps define its visual quality. Conceptual representations are even further distilled (processed, transformed) away from the world of objects. These more complex and abstract symbols are thought to emanate from the activity of the neocortex. Linguistic representations—words and their various elements and combinations—constitute the modality of specific regions in the left hemisphere. The nonverbal intonations or prosody of spoken language are thought to emanate from the activity of the right hemisphere. Overall, *the localization of processing lends a unique qualitative sensation to our experience of mental representations.*

Cognitive neuroscience describes the notions of mental "modules," "modes," "systems," and "processes." These ideas (which are discussed in greater detail in Chapter 6) imply a separateness that may emanate from the neuroanatomically distinct sites in which mental representations are created and processed. Like the intricate interconnections within the brain itself, which interrelate the functions of numerous circuits, so too do the mental modules of the mind act interdependently. For example, representations within implicit memory may often act upon us without conscious awareness.[12] The generalizations of *implicit* memory, our mental models of the past, can directly shape our active perceptions and *explicit* memory. Here we see two "independent" modes of processing having an influence on each other. Undoubtedly such influences reside in not-yet-determined neural connections between these two complex systems of the brain.

DEVELOPMENTAL PROCESSES
AND BRAIN ASYMMETRY

We have seen how mental experience emerges from the activation of different circuits within the brain. Emotion has been defined as a set of processes involving, most importantly, the appraisal of information and the arousal of energizing activations. How the mind creates representations and places value on them is inextricably linked with emotional processes. Though we use these terms for didactic purposes, there is no true dichotomy between "cognition" and "emotion." Brain structure and function give rise to the integrated complexity of mental life. In fact, infant studies suggest that we can examine how the intrinsic features of the developing brain may create specific forms of representations via neural specialization present at birth, such as brain asymmetry.

Colwyn Trevarthen, who has studied infants and brain asymmetry for decades, suggests:

> Psychology and brain science come together in the scientific analysis of cerebral localization of function. Asymmetries of function, correlated with the deeply separated left and right cerebral hemispheres, have particular value in the opening up of an approach to mental activities at the highest level. Cognitive and voluntary processes that attain maturity only after many years and that have special importance in cultural life tend to be asymmetric in the brain. The basis for this asymmetry seems to be set down very early, probably in fetal stages. It becomes elaborated in the subse-

quent development of the brain. Throughout childhood, as the brain takes up the lessons of experiences, and even in the moment-to-moment adjustments of adult consciousness, structures beneath the cortex continue to exercise their regulations. They assist in the development of a bihemispheric system in which the two sides have complementary roles.

Finally, completing the picture, we find evidence that the intrinsic regulators of human brain growth in a child are specially adapted to be coupled, by emotional communication, to the regulators of adult brains of people who know more. This seems to be the key generic brain strategy for cultural learning that takes place not in single brains, but in communities of them. Developmental brain science will have great importance in future efforts to understand the growing human mind, and the life of ideas and beliefs in human communities.[13]

Trevarthen proposes an "intrinsic motive formation," which emerges in the embryo brainstem and regulates asymmetries in the development and functioning of the cerebral cortex.[14] Within the brainstem are interneuronal systems that carry out aspects of sensory integration; that coordinate motivational states and motoric action patterns; and that develop linkages to the important regulatory structures of the hypothalamus, basal ganglia, and amygdala. These are the brain circuits that constitute the intrinsic motive formation, which is proposed to exist even before cortical neurons develop. These essential and asymmetric elements of the emotional, motor, and motivational systems are in place long before the "higher" representational neocortex is formed.

Indeed, the cognitive systems exhibiting the most distinct asymmetry are thought to exist between intake and output circuits and the emotional processing limbic region of the brain; again, this view emphasizes the interweaving of emotion and cognitive processing. Trevarthen goes on to state:

Human cerebral asymmetry at the level of neocortical cognitive processes that take up and store experience develops from a deeper and more ancient asymmetry in regulatory motive structures that both control morphogenesis of the brain in the embryo and guide the infant into skilled action and an understanding of the motives and ideas of other members of the cooperative community. Expression of motives and emotions between young children and their caregivers and companions regulates the acquisition of sense in the human world.[15]

Numerous lines of research suggest that the hemispheres differ in the predominance of those neurotransmitters that regulate attention, motor behavior, approach–withdrawal, and self-regulation. From the embryonic stage onward, there appear to be remarkable differences in "intrinsic motives," the driving forces behind both in-the-moment processing and developmental trajectories. Trevarthen proposes that *the left hemisphere tends to have an "assertive" motivational state* governing active engagement with the world of others, as seen in the finding of the infant's right-hand gestures and cooing vocalizations in response to the mother's speech (each of which is left-hemisphere-mediated). In contrast, *the right hemisphere is proposed to be more "acceptive"*—that is, receptive and self-regulatory—as evidenced by the infant's left handed self-touching and the right hemisphere's being better developed than the left and responsive to the prosody of "motherese" (nonverbal, sing-song quality of tone of voice). These findings are supported by the notion that the left hemisphere is more active in motor expression and "approach," mediated by activity of the neurotransmitter dopamine. The right hemisphere, in contrast, mediates "withdrawal" in social situations and is more involved in attentive and reflective states, mediated by activity of the neurotransmitter noradrenaline.[16]

Tucker, Luu, and Pribram offer a complementary view of the relation between circuitry and representational asymmetries. These authors review the development of two "streams" of information that have evolved between the cortex and deeper structures via the frontal lobes. In an "archicortical trend" or "dorsal pathway," there is an emphasis on certain types of cells and on noradrenergic activity. In a "paleocortical trend" or "ventral pathway," there is the involvement of different regions and a predominance of dopaminergic activity. Though each of these trends is present on both sides of the brain, *the dorsal pathway appears to be predominant on the right side of the brain, and the ventral pathway on the left side.* Tucker and colleagues suggest that

these two limbic–cortical pathways apply different motivational biases to direct the frontal lobe representation of working memory. The dorsal limbic mechanisms projecting through the cingulate gyrus may be influenced by hedonic evaluations, social attachments, and they may initiate a mode of motor control that is holistic and impulsive. In contrast, the ventral limbic pathway from the amygdala to orbital frontal cortex may implement a tight, restricted mode of motor control that reflects adaptive constraints of self-preservation. In the human brain, hemispheric specialization appears to have led to asymmetric elaborations of dorsal and ventral pathways. Understanding the inherent asymmetries of corticolimbic architecture may be important in interpreting the increasing evidence that the left and right frontal lobes contribute differently to normal and pathological forms of self-regulation.[17]

Tucker and colleagues review the findings that the ventral pathway (dominant on the left side) has a motivational bias toward specific details of objects and involves a feedback system whereby representations of present perceptions have a high degree of tight monitoring of the generation of behavioral output. Such a feedback process lends itself to object perception and competence in analytic processing, which may "be especially involved in object memory and the fine-tuning of the neocortical representation of objects whether the objects are conceptual or perceptual."[18] In contrast, the dorsal stream of information (dominant on the right side) involves spatial and context representations that rely on a "feedforward" or projectional mode of motor control, which activates arousal of attention and memory processes in response to novel situations and favors "impulsive" or spontaneous behavioral output. Such a projectional mode is also thought to involve representations of the future. This dorsal stream incorporates information from the body itself (autonomic activity and the state of viscera and smooth muscles), which makes it "well suited to evaluate stimuli for their motivational significance in relation to internal states."[19]

We therefore see a parallel in viewpoints that the right hemisphere plays a dominant role in autonoetic consciousness, which involves a sense of self (internal states, state of the body), context, and time as these can be represented in the past and projected into the future. The predominance of the dorsal stream in the right hemisphere in this way establishes the motivational formation that drives the creation of autonoetic representations of the self through time. These views allow us to understand the notion of "cognitive representations" in a developmental light: Neocortical capacities to represent reality between perception and action emerge in the setting of powerful and asymmetric intrinsic motivational factors built into the structure and function of the brain. These motivational systems influence embryonic growth and postnatally depend on interpersonal experiences for their continued differentiation. We shall see that these genetically driven asymmetries create their own subjective and interpersonal effects on human experience.

MODES OF PROCESSING: CEREBRAL ASYMMETRY AND "DICHOTOMANIA"

Literature on the two hemispheres of the brain reveals the fascinating origins of the awareness of our distinct ways of knowing about the world.[20] An early form of research into these modes focused on the experiences of patients with epilepsy who had to undergo a procedure that cut the connections between the two hemispheres in order to control their seizures. In these people, called "split-brain patients," the corpus callosum was severed, resulting in the functional isolation of the left and right halves of the brain. Researchers were then able to present either half of such a patient's brain with stimuli and study the patient's responses. A second prevalent source of information has been research on patients with anatomic lesions (tumors, strokes) in one hemisphere or the other. Their deficits demonstrate patterns of disrupted functioning implicating the central importance of processes specific to a particular side of the brain. A third source of insights has been ingenious experimental designs devised to expose only one hemisphere of the brains of normal subjects to stimuli. The "unilateral" response in these situations has provided more data supporting the notion of hemispheric specialization. More recently, a fourth type of research utilizing brain imaging studies has contributed to the examination of hemispheric laterality by following the activity of normal subjects' brains during various procedures. These studies have revealed patterns of activation that tend to confirm the findings from the earlier forms of investigation.

Springer and Deutsch, in reviewing the scientific studies investigating bilaterality, approach this topic by examining the methods and results from an array of research approaches in order to offer the data prior to any unwarranted generalizations.[21] They caution against a trend they call "dichotomania," in which popular writers have extended the scientific findings far beyond even the implications of the data. For example, whole cultures have been accused of being only "left-brained" or "right-brained," without an acknowledgment of the usual bilateral participation of the hemispheres in the vast array of mental processes. The temptation to focus on two distinct modes of processing has its historical roots. Philosophers have long noted the differing styles of knowing about the world; they have contrasted creative, synthetic, emotional, intuitive, and nonconscious patterns with those of critical, analytic, intellectual, rational, and conscious modes of thought.

There may be a very basic reason for this long history of seeing dichotomies in human experience. As we've discussed, the anatomic structure and neurochemistry of the two halves of the brain are somewhat distinct.[22] But even more than mere anatomy and physiology, the processes that have now been identified to be dominant in the functioning of each hemisphere generally support the philosophers' observations. The essence of the findings from the varied and careful studies of laterality is as follows. The brain, including the amygdala and orbitofrontal cortex (responsible for the assignment of meaning to stimuli), the hippocampus (the major center for conscious, declarative, explicit memory processing), and the lateral prefrontal cortex (thought to be a primary center for focal, conscious attention), is divided into two halves. At various points, bands of tissue, including the corpus callosum and the anterior commissures (and, indirectly, the cerebellum), connect the left and right halves of the brain. The uppermost part of the brain is called the cerebrum and includes the area called the neocortex, where complex thinking is believed to reside. Each half of the upper brain can be referred to as a "cerebral hemisphere." In this book, the terms "right" or "left" as applied to brain, cortex, hemisphere, side, or mode refer in general to the specialized anatomy or functions of that side of the entire brain: from the abstract processes at the top of the brain, to the more basic physiological and sensory ones lower down, emanating from the brainstem. As we've discussed above, asymmetries exist within the brainstem and limbic system long before neocortical development. These intrinsic differences may have direct effects on the unfolding of asymmetric representational capacities, including the more abstract processes of the neocortex. The predominance of the ventral or dorsal pathways within each hemisphere may shape the motivational bias of attention and memory within that stream of information. Although certain functions appear to be specialized in each half, the normal functioning of the mind involves "cross-talk" between the two sides of the brain. The connecting tissue between the hemispheres appears to be important for both mutual activation and inhibition of corresponding ("homologous") cerebral centers on either side of the brain. As we'll explore, the way in which modes of processing interact with each other cooperatively, interact conflictually, or remain rigidly dis-associated may play a large role in the qualitative experience of mental functioning and well-being.

The following is a generally accepted description of the processes in which each cerebral hemisphere specializes. In the right hemisphere are fast-acting, parallel (simultaneously active), holistic processes. The right side specializes in representations such as sensations, images, and the nonverbal polysemantic (multiple) meanings of words. These nonverbal representations are often called "analogic." Visuospatial perception is an example of such an analogic function specialized on the right side. Note that the traditional verbal–nonverbal distinction between the left and right hemispheres is not completely accurate. Examples of this include the contribution of the right hemisphere for understanding metaphor, paradox, and humor. Also, the reading of stories activates both left- and right-hemisphere processes more readily than the reading of scientific texts, which primarily activates the left hemisphere.[23]

On the left side of the brain are more slowly acting, linear, sequentially active, temporal (time-dependent) processes. Verbal meanings of words, often called "digital" representations, are a primary mode of processing for the left side. The left hemisphere is thought to utilize monosemantic "packets" of information as basic representations, which are then processed in a slower, linear mode. Examples of linear processing are reading the words in this sentence, aspects of conscious attention, and determining the sequence of events in a story. Our language-based communication is dominated by this linear mode of expression and reception of "bundled" bits of symbols, which carry restrictive definitions and relatively clearly demarcated chunks of information. This is quite distinct from the analogic representations seen, for example, in an artist's painting or in a photograph. We can translate these analogic components of the world into digitalized forms within words, but the translation is never complete. In this way, some authors argue that the right hemisphere more fully "sees the world for what it is," whereas the left hemisphere must reduce the world much more into mentally defined, often socially constructed chunks of information.

These distinctions have their developmental origins in infancy, as we've discussed above: The right hemisphere is dominant for the prosodic aspect of "motherese" and appears to be more involved in acceptive, receptive, and self-regulatory motor activity. In contrast, the left hemisphere is involved in actively asserting communications via the right hand; these are more outwardly oriented, approach/ assertive motor activities.[24] One can propose a perhaps simplistic but useful generalization here that the left hemisphere is motivated for externally focused attention and action, whereas the right is motivated for internally focused attention and action. As neocortical representations emerge between perception (input) and action (output) in the form of thought and memory processes, we can see that such core asymmetries in motivational factors will bias each hemisphere to develop distinct capacities for complex representations. On the left are the semantic memory representations of objects in the world, which can be manipulated and communicated to others as distinct packets of information. On the right is the internal world of the mind—both of the self and of the other—as the primary subject of memory representations within episodic memory and social cognition. The "theory of mind," or capacity for "mindsight" and for representing mental states of others and the self, is the stuff of right-hemisphere representations. Intentions, beliefs, attitudes, perceptions, memories, and feelings are represented in analogic forms that are not easily reduced to digital packets of information.

Studies of laterality have also suggested the following findings, which have a bit fewer numbers of subjects and therefore fewer available data supporting their universal acceptance. The right hemisphere is considered to work as a pattern recognition center, assessing the gestalt and context of input from a synthetic mode of processing. The left, in contrast, uses logical and analytical processing to construct its detail-based representation of reality. Because of these differences in processing, writers have often summarized the contrast between right and left as that between the intuitive and the rational, between context and text, and between the monosemantic and the polysemantic meanings of words.[25]

Michael Gazzaniga and colleagues suggest that the left hemisphere is primarily responsible for "syllogistic" reasoning, in which the mind searches for causal explanations about events and reaches conclusions based on limited information.[26] The right hemisphere lacks such a drive to explain; rather, it "sees things as they are with little alteration."[27] Gazzaniga has used the term "the interpreter" to describe the process of the left hemisphere's attempts to use reason to explain cause–effect relationships in the limited pieces of information with which it is provided. In split-brain patients, the left hemisphere has been shown to weave fanciful tales to explain its perceptions.

Such narratives, Gazzaniga and colleagues argue, are driven by the interpreter's need to create an explanation even in the face of quite limited data. Under normal conditions, such sustained syllogistic reasoning allows us to try to explain how things function and why the world is the way it is. In this manner, the left hemisphere is the center of the cognitive machinery that attempts to explain events and therefore, in Gazzaniga's view, is the primary motive to narrative thinking. In later chapters, we will return to this notion of an "interpreter" and its contribution, together with that of right-hemispheric processes, to the production of autobiographical narratives and attachment patterns.

More fanciful authors have extended these general dichotomies to less well-accepted philosophical notions such as that of the right hemisphere as the origin of Eastern thought and the left hemisphere as the source of Western philosophical views. Psychological works have suggested that the right hemisphere is the center of the "unconscious" and that the left hemisphere is the origin of "consciousness."[28] Although these views indeed may be useful and perhaps have an essence of truth, their blind acceptance can limit a more careful application of the scientific findings to understanding subjective experience. An important example is in the generalizations of laterality and emotion.

ASYMMETRY AND EMOTION

The most common (and oversimplified) notion in the popular literature on psychology is that the intuitive, nonverbal right hemisphere is the source of all emotion. If this idea is taken literally, it does not leave much room to explore the various shades of emotional response woven throughout all internal processes on each side of the brain. Emotion exists on both sides of the brain. Research on emotion, for example, demonstrates the intimate influence of emotion on all cognitive processes, from attention and perception to memory and moral reasoning.[29] Examination of the actual scientific data available on the nature of emotion and laterality can shed some fascinating and useful light on the topic, and can help us move further in understanding the development of the mind.

In the various studies of emotion and hemispheric specialization, the right hemisphere appears to be primarily responsible for the reading of social and emotional cues from other people, and for the external expression of affect by the individual. For example, the left side of the face, controlled preferentially by the right side of the brain, has been shown to express more emotion than the other side.[30] Studies of patients with right-hemisphere deficits also suggest that attentional mechanisms may be dependent on the right prefrontal cortex.[31] Recall that appraisal and arousal, which constitute the second and central phase of emotional response, alert the brain to focus attention on stimuli labeled as "important." Anatomically, the right side has a slightly higher density of neuronal interconnections than the left. As discussed earlier, what is particularly fascinating is that the right cortex also contains a more integrated somatosensory representation of the body, including the state of tension of the body's voluntary muscles and positions of the arms and legs. This finding, plus the presence of representational input from the body's viscera (heart, lungs, intestines)—the somatic markers—in the right orbitofrontal cortex, suggests that the right hemisphere is more capable of having a sense of the body's state. It may indeed be the right hemisphere that is capable of sensing a "gut reaction" to something.[32] Emotions are directly influenced by the right brain's representations of the body's changing states. The sensations experienced as visceral representations in the right hemisphere may be quite difficult to translate into the words of the left hemisphere. The "language of the right hemisphere," the nonverbal representations, may be a more direct means of both being aware of and expressing primary emotional reactions.

The right hemisphere, via the orbitofrontal cortex, also appears to be more capable than the left hemisphere of regulating states of bodily arousal.[33] This suggests that whatever factors directly impinge on right-hemisphere processing, such as bodily input or nonverbal emotional expressions in the voices, body signals, and facial reactions of others, may have a direct impact on a person's own emotional state before the involvement of a linguistically based consciousness or a rational, linear analysis of an ongoing experience.[34]

The right brain will thus be more immediately involved in the registration of the somatic markers that make up part of an emotional experience. Control of the body's response will also be located primarily on the right side. For these reasons, primary emotions—the textured emotional states resulting from initial orientation, appraisal, and arousal—are likely to be experienced more immediately and intensely on the right than on the left. However, appraisal and arousal circuits, the value centers of the brain, are located on both sides. For these reasons, it is fair to say that both sides of the brain are filled with meaning and emotional processes. *The qualitative ways in which each hemisphere is influenced by these neuronal activations—the essence of primary emotions—may be quite distinct because of the representational processes that are unique to each side.*

Studies of emotion and bilaterality have led to several different theoretical models. At this point, there is no clear view of some simple way in which emotion is asymmetrically processed. One view is based on emotional intensity: It holds that the right hemisphere is able to generate and experience more intense emotion than the left. States of high arousal, ranging from intense joy to rage, are thought to be products of the right hemisphere. More regulated, even-keel emotional states of mild interest and calm are thought to be the left hemisphere's range of affective experience.[35]

Another model of emotion and asymmetry is based on *hedonic tone* or *valence.* Studies have suggested that negative, uncomfortable emotions are the products of the right hemisphere.[36] For example, patients with overactive right-sided functioning may experience intense sadness, anger, or anxiety. Left-sided overactivation, in contrast, yields states of happiness and contentment. Popular extensions of these studies might call the right hemisphere pessimistic and the left optimistic. There is much controversy over this distinction, in that studies suggest a role of inhibition of the asymmetric cortico-limbic dorsal and ventral pathways, rather than merely an activation of one side or the other.[37] Furthermore, each hemisphere may be involved in contralateral inhibition—and thus lesion studies that have been interpreted to reveal, for example, negative affect on the right side may actually be demonstrating release of the inherent emotion of the opposite side of the lesion. Nevertheless, there is some agreement that emotions eliciting approach behaviors are experienced on the left side and emotions producing avoidance are processed on the right.[38] This view is supported by the notion that motivational factors are asymmetric from prenatal development onward, and that the value systems on each side of the brain push experience and development in specific directions.

Another view is based on a distinction between "social" and "basic emotions."[39] Social emotions—adaptations of emotional states to meet the needs of social situations—are thought to be functions of the left hemisphere. In this model, basic emotions include both primary and categorical emotions as these have been defined in Chapter 4; they are the value responses to internal or external events and are thought to be products of the right hemisphere. In this view, sadness, anger, fear, disgust, surprise, interest/excitement, enjoyment/joy, and shame are all part of the right hemisphere's processing. Display rules—the culturally transmitted lessons about which, and how, emotions can be expressed in social settings[40]—determine the social appropriateness of affective expression and are presumably mediated by the left hemisphere. This view is consistent with the notion proposed earlier that the left hemisphere has an inherent external bias toward attention and memory processing, whereas the right is biased toward internal mental experience. Spontaneous motor output, the direct expression of internal states via affective signals, is a product of the right hemisphere. The tightly controlled, routinized output of social display rules is a product of the left hemisphere in this model.

CONSCIOUSNESS AND LATERALITY

Though the popular literature and other publications sometimes call the right hemisphere the "seat of the unconscious," *each hemisphere may have its own conscious and nonconscious processes.* Both hemispheres may sometimes function in a quite distinct and isolated fashion; at other times there may be an integration within bihemispheric functioning. Consciousness in general may be qualitatively different on the left and on the right, because the connection of working memory within the lateral prefrontal cortex and the 40-Hz thalamocortical sweeping process will recruit and have available to it representations which are distinct in character within each hemisphere. The associational processes thought to underlie conscious experience may also be quite different on each side of the brain. It is therefore reasonable to suggest that there may be a right-brain and a left-brain form of consciousness. Both hemispheres can become involved as a "supersystem" in which consciousness recruits various neuronal groups across the hemispheric connections, leading to a bihemispheric form of consciousness. We can call this a form of "interhemispheric resonance."

The left hemisphere is the center of logical, linguistic, linear processing. (It may help your explicit memory to notice all the L's in this left-sided list.) This sequential set of one representation leading to another and then another is inherently slower than the rapid, parallel processing of the right side. The basic form of conscious representation in the left hemisphere is the word: Thoughts filled with linguistic representations fill our consciousness from left-hemisphere activity. What we call "thinking" often refers to the conscious verbal processing of the left hemisphere. When we are conscious of sensations and images, these may be likely to emanate from the right hemisphere.

Of note is that *the left hemisphere appears to be inept at reading nonverbal social or emotional cues from others.* Facial recognition centers are primarily in the right hemisphere. What this suggests is that *right-hemisphere "reality," its constructed representational world, will contain the information derived from the emotional states of others.*[41] The right hemisphere's language is one of nonverbal sensations and images. In sum, the general impression of the right hemisphere as being "more emotional" is somewhat oversimplified; it is more accurate to state that the emotional experience in the right hemisphere may be more attuned to the emotional states of others. The right hemisphere's nonverbal representations involve the essence of affect, whereas the left hemisphere may have little innate ability to construct or be conscious of such a nonverbal, nonlogical view of the world. However, the left hemisphere is able to mediate social display rules and can assess complex social situations to some degree.[42] Emotional processes are a fundamental part of both hemispheres and are not restricted to only one side or one area of the brain. Our abilities to perceive primary emotional states, and to become both conscious of them and able to translate them into expressions to others, may be at the heart of the qualitative difference in the experience of emotion between the hemispheres.

The whole brain creates the mind. In neurologically intact individuals, the activity of both sides of the brain contributes to the functioning of the brain as a whole with greater or lesser degrees of interdependent activity. Just as we've seen that certain mental systems can function in association (such as explicit and implicit memory), in some conditions there is a dis-association in functioning. The mental systems, modules, or modes carrying out the functions of the mind probably emanate from the activity of the intricate circuitry in specific regions of the brain.[43] Examining the location of these modules can only help us understand human experience. The studies of laterality offer a powerful tool in understanding the mind.

ATTACHMENT, LATERALITY, AND REPRESENTATIONAL PROCESSES

Because emotions are fundamentally linked to appraisal–arousal mechanisms in both the right and left hemispheres, they influence all aspects of cognition, from perception to rational decision making. As we've seen, attachment experiences early in life appear to have direct influences upon various basic processes, including forms of memory, narrative, emotional regulation, and interpersonal behavior. No formal studies exist at the present time examining how these early emotional relationships may preferentially influence the function and development of each hemisphere. Given that studies do suggest that the left and right hemispheres may experience different aspects of emotional response, we can ask how intimate affect attunement—the resonance of states of mind between child and caregiver—might influence the two hemispheres in unique ways in the different attachment relationships. The proposal being made here is that the different patterns of attachment relationships can be understood in part as differentially involving communication between one hemisphere of the parent and the similar hemisphere of the child. The conceptual basis for this proposal is that the more mature adult parent's state of mind will tend to recruit similar brain processes in the child. If this occurs repeatedly and during the crucial early years of development, it is plausible that these shared states may become engrained within the child.

What is the evidence that parent–child relationships may involve asymmetric effects on the developing child's brain? Studies by Geraldine Dawson and by Tiffany Field and colleagues suggest that the left hemisphere's involvement in positive emotions, such as joy and excitement, make it particularly vulnerable to dysfunction in cases of maternal depression.[44] In Dawson's studies of mother–child dyads with prolonged maternal depression, EEG findings were suggestive of dampened left-hemisphere functioning with relative increases in right-hemisphere activation in both mothers and children. If a mother's depression lasted beyond one year, then the child was more likely to have prolonged impairment in left-hemisphere activation in the future. Maternal depression involves decreased affective attunement and diminished sharing of heightened moments of state-to-state resonance around feelings such as excitement, interest, and joy.[45] The right hemisphere, in this view, is involved in negative emotions, such as fear, sadness, and anger. These findings support the valence-based view of emotional laterality, in which asymmetry determines the hedonic tone of emotional experience.

Other types of studies suggest that the form of parent–child communication during the early years of life may directly shape the lateralization of brain function. Bavellier, Corina, and Neville have revealed that the mediation of American Sign Language (ASL), a visual display of signals used to communicate with hearing impaired individuals, is carried out in different areas of the brain depending on when it was learned.[46] For example, congenitally deaf individuals who have learned ASL utilize the left hemispheric regions usually involved in spoken language. Bavellier and colleagues also elected to study normal-hearing children raised by deaf parents who learned sign language as their first "language" and to compare them to individuals who learned ASL later in life. In individuals who learned to communicate with ASL early on, the left hemisphere centers that usually mediate "spoken" language subsumed this role for the manually based visual language. However, in normal-hearing adults who learned ASL after adolescence, the left hemisphere did not subsume this role.[47]

These studies suggest that the brain is capable of devoting its circuitry to alternative sensory modes depending on stimulus input, and that the timing of exposure to stimuli has a direct influence on how "plastic" the brain is in adapting its circuitry. We can further propose that the social nature of information processing—the form in which interpersonal communication takes place—may be an important determinant in brain differentiation. This latter possibility highlights the notion that whether language is mediated by visual or by auditory means early in life, similar brain regions will take on the task of language processing. Could it be that forms of emotional communication—or the lack of them—that involve nonverbal aspects of communication can also directly shape brain development in these lateralized ways by experience-dependent developmental processes as well? Future studies will be needed to explore this possibility.

The right hemisphere is dominant in its activity and development during the first three years of life.[48] Children who experience severe emotional deprivation during this period may be at most risk of having losses in the structural components of their right hemispheres, especially in the region of the orbitofrontal cortex.[49] This vulnerability may be understood as a function of the primary role of the right hemisphere in mediating the affect attunement that serves as a major form of connection and communication between the child and caregiver. This view also supports the notion that primary emotions, which give rise to vitality affects, may be more closely linked to right-hemisphere function. When we examine the functional properties of each hemisphere, especially the right hemisphere, we can begin to appreciate some possible insights into the differences between individuals with different attachment experiences.

These issues also raise the point that the timing of experience, be it optimal or traumatic, may have the largest impact on those parts of the brain that are in the most active phase of development. These are times of maximal opportunity as well as vulnerability. As Robert Thatcher and colleagues have demonstrated, the brain may undergo a cycling of phases throughout childhood, in which one and then the other hemisphere is in an active phase of growth and development.[50] Clinicians and researchers may benefit from awareness of the possibility that the correlation of overwhelming experiences with the natural oscillations in hemisphere maturation may lead to differing outcomes for development.

If a child has had little resonance of the activity of his right hemisphere with that of his caregivers during the first three years of life, an underdevelopment of that hemisphere's functioning may result. Nonverbal communication, facial expressions, subtleties in tone of voice, and emotional attunements will all be minimal in the "experience-dependent maturation" of this child's right hemisphere. These are the experiential food for the right hemisphere during early development, as well as in adult life. A parent's attachment model may directly influence the nature of her emotional attunement, selectively reinforcing the activity of certain emotions and disavowing (by nonattunement) other ones.[51]

Fonagy and colleagues' findings that certain attachment dyads do not foster the development of elements of the "theory-of-mind" module of processing information[52] can be extended here to support the idea that attachment has lateralized effects. We can propose that "reflective function," in which the mind of one person is able to "mentalize" or create the mind of another, is probably dependent upon processes mediated primarily via the right hemisphere. The reflective function also serves as the substrate for self-awareness and the ability to process information about the self and the self with others. Recognizing facial emotional expression, having cognitive representations of others' minds, having self–other relationship representations, and having the capacity to respond to the mental state of others can all be proposed to be mediated by the social-emotional processing of the right hemisphere. However, the integration of these modules of processing into a coherently functioning reflective mode may require a well-developed coordination of right-hemisphere and left-hemisphere processing, as discussed below. Attachment studies by Fonagy and his coworkers support the notion that interpersonal experiences within early caregiver-child relationships can facilitate, or impair, the development of such reflective capacity.[53]

Adults who have insecure states of mind with respect to attach-ment can be proposed to reveal, within their AAI narratives, frames of mind in which such integration of the hemispheres has not been achieved. Such a restricted parental state of mind may impair the parent's ability to achieve resonance of states with the child. Spe-cifically, the parent will be unable to foster the activity of each hemi-sphere and will have difficulty enabling the child to achieve some form of interhemisphere integration. We can further suggest here that the coherent AAI narratives of securely attached adults reveal a coor-dinated functioning of the "mentalizing" right hemisphere and the "interpreting" left. We shall see how the integration of right- and left-hemisphere representational processes and motivational states leads to a "bilateral form of coherence" and can be revealed within coherent life narratives. The ways in which the mind may come to integrate these processes and achieve such coherence will be explored in greater detail in Chapter 9.

The right hemisphere has a nonverbal "language" of its own, focusing on the gist, context, or social meaning of experiences. Just as the left hemisphere requires exposure to linguistically based lan-guage in order to grow properly, one can propose that the right hemisphere may require emotional stimulation from the environment in order to develop properly. Attachment research clearly demon-strates that communication between caregiver and infant shapes the ways in which the child's developing mind learns to process informa-tion. As Aitken and Trevarthen have stated, "Human cognition developments, and their pathologies, are regulated, from birth, by highly specific motives in the child's brain for engaging with motives in other brains. Emotions constitute an innate system by which func-tions of attending, purpose, and learning may be coordinated between subjects."[54] In this manner, emotional communication and affective attunement become the medium in which the child's cogni-tive capacities develop.

As the organization Zero to Three's logo reads, "To grow a child's mind, nurture a baby's heart." This view is supported by the writing of Stanley Greenspan, who suggests that early emotional relationships form the building blocks for the development of all other representa-tional processes.[55] Aitken and Trevarthen also suggest this view:

> Subjective and intersubjective processes are mutually regulating, and, in early infancy, before manipulative investigation of objects is under efficient volitional control, the regulations of communica-tion with a caregiver who offers affectionate, emotionally available

company appear to dominate in the discovery and learning of real-ity. . . . There is abundant evidence now that neonatal brains are embarking on changes in organization that are highly responsive to stimulation from caregivers. The effects of this experience, while demonstrating the adaptive plasticity of the newborn brain, also give proof of highly elaborate and highly selective systems in the infant for engaging with the processes that motivate expressive behaviors in caretaking individuals.[56]

In other words, the infant both responds to the world of others and plays an active role in influencing how others respond. This process can be seen as a form of "recruitment," in which neuronal processes selectively activate patterns of firing of other neural pathways—in this case, within other brains.

Recall that when neuronal circuits become activated, they create and reinforce their connections with each other. With this in mind, we can see why an avoidantly attached child's conscious experience of life, his subjective sense of daily living, may be quite different from that of a securely attached child whose right hemisphere has been encouraged to develop. Once established, such a pattern in neuronal activations will tend to recruit similar patterns in the future. Within the avoidantly attached individual, there may be a disconnection in the integrative functioning of the two hemispheres that parallels the emotional disconnection within the attachment relationship. Studies of avoidant mother–child pairs have shown that words are used without correlation with nonverbal components of communication.[57] Such an interactive disconnection becomes repeated within a child's own mind. In this way, one hemisphere may begin to act as an autonomous subsystem of the brain. At the extreme, one might predict that such a person may feel more comfortable with abstract ideas and the sharing of intellectual views about the world than with intense emotional exchanges involving the sensation of "feeling felt" or the content of others' minds. Over time, the relative dominance of one hemisphere over the other and the functional isolation of the lateralized modes of processing may begin to dominate the subjective experience of life for that individual.

GENETICS, GENDER, AND EXPERIENCE

Before we can accept the proposal being made here that certain attachment experiences preferentially reinforce the development of one hemisphere over another and lead to impaired bilateral functioning, we need to take a more global perspective on what is known about the effects of innate, nonexperiential factors on the developing individual. Studies have found, for example, that gender plays a large role in determining hemispheric strengths.[58] On the average, females are better than males in a broad range of skills involving the use of language, such as verbal fluency, articulation speed, and grammar. They are also superior to men at tasks involving perceptual speed, manual precision and arithmetic calculations. Males, in contrast, are generally better at tasks that are spatial in nature, including picture assembly, block design, mental rotation, maze performance, and mechanical skills. Men are also superior to women in mathematical reasoning, in intercepting a moving object, and (believe it or not) in finding their way along a route. As you can see, these differences demonstrate a trend that may be surprising: Women have more facility in classically left-hemisphere processes, and men in right-hemisphere ones.

Exposure to hormones during fetal growth is felt to be one factor that directly influences the specialization of hemispheric function. Studies have found that lateralization probably occurs before birth, reinforcing the notion that innate genetic and other constitutional factors (produced by conditions *in utero*) may play a large role in the initial differentiation of the two hemispheres.[59] As the newborn grows, specialization appears to continue for the first few years and is held by some to be complete by the end of the second decade of life. The role of socialization in hemispheric specialization has not been clarified as yet. How the known distinctions in the rearing of boys versus girls serve to elaborate and reinforce these inborn differences is an important but unclear issue.

One generally accepted finding is that females tend to have more processes that are *bilaterally* distributed. For example, women often have words represented in both the (usual) left and the right hemisphere. This finding of more integrated functions across the two sides is supported by anatomic studies demonstrating a number of differences between women and men that support, but do not prove, the notion of increased similarity and accessibility of the left and right hemispheres to each other in women. Cerebral blood flow findings also support the view that men have greater asymmetry in function than women. One way of summarizing these suggestions is that women are "less lateralized" than men. For both men and women, however, the left and right hemispheres are anatomically quite distinct.[60]

One proposal we can make is that perhaps men and women differ in the way the dorsal and ventral circuits develop within each hemisphere. As discussed earlier, Trevarthen has suggested that the dominance of each circuit may act as an "intrinsic motive formation" that shapes the development of more complex representational processes.[61] Could it be that in men there is a more predominant development of the dorsal stream in the right hemisphere and the ventral stream in the left? Likewise, women may have a more evenly contributing influence of dorsal and ventral streams on each side of the brain, leading to the finding of less lateralization. These possibilities will need to be explored in future research.

Why would the brain be genetically programmed to differentiate left from right in the first place? Why do we have two hemispheres with differential functions anyway? There are many speculative answers to these questions. One view holds that the functions of one hemisphere can conflict with those of the other. This is called the "cognitive crowding hypothesis" and specifically highlights the idea that if each hemisphere performed the same function, then the ensuing competition would lead to cognitive dysfunction.[62] Having two separate hemispheres with distinct forms of processes allows for the preservation of the functions of each side. Those organisms that developed bilateral specialization had increased survival ability and were able to pass on the trait generation after generation. Asymmetry actually appears to have a long history in many species of animals.[63]

And why do women and men differ in their laterality? One view is that proposed by Jerre Levy, who suggests that the greater lateralization in men would have been necessary to preserve the high level of visuospatial skills necessary for hunting. In women, the role of child rearing would have necessitated more bilateralization of functions such as the use of language for communication of internal states, as well as social sensitivity and facility with nonverbal modes of communication.[64] This hypothesis combines an anthropological view of gender roles with cognitive findings on the relationship between sex and asymmetry. It speaks directly to the idea of how generations of humans exposed to evolutionary pressures may have been selected for particular patterns of hemispheric specialization. It does not focus on how an individual's experience will "pull" for particular functions. Gender differences in cognition may change as cultural roles in future generations continue to evolve.

HOW DOES EXPERIENCE INFLUENCE HEMISPHERIC SPECIALIZATION?

There are developmental phases in which primarily one, then the other, hemisphere grows and expands.[65] In the first few years of life, as described earlier, the right hemisphere is both more active and growing more rapidly. After these first years, the left hemisphere becomes more dominant in activity and development. By the end of the third year of life, the corpus callosum allows for the transfer of information between the two hemispheres. But before this time, one can almost view the child as a "split-brain" subject, in which the world of words may often be quite separate from that of intense emotional reactions. The mind is created from the whole brain within the activity of its disparate circuits and their interactions with each other. As we've seen, the intrinsic motive formation system may exist before the neocortical capacity to construct representations even begins. The developing mind of the child reflects the manner in which it is anatomically predisposed to processing information. After four years of age, children usually become much more facile at using words to describe their inner states and impulses. Preschools take advantage of this developmental capacity in helping children learn to socialize with their peers by utilizing language to express what they feel and want. Such accomplishments require the joint cooperation of both hemispheres and may not be possible at an earlier age in most children.

We know from studies of children and adults with neurological lesions that the brain can adapt to experiential pressures.[66] For example, in young children with severe forms of epilepsy who have had to undergo treatment involving removal of an entire hemisphere, the remaining half of the brain appears to be able to take on the functions (such as language) of the now missing hemisphere. In adults suffering from strokes, however, the brain may not be so "plastic" or able to adapt to loss of specialized functions. Through lengthy rehabilitation efforts, however, experience can result in the emergence of needed old functions within new circuits. The same appears to be true in cases of congenital impairment of certain sensory modalities, such as sight, in which other modalities (such as touch) utilize the anatomic zones usually specializing in the impaired mode.[67]

In professional musicians, the study of music appears to involve the growth and development of parts of the brain in a different manner from their development in the casual music listener. Specifically, the left brain's language-based, analytic mode becomes a more dominant part of the music experience with education and formal training. This appears to involve judgments about duration, sequence, and rhythm. In contrast, the right side's ability appears to be stronger in the areas of tonal memory, melody recognition, and intensity.[68]

The repeated activation of specific neuronal pathways reinforces the strength of connections between groups of neurons. Those neuronal circuits that are not activated do not get reinforced and can die away. Some researchers suggest that there are "windows of opportunity" during which time activation of specific functions is essential for continued development in that area. If kittens are not exposed to horizontal lines during a certain critical period, for example, the visual cortex may lose the ability to process such input later in life.[69] Infants who are not exposed to any spoken language may lose the ability to acquire normal linguistic functions after the first few years.[70] Similarly, infants who have no attachment relationships (for example, who are in orphanages with so few staff members that attachments do not develop) before the end of the third year of life, at the latest, may have extreme difficulty forming attachments later in life.[71] The motivational system of attachment—its circuits and potential for development—may have died away and be unavailable for maturation in the future.

How "plastic" is the brain after the early years of childhood? For example, if it is true that certain attachment experiences lead to the underdevelopment of the right-hemisphere processing of nonverbal aspects of emotional signals, how much can new experiences alter such a condition in an adult? Research on humans has provided no data as yet to answer this question. Research on other primates, however, suggests that there is far more plasticity in the brain of adults than was previously believed to be possible.[72] These studies suggest that alterations in input from the environment, such as those resulting from amputation of a limb, lead to restructuring of the representational processes in certain regions of the brain. Even in an adult, therefore, the brain appears to be capable to some degree of responding to changes in experience with further development of brain structure and function.

Another reason for optimism about catalyzing further development in adults is that some psychiatric disturbances may be due to impairments in integrative functioning among widely distributed, sometimes bilateral processes. These impairments may be due to the failure to develop associative neural pathways linking relatively autonomous modules of processing. However, the creation of new neural integrative links may be a learning process that remains possible into adulthood. Addressing the issue of the emergent properties of neural systems in development, Post and Weiss suggest, "The synaptic networks are in a state of continual rearrangement on both a micromolecular basis at the level of neurotransmitter and receptor subtype, as well as on a larger integrative basis for the synthesis of objects in the environment, including food and individuals such as self and others."[73] Our brains may retain the ability to continually reshape, in some fashion, emergent properties that allow us to learn and grow with new experiences.

Informal clinical observations suggest that some individuals do remain capable of activating the inherent capabilities of the right hemisphere well into adulthood. Learning to integrate these nonverbal functions into an active contribution to both internal and interpersonal experience can be a major challenge, however, especially for those with avoidant attachment histories. Other individuals seem much less able, or at least willing, to experience such transformations. One question is how impairments in integrative functioning may be a result of underdevelopment or an adaptive underutilization. For example, allowing the mind to begin to process the less definable, predictable, and controllable information inherent in nonverbal representations can be frightening for some people. At times, having unilateral dominance may be a defensively adaptive function. In this situation, attempts to improve bilateral functioning may involve efforts both to catalyze new development and to support the lowering of defensive avoidance tactics.

The blockage of right-hemisphere processes from consciousness and from engagements in interactions with others may be an adaptive "defense" against feeling anxious and out of control. Moving toward the left hemisphere's more detail oriented, routinized, top-down processing and its "even-keel" emotional style may be a mental system that is eagerly welcomed if the world is otherwise filled with uncertainty and excessive overstimulation. Such may be the case for individuals with certain highly reactive temperamental styles or for those raised in chaotic homes.

In fact, bilateral asymmetries have been associated with certain temperamental, affective, and cognitive styles.[74] For example, as discussed in Chapter 4, right-hemisphere dominance has been found in young infants who later are found to have shy temperaments.[75] The behavioral inhibition that accompanies such a constitution can be thought of as due to an excessive reactivity of the right hemisphere, which has been proposed to mediate withdrawal behavior. In the face of novelty, such activation may lead to a turning inward and avoidance of engaging in the world. Recall that the dorsal cortico-limbic pathway is dominant in the right hemisphere, and that this pathway is involved in the orienting to novel stimuli, the activation of internal self-regulatory mechanisms, the representation of the self and the body, and the "feedforward" representation of the future.[76] As we put these elements together here, we can propose that an individual with an overly active dorsal pathway/right hemisphere early in life may experience not only increased attention and reactivity to novel situations, but also representations of the self in distress, which may create further caution and withdrawal. As such a child matures, the active representation of the future within the dorsal stream may extend such a cautious stance as the mind attempts to anticipate the world of uncertainty by matching actual experiences with well-elaborated expectations. Such an attempt to anticipate the world can be seen in the behavior of the slow-to-warm up, shy child clinging to a parent's side at a friend's birthday party. What has begun as an initial overdominance of right-hemisphere functioning may now have blossomed into a significantly impairing behavioral inhibition. Interactions with parents and other caregivers during the early years of such a constitutionally shy child's development can help ameliorate such a trajectory. As discussed earlier, Kagan has demonstrated that interactions supporting a shy child's emotional experience but nurturing attempts to "push the envelope" into tolerable levels of uncertainty and exploration may be the most helpful in enabling the child to grow and develop.[77]

WAYS OF KNOWING

What are the implications of asymmetry for our experiential ways of knowing about reality? One view is that with the advent of language, the brain has to preserve a way to continue to process things quickly and more directly in relation to the body and the external world. This becomes the continued work of the right hemisphere. The left, in contrast, has fewer inputs from the body and is able to use the abstract manipulations of linguistic representations to allow us to experience a "higher-order consciousness": Linguistically, we are able to reflect on the past and the present, and to anticipate and plan for the future. Such abilities also allow us to create new combinations of things, in our minds and in the world. We can build buildings, fly airplanes, and write books of poetry (or books about the brain). The logical, linear, detail-focused, linguistic left brain is crucial for human creativity as well as technology. It is essential for getting the message into shareable packets of socially transmissible information. What is the right brain for?

The right brain appears to be able to perceive patterns within a holistic framework, noting spatial arrangements that the left is unable to sense. The right brain is able to create the gist or context of experiences and the overall meaning of events. The nonverbal "language" of the right hemisphere is based on sensations and images. These rapidly associated images give us a more direct and immediate representation of the world and of ourselves. This gives us a perceptual advantage: We can perceive the world for "how it is" from a bottom-up perspective. The left hemisphere, in contrast, is able to categorize perceptions based on prior experience from a top-down view. In their essential features, Levy argues, the spatial abilities of the right hemisphere are directly conflictual with the linguistic representations of the left.[78] According to this "cognitive crowding hypothesis," *keeping the right mode separate from the left allows for the existence of two extremely different but vital and important ways of knowing.* In this manner, the isolation of the two hemispheres is required in order to achieve the unique information-processing modes of each side of the brain.

Memory processes are also specialized in each hemisphere.[79] The memory researcher Daniel Schacter notes,

> Neurologists and neuropsychologists have known for over a century that language and verbal abilities are heavily dependent on the left hemisphere, whereas nonverbal and spatial functions are more dependent on the right hemisphere. Memory is similarly lateralized. Patients with damage to the left hippocampus and medial temporal lobe tend to have difficulties explicitly remembering verbal information but have no problems remembering visual designs and spatial locations. Patients with damage to the right hippocampus and medial temporal lobe tend to show the opposite pattern.[80]

Goldberg and Costa extend this argument by suggesting that the functional and anatomic studies of specialization support the view that the right hemisphere is better equipped to deal with *interregional* integration.[81] That is, the right hemisphere has more associational links, integrating information within the right brain in a "horizontal fashion" across modalities and attaining a contextual pattern of the world. The right hemisphere has a greater capacity for dealing with context and informational complexity and for integrating across various modes of representations (such as sight, sound, and touch) within a single effort or task. Some consider that the right hemisphere is in this way better equipped to perform parallel processing.

The left hemisphere, in contrast, is built for "vertical integration," with *intraregional* linkages allowing for detailed assessment of a single mode of representation. For example, when a perceptual representation matches a linguistic category, it allows the left hemisphere to move deeply into routinized responses in its top-down processing. These linear relationships are well established and link specific inputs with particular outputs. The left hemisphere is therefore said to be built for a categorical response to routine stimuli. In other words, the left hemisphere's experience of reality is literally created by the more rigidly established definitions of its linguistic packets of representations: words. The right hemisphere, in contrast, is designed for newly assembled responses to novel stimuli. This asymmetry of the brain creates a functional contrast between familiarity on the left and novelty on the right.

A practical and intriguing example of experiencing the difference in these two modes of seeing reality is provided by Betty Edwards's book *Drawing on the Right Side of the Brain*.[82] In this practical workbook, the educator/author introduces the reader to the notion of cerebral lateralization and provides exercises in which the differences between the two ways of knowing can be personally experienced. Essentially, when the left brain is told to "be quiet" and is not allowed to categorize what it sees, the right brain is able to assert its bottom-up mode of constructing visual reality. The results can be staggering; for instance, those who have forgotten since childhood how to draw may be happily shocked at how active their right hemispheres can still be. As Edwards's book demonstrates, many individuals have found a way to live primarily in a left-hemisphere mode of top-down categorizations with routinized perceptions and behaviors. The timeless and direct quality of experience that the book facilitates—the right hemisphere's mode of knowing the world—can make the reader feel quite alive.

Such an experience often leaves the individual with a clear view of how distinct these two ways of knowing are. Though supported by a wealth of research data on laterality, the issue of "left brain or right brain" is not even really important in the final analysis. What we are concerned with is the subjective experience of minds, not merely the functional anatomy of the brain. It is indisputable that there are two profoundly different modes in which the mind processes information. One or the other mode can dominate our conscious experience at various times. The finding that these modes of the mind do indeed have robust correlations with the sides of the brain just helps us to understand the probable neurophysiological mechanisms underlying what has been known for hundreds of years.[83]

Neuroscience can also help us avoid excessive generalizations about bilaterality. Our different ways of knowing intermingle in our daily lives. Creativity does not come from only one mode or the other. Happiness or other emotions do not emerge from living only in the timeless, nonverbal mode of constructing reality. Success does not emerge solely from the linguistic, controlled, and well-defined rules of the other mode. What research findings can be synthesized to suggest and what we can propose, in fact, is that an emergent quality of living a vital and flexible life may come from an openness to bilateral functioning involving many ways of knowing.

THE DEVELOPMENT OF MINDSIGHT: MINDS CREATING MINDS

One of the basic forms of information that the mind constructs and processes is that of the sense of mind itself. The "mind-creating" module of the mind appears to be a function of the right hemisphere and develops early in life.[84] Children during the first years of life are able to detect the difference between animate and inanimate objects and to attribute qualities of mind, such as intentions, attentions, and feelings, to the former ones. By their third year, they are able to engage in symbolic play, in which they can invest inanimate objects with animate qualities of intentionality and emotional response.[85] This immersion in pretend play involves the creation of social interactions and stories that involve the subjective, mental lives of the interacting characters. As Fonagy and Target have noted,

> The child's development and perception of mental states in himself and others thus depends on his observation of the mental world of his caregiver. He is able to perceive mental states, to the extent

that his caregiver's behavior implied such states. This he does when the caregiver is in a shared pretend mode of playing with the child (hence the association between pretend and early mentalization), and many ordinary interactions (such as physical care and comforting, conversation with peers) will also involve such shared mentation. This is what makes mental state concepts such as thinking inherently intersubjective; shared experience is part of the very logic of mental state concepts. . . . We believe that most important for the development of mentalizing self-organization is that exploration of the mental state of the sensitive caregiver enables the child to find in his mind an image of himself as motivated by beliefs, feelings, and intentions, in other words, as mentalizing.[86]

The initial sharing of mental experiences therefore lays the groundwork for the rest of mental development, including the acquisition of complex cognitive abilities. How does this occur? As with other aspects of mental functioning, looking toward information processing helps us to understand the "mentalizing" module of the mind.

The normal child's brain is able to take in information about the subjective mental state of another person. These signals are those of the nonverbal realm, which we've discussed: eye contact, facial expression, tone of voice. An important aspect of communication involves "joint referencing" signals (such as looking at a third object or pointing), which contain the information that the sender is focusing her attention in a certain direction or on a particular object. During the first year of life, joint referencing becomes a shared form of communication. It is during this phase that the child begins to sense the intention of another person; this permits jokes, such as pretending to jump in a sink or to eat a book, to be understood and enjoyed. During this phase of life and onward, *the mind has the ability to detect that another person has a mind with a focus of attention, an intention, and an emotional state.* To put it simply, the child has a concept of others' minds. This is also referred to as the child's "theory of mind." As we've discussed earlier, the theory-of-mind module is a component of the larger capacity of "reflective" functioning hypothesized to be an essential parental feature of secure attachments.

In the pervasive developmental disorder of autism, one sees the dysfunction in this mind-creating mental module of the mind.[87] Simon Baron-Cohen has used the term "mindblindness" to refer to this inability to see others' minds.[88] We have used the opposite term, "mindsight," to refer to this innate capacity for perceiving the minds of others. Baron-Cohen discusses the central role of the right orbitofrontal cortex in mediating this fundamental process, which is constitutionally abnormal in children with autism.

We can also use the information-processing framework to suggest what mindsight means for the mind. We can create representations within our own minds of the elements of others' subjective experiences: their intentions, emotions, focus of attention, beliefs, attitudes, thoughts, perceptions, and memories. Of course, these attributes exist in other persons without our creating them. But in a mind that does not have the capacity to process the signals from another person, or to create the mental representations of another's mind, there is literally an absence of such a reality. In this case, the mind of the other does not exist. Within the perceiver's mind, the other's mind has not been created by the necessary representational machinery of the mind itself. It may also be that the perceiver lacks the ability to reflect upon her own mind because of this impairment in the ability to form representations of minds.

How can a mind not be able to conceptualize a mind? If we view the mind as a processor of information, the answer is straightforward. Without the representations of mind within the neural symbols of the mind, there exists no information about the mind within the mind. Others' subjective experiences, their minds, do not exist.

In most individuals without autism, the mind-creating or mindsight module is presumably neurologically intact. We would be advised to remember that mindblindness, though, is not like being pregnant: There appear to be mild degrees of impairment in mindsight that may have neurologically constitutional underpinnings.

Can impairments to mindsight be created by experience? Fonagy and Target suggest that the answer is yes: Specific forms of insecure attachment in which the parent does not focus on the mental states of the child and in which parental states are intrusive or disorganizing can lead to an impairment in the acquisition of theory of mind.[89] How are such impairments to mindsight mediated? Are the dulled mindsight abilities of a dismissing adult a form of such impairment? Are they established by their lack of activation during childhood? Do such developmental impediments respond to future interventions? These are questions that researchers of the future may attempt to answer.

ADAPTIVE IMPAIRMENT OF MINDSIGHT

Psychosocial context can permit the activation or deactivation of reflective function.[90] To mediate this context-specific use of the reflective, mentalizing function, we can propose here that the mind may be capable of dis-associating component modules by impairing the integrative function of essential associative neural pathways. Relationship histories can impair the development of the integrative reflective function. This impairment can be pervasive and can lead to a child's generalized inability to mentalize, as revealed in impaired symbolic play and joint referencing.

We can also suggest that an impairment to mindsight may be state-dependent. That is, under specific conditions, a child (or adult) may be able to disengage the components essential for reflective function, shutting down this important capacity. How does the mind achieve this? In this instance, we can propose that blockage of the corpus callosal fibers interconnecting the two hemispheres, and of interconnections within the right hemisphere itself, may be a mechanism that allows mindsight to be impaired as an adaptation to certain overwhelming situations. Developmentally, this may be the situation in avoidant or disorganized attachment, in which communications are emotionally empty or terrorizing, respectively. In either of these situations, a child adapts to a particular relationship context with the inhibition of reflective function.

This finding may help explain why some individuals, such as those who commit war crimes or genocide, are capable of empathic relationships with their family and friends but can enter cold, disconnected states when involved in crimes against individuals or humanity. This ability to dis-associate thinking and behavior from the creation of the subjective mental experiences of others within our own minds may help us to understand various aspects of antisocial behavior. The fact that such state-dependent impairment or more pervasive lack of development of mindsight exists is too often revealed in the increasingly violent society in which we live.

This impairment in reflective function in the setting of limited but functioning logical language-based thinking reveals how the separation of the hemispheres can allow for the dis-association of normally associated modes of processing information. As an example, let me offer one possible explanation for the phenomenon of intellectualization seen within some members of the medical profession, especially during training, as an illustration of an adaptation to stressful conditions. This example helps explain how under certain conditions it may be prudent to develop at least partial impairment of one's mindsight abilities. Working for the first time with acutely ill patients in a medical setting may call for a medical student to use a nonmentalizing mode of processing—an adaptive inhibition of empathic, interpersonally connecting processing. This allows the student access to the linear, logical sequences of factual knowledge and the ability to focus on the details of patient care, while avoiding the mulitlayered emotional meaning of a patient's illness. At the oversimplified level, this could be explained by a shutting down of the right hemisphere's capacity to reflect on mental experience, while at the same time maintaining the syllogistic reasoning of the left hemisphere's mode of cognition.

If the medical student can't reintegrate the information-processing modules of her right hemisphere after a work day, or after a week, month, or year, then we can predict that certain features may then become missing from her life. These adaptations can be seen as a function of the student's present hemispheric adaptations, but they may be shaped in part by the patterns from an earlier attachment history. That is, these learned adaptations may result in part from patterns of disconnection that may have been established and made readily accessible by prior experience. For the student, the present disconnection may lead to a loss of readily accessible autobiographical memory and of intense primary emotional states whose appraisals create a sense of meaning in life. Personal relationships may become strained as communication becomes dominated by context-independent details and logical, linguistically based talk, rather than also including emotional messages between two relatives or friends. For this medical student, or for others engaged in emotionally challenging work, shutting down the right hemisphere temporarily may be a needed adaptation in order to perform a job efficiently. Living in an isolated, left-hemisphere-dominated internal world, however, can be experienced as filled with highly categorized routines or top-down processes that lack a feeling of spontaneity and vitality. If the right hemisphere does not become integrated with the left later on, then such adaptations may prove to be dysfunctional and lead to serious problems outside, or even inside, the workplace. The medical student, and others learning to cope with overwhelming experiences, may be aided by understanding this adaptive dis-association of integrative processes.

In this example, the adaptive need under stress to diminish (at least conscious) access to the representations of others' minds may lead to the isolated restriction of the mindsight module of the right hemisphere. As with any form of dis-association, anatomically dispersed processes can become functionally isolated if the integrating neural pathways making associations become blocked. Such a process may occur either at the level of the interhemispheric transfer of information or in the form of dis-associations within the information processing of one hemisphere—in this case, that of the right. As with other forms of dis-association, blockage of certain modes may also involve the impairment of related functions. In this example, the orbitofrontal cortex is the primary site for integrating a wide range of fundamental processes, including mindsight, stimulus appraisal, somatic representation, autonomic activity, affect regulation, and autonoetic consciousness. The adaptive blockage of mindsight representations may tend to be associated with the unintentional impairment of a number of these anatomically and functionally related orbitofrontally mediated processes.

Just as the mind can isolate implicit recollections from explicit ones, so too can it isolate right- from left-hemisphere functions. Hemispheric dis-association can be understood as a domination of one mode over the other. The monosemantic, linguistic left hemisphere—filled with modes of information processing that rely upon the rules of logic and reason, and able to negotiate in an external world of symbols and language—can often find its active place in interacting with the outside world. The left hemisphere's experience of consciousness may be better equipped to deal with the world in abstract concepts independent of emotional context. The right hemisphere, in contrast, is filled with polysemantic images of the world, perceptions of others' emotions, sensations of the body, and holistic patterns of intuitive insights that often defy words. These mental representations are context-dependent, filled with horizontal, multilayered associations to a wide array of bodily sensations, sense of self and other, autobiographical memories, and emotional meaning. There is often no easy way for the right hemisphere to "speak," especially if only the left hemisphere of oneself or another is listening.

REFLECTIONS: REPRESENTING REALITY AND PSYCHOLOGICAL WELL-BEING

The mind constructs its own experience of reality. Emanating from the interface of the brain and human relationships, the mind creates connections among the various elements of representations, ranging from sensations and images to concepts and words. The connections among the layers of neural activity weave a fabric of subjective life: They enable us to feel, behave, think, plan, and communicate.

Living in a world constructed by our own minds makes knowing about these representational processes essential in deepening our understanding of human experience. Patterns of representations differ markedly between the left and right halves of the brain. An important distinction, often underrecognized within the fields of clinical psychiatry and psychology, is the distinction between the modes of representation within the two hemispheres of the brain. The left hemisphere has been described as having a logical "interpreter" function that uses syllogistic reasoning to deduce cause–effect relationships from the representational data it has available to it. The right hemisphere specializes in the representation of context and of mentalizing capacities. It is therefore uniquely capable of registering and expressing affective facial expressions, developing a "theory of mind," registering and regulating the state of the body, and having autobiographical representations.

How are these bilateral processes relevant to relationships? Communication is crucial in establishing neural connections early in life and involves the sharing of energy and information. Levels of arousal (energy) and mental representations (information) are very different on each side of the brain. The sharing of arousal and representations from one brain to another—the essence of connecting minds—will thus differ between the hemispheres. One can propose, in fact, that the right brain perceives the output of the right brain of another person, whereas the left brain perceives the left brain's output. In intimate, emotional relationships, such as friendship, romance, parent–child pairs, psychotherapy, and teacher–student dyads, what does this look like? The left brain sends out language-based, logical, sequential interpreting statements that attempt to make sense of things. The left brain receives these messages, decodes the linguistic representations, and tries to make sense out of these newly arrived digital symbols. At the same time, the right brain is sending nonverbal messages via facial expressions, gestures, prosody, and tone of voice, which are perceived by the other's right brain. OK. So what?

The "what" of it is that the right brain takes this information and uses its social perceptions of nonverbal communication to engage directly in a few very important processes. It creates an image of the other's mind ("mindsight"). It regulates bodily response while at the same time registering the somatic markers of shifts in bodily state. It creates autobiographical representations within memory. It appraises the meaning of these events and directly affects the degree of arousal, thus creating primary emotional responses. Intense and primary emotional states are therefore likely to be mediated via the right hemisphere.

When we examine these findings alongside the independent set of data from attachment research, certain patterns are suggested. The early affect attunement and alignment of mental states can be seen as a mutually regulated hemisphere-to-hemisphere coordination be-stween child and parent. In this view, we can propose that avoidant attachment involves a serious lack of this form of communication between the right hemispheres of child and parent. The extension of this finding to laterality research raises the possibility that the left hemisphere serves as the dominant mediator of communication between an avoidant child and a dismissing parent. In support of this perspective, it turns out that in 1989, Main and Hesse examined exactly this hypothesis in two large-scale samples of Berkeley under-graduates, each of whom were asked about their degree of right (or left) handedness, as a rough approximation of brain dominance.[91] At the same time, Main and Hesse had devised a set of self-report items that they considered indicative of a "dismissing" state of mind. Although this type of scale was not ultimately able to predict AAI classifications statistically,[92] and therefore these findings were never published, in keeping with the hypothesis both studies found that the degree of right handedness was significantly correlated with elevated scores of the scale for "dismissing" state of mind.

Further extensions of these ideas to relationships allow us to look more deeply into why certain couples may be "unable to com-municate" with any emotional satisfaction. When we know about the different languages of the right and left hemispheres, it is possible to make hypotheses about why interactions may be frustrating: Indi-viduals may not know how to understand the particular language being expressed by their significant others. If we then integrate past attachment history in understanding the pattern of these difficulties, it is possible to create a framework of understanding that can help the partners in such relationships escape their well-worn ruts.

If this laterality–attachment hypothesis is correct, then a logical implication would be that any experiences that help to develop the processing abilities of each hemisphere and/or the integrated activi-ties of the two hemispheres may improve certain individuals' internal and interpersonal lives. Such movement toward more coordinated interhemispheric functioning would be quite welcomed by many people (especially by the lonely and frustrated spouses of dismissing individuals). The developmental and experiential histories that have led to a lack of integration of the functioning of the two hemispheres may leave individuals vulnerable to emotional and social problems. Unresolved trauma and grief, histories of emotional neglect, and restrictive adaptations may each represent some form of constriction in the flow of information processing between the hemispheres. This proposal of the central role of dis-associated hemispheric processing in emotional disturbances is supported by the finding that insecure attachments in childhood may establish a vulnerability to psychological dysfunction.

Emotional relationships that enhance the development of each hemisphere and its unrestricted integration with the activity of the other can thus be proposed to be likely to foster the development of psychological well-being. In this way, a secure attachment can be seen as a developmental relationship that provides for an integration of functioning of the two hemispheres, both between child and caregiver and within the child's own brain. At the most basic level, right-hemisphere-to-right-hemisphere communication can be seen within the affectively attuned communications that allow for primary emotional states to be shared via nonverbal signals. Left-hemisphere-to-left-hemisphere alignment can be seen in shared attention to objects in the world. Reflective dialogues, in which language is used to focus attention on the mental states of others (including the two members of the dyad), may foster bilateral integration between the two hemispheres of both child and parent. The resilience of secure attachments can thus be proposed as founded in part in the bilateral integration that these relationships foster.

CHAPTER 6

——

States of Mind

Cohesion, Subjective Experience,
and Complex Systems

DEFINING STATES OF MIND

States of Mind and Activity of the Brain

How does the mind coordinate its many modules of information processing in order to construct reality in the moment? How can we begin to understand how the billions of neurons with trillions of interconnections within the brain become activated in organized patterns that create the mind? How is the flow of energy within the widely distributed activations of neurons regulated? An answer to each of these questions is in the idea of a "state of mind." *States of mind allow the brain to achieve cohesion in functioning.*

A "state of mind" can be defined as the total pattern of activations in the brain at a particular moment in time. Patterns of activation reveal the neural net profiles within the various circuits that mediate the mental modules of information processing. These circuits are distributed in a widely interconnected web, with profoundly complex inputs and outputs linking various clusters of cells that carry out particular functions.[1] At a very basic level, for example, we can suggest that a fearful state of mind is the clustering of related processes in a cohesive whole. A state of heightened caution, focal attention, behavioral hypervigilance, memories of past experiences of threat, models of the self as a victim in need of protection, and emo-

208

tional arousal alerting the body and mind to prepare for harm are all processes that become functionally primed or readied for activity. A state of mind therefore involves a clustering of functionally synergistic processes that allow the mind as a whole to form a cohesive state of activity. The benefit of cohesion is to maximize the efficiency and efficacy of the processes needed in a given moment in time. Cohesive states of mind are highly functional and adaptive to the environment.

As we've seen in Chapter 5, one of the most basic processes of the mind is the representation of information. As neural symbols, representations both contain information and make further processing events happen. In this way these dynamic representations cause further neural excitation, which itself carries information.[2] The links among such a changing, distributed system of processes are overwhelmingly complex. To understand the notion of these complex processes—of states of mind—we must look at some ideas about how systems function.

States, Traits, and Cohesion

How can we conceptualize the systems that make up the mind, and the mind itself as a complex system? One framework can be derived from the mind's central function as an information processor. Mental activity stems from basic processing modules. A "module" can be defined as a set of neural circuits carrying a certain type of information and utilizing a similar form of mental signal or code. For example, a module for processing visual input involves the signals sent from the eyes to the visual cortex. This sensory module may include circuits that detect certain shapes, contrasts, or angles. Another type of module, a visual perception module, may consist of circuits that cluster these sensory representations into perceptual patterns (such as "form of furniture" or "face"). Taken together, these and similar modules process visual data as a collection of circuits with representational processes, forming the visual "mode." If the information is then coordinated with other perceptual modalities (modes), then we have the perceptual "system." Examples of other systems of the mind include the various forms of implicit and explicit memory. Within explicit memory, there is a system composed of the modes of autobiographical versus semantic memory. Within the autobiographical mode are the modules encoding specific episodes, gists, and generic autobiographical knowledge. For example, when we ask someone to tell us what he remembers about last year, he will activate his explicit memory system's subcomponent mode of autobiographical memory and its basic modules. As we've discussed, these components have specific neural circuitry involved in the encoding and retrieval functions of autonoetic consciousness.

So we are using a vocabulary of modules, modes, and systems to describe one way in which the system of the mind can be conceptualized. What is the point? The point is that the activities of the brain, these layers of increasingly complex information processing, become organized in a patterned fashion. We experience these patterns of activity as states of mind. We will see that a state of mind does two fundamental things: *It coordinates activity in the moment, and it creates a pattern of brain activation that can become more likely in the future.* That is, a state of mind can become a remembered brain activity configuration or neural net profile. Repeated activation of particular states— for example, a shame state or a state of despair—can become much more likely to be activated in the future. In this manner, states can become traits of the individual that influence both internal and interpersonal processes.[3]

A state of mind clusters the activity of specific systems of processing. The degree to which this clustering is effective and useful determines the state's cohesiveness. What coordinates such a clustering process? We can propose here that part of the answer is emotion. The regulation of emotion directs the flow of energy through the changing states of activation of the brain. Recall from Chapter 4 that there are convergence zones in the brain, such as the orbitofrontal cortex, thought to be responsible for the coordination of the activity of widely distributed systems: bodily state, arousal–appraisal centers, attention via the lateral prefrontal cortex, perception from the sensory cortices, abstract representations within the associational neocortex, memory processes via the medial temporal lobe, and motor responses via the basal ganglia.[4] The activation (energy) of these circuits determines their contribution to the overall state of the brain at a given point in time. When activated, these circuits create and process representations (information) within their specialized computational modes. The regulation of emotion is mediated by the limbic region of the brain, with its structural interconnections and functional capacity to coordinate a wide range of brain activity.

What does "to coordinate a wide range of brain activity" actually mean? Literally, this means that the various systems that make up the brain, from "lower" or "simpler" ones (such as the registration and regulation of the autonomic nervous system's control of bodily states) to the "higher," more complex ones (such as the neocortical conceptual representations of thought), can be functionally linked and temporally associated with each other in a given state of mind. In this context, "linked" means that the systems are simultaneously activated and have functional influences upon each other. This is a state of mind.

Each moment brings a combination of activations creating a unique state of mind. However, repeated patterns of activation may become "engrained," meaning that they are made more likely to be reactivated in the future (as noted above). Particular states of mind may develop cohesion through their repeated activation, as well as through the functional benefits of their internal linkages.

At times, the mind cannot organize itself effectively in response to experiences. Such experiences are traumatizing, in that they overwhelm the mind's ability to adapt.[5] As we've discussed in the case of disorganized attachment, some interpersonal experiences result in the mind's becoming unable to form a cohesive and adaptive state. In this situation, the mind enters a chaotic, disorganizing state of activations lacking in cohesion. The noncohesive characteristic of such a state may itself actually become a trait of the individual. Disorganization or disorientation becomes a repeated pattern of activation or state of mind. This may explain the acquisition of dissociation as an adaptation to stress seen in those with histories of disorganized attachments.

Organizing States of Mind

A state of mind can be proposed to be a pattern of activation of recruited systems within the brain responsible for (1) perceptual bias, (2) emotional tone and regulation, (3) memory processes, (4) mental models, and (5) behavioral response patterns. A state of mind can have enduring clusters of activation of each of these basic elements. One can discover the elements of an individual's state of mind by focusing on the elements of her perceptions, feelings, thoughts, memories, attitudes, beliefs, and desires—and how these may be influencing her behavior and interactions with others. Also, because states of mind are dynamic processes, trying to understand them also requires that we look at the changes in the individual's mental processes over time.

For example, if an individual has been exposed to repeated neglect as a young child, a state of despair may have been activated and engrained. In this excessively low energy state, perceptions of the world are marked by a sense of rejection; emotions are filled with shame and hopelessness; memories may evoke previous experiences of being rejected; a model of the self as unlovable and of others as unavailable may be activated; and there may be a behavioral tendency to withdraw. Because this state of despair has been repeatedly activated, it will be more likely to be activated in response to even minor signs of rejection, such as a friend's or therapist's not returning a phone call on time. The change in state in response to this environmental context is a function, in part, of this individual's history. The entire cluster, however, can quickly become the dominant information-processing mode at such a moment, giving the individual a sense of massive rejection and despair far exceeding the initial stimulus and not having any clear, consciously accessible connection to experiences from the past.

Our subjective lives emerge from mental states that are exquisitely sensitive to social interaction. Recall that as open, dynamic systems, we are composed of lower levels of subcomponents as well as being ourselves subcomponents of the larger systems of social connections in which we live. Our brains have circuits specifically designed to receive and send social signals. Our minds are thus able to process this information and utilize it so that we can be active participants in social communication. In the example above of a despair state, this individual's prior history has engrained a tendency to be excessively sensitive and responsive to social signals containing information about another's lack of interest. In simpler terms, the person can easily feel rejected. When not in such a state of mind, the individual may function perfectly well. However, the regulation of her state of mind—her modulation of emotion—is such that she can quickly (and maladaptively) enter a paralyzing state of despair, which influences the rest of her mind's information processing in the direction of reinforcing that state. She perceives, feels, remembers, conceives, thinks, and behaves in ways that even more deeply engrain the state of mind at that time. Such are the organizing and self-reinforcing effects of a state of mind.

In this chapter we'll explore some ways of thinking about the organization of complex systems to understand how the brain can create a state of mind. We'll also look into the idea of how the state of mind of one person can influence the organization of the state of mind of another. First, let's look at an example of how the state of mind can change rapidly in response to environmental cues.

Context Sensitivity

If a man is walking with his romantic partner on a beach, enjoying the breeze and the sound of the waves, he will be in a certain state of mind that may be characterized by an attentional focus on the water and sky and on his lover's hand in his own; an awareness of a deep sense of calm and connection; easy access to other similar romantic moments; a mental model of life as simple and rewarding; and a behavioral set of gentle, easy responses to others as he strolls down the sand. He may have a model of himself as a lovable person deserving of such a tranquil and connecting experience.

If someone suddenly grabs this man's shoulder and roughly says, "Hey, give me your money!", his state of mind is likely to be suddenly transformed. This encounter with the environment will create a new context. The state of his mind is extremely sensitive to external conditions. This change in the environment creates a shift in his brain. He perceives the sound of the intruder's tone of voice, the content of his message, and the bodily contact. All of his sensory processing systems, including auditory, visual, and somatosensory (bodily sensations), take in the data. At an early, "lower" level—before complex processing and long before conscious awareness—his alarm/ defense system, including the amygdala, fires an internal signal of "Danger!" This subcortical processing takes rapid effect in shifting his state of mind. This shift in state leads him to have a perceptual bias to interpret stimuli in the environment as threatening. A behavioral response pattern of fight or flight will become activated, with his heart beginning to race and muscles tightening. These sensations may feed back to his emotional processing centers, especially the orbitofrontal cortex, and let his mind know that he is feeling scared and/or angry. His attentional mechanisms may be mostly focused on the intruder's actions, but he may also become aware of his bodily response and altered mental state within working memory, which (as we've discussed) has been proposed as a possible mechanism for conscious experience. Memories, explicit and implicit, of other moments of danger and fear may become more readily accessible via the mechanism of state-dependent retrieval. This is useful in accessing knowledge of what he did and skills he exercised in similar past situations. A mental model that the world is a dangerous place may now become active. A model of the self may include anything from "I can protect myself" to "I knew this would happen to me; I am such a vulnerable and helpless person."

Often the shift between states of mind is not so dramatic as in this example. Context changes can be quite subtle; they may be induced, for example, by alterations in a companion's tone of voice or facial expression. Our minds are continually responding to external cues, especially from the social environment.

An example of a more common situation is that in which state shifts occur during an adult's visit "back home" for the holidays. Returning to the physical and social environment of one's youth can provide context cues that activate old states of mind. A person may find herself, unwillingly and initially unknowingly, suddenly feeling "like a child" again. Sensations of dependence, inadequacy, or anger may dominate her emotional experience. She may begin acting in ways as if she were a teenager again, taking part in minor (or major) battles with parents with whom she hasn't lived for years. As this person watches herself taking part in these old behavioral patterns, she may notice that her parents are also acting as if she is their renegade adolescent again! Which came first, their treatment of her or hers of them? How does this process occur? To understand states of mind and the rapid and intricate ways they are influenced by our present experiences and past encounters, we need to turn now to the study of complex systems.

COMPLEX SYSTEMS

Complexity, Natural Selection, and Connectionism

A state of mind allows disparate activities of the brain to become cohesive in a given moment in time. A single brain functions as an elaborate system that can be understood by examining the "theory of nonlinear dynamics of complex systems" or, more briefly, "complexity theory."[6] This perspective has been applied to a range of inanimate and living systems in an attempt to understand the often unpredictable but self-organizing nature of complex clusters of entities functioning as a system. The human brain has recently been examined by a number of theoreticians as one such nonlinear dynamic system, also called a dynamical system. Though a detailed review is beyond the scope of this chapter, some of the basic ideas of this approach are described here. Moreover, applications of these principles not only to the single mind, but to the functioning of two or more minds acting as a single system, are proposed. These applications allow us to deepen our earlier discussion of states of mind and their fundamental importance in creating internal experience and shaping the nature of interpersonal relationships.

The brain is a complex system whose processes organize its own functioning. This property is called "self-organization."[7] We have stated from the beginning that the mind emanates from the activity of the brain, and thus it is fair to say that the mind itself is complex and has self-organizing properties.[8] Despite the huge number of neurons involved and the nearly infinite variety of states of mind that can be created, this conceptual approach helps us to make sense of the self-regulating processes of the mind. The following brief overview draws on a variety of related theories about systems, complexity, and "parallel distributed processing" or "connectionism."[9]

Complexity theory is a mathematically derived collection of principles governing the behavior of physiochemical systems, such as groups of molecules or patterns of clouds.[10] The application of this theory to biological systems, including the mind, has some fascinating implications. How can we equate clouds with the human psyche? Aren't inanimate objects and life forms fundamentally different? Remember, however, that biological systems are composed of basic atoms that are not alive. Complexity theory has been applied to an understanding of systems from molecules to societies, with extremely useful and unique applications.[11] What makes living systems unique is that they have evolved through natural selection into the adaptively complex forms that make up life on earth. Evolution has yielded complex designs without a formal designer; the function of the complex forms has allowed them to be open to the external environment and to adapt to it over generations.[12] In this way, *living systems are open systems capable of responding and adapting to the environment.*

What have these complex systems evolved to do? Given enough diversity and the passage of time, organisms have evolved in ways that enable them to survive and reproduce. This is the fundamental principle of natural selection. How well a trait works within a particular environment determines whether a species will maintain the trait in subsequent generations. In this way, a living system is organized to attain goals: to maintain itself and to pass on its genes. The human nervous system, particularly the brain, has evolved to be specialized at solving problems. These problems can range from how to avoid drowning to how to find food or a mate. The adaptive design of the brain allows it to process specific forms of information in the service of achieving the fundamental goals of natural selection: survival and reproduction. The mind, as a product of the activity of the brain, in many ways reflects this evolutionary process.[13]

But the brain has a physical structure of its own that is unique to its evolutionary history. Certain regions, such as those for smell and vision, have become relatively smaller than those of our ancestors. Other regions, such as the neocortex, have become larger. It is clear that the brain itself is composed of an intricately interconnected set of neurons distributed in a parallel, spider-web-like fashion.[14] Studies of this "parallel distributed processing" are part of a perspective called "connectionism."[15] The theory of natural selection does not in any way contradict a connectionist view of the brain. Nor do either of these two views preclude our understanding of the brain as an information processor. In fact, creating computers as parallel processors, rather than as the serial processors of early computer design, has resulted in learning capacities far more similar to those of human brains than could have been imagined. The issue is that the innate structure of a connectionist set of interconnected processors, such as neurons, yields the ability to remember, compare, and generalize. This helps us understand how the brain carries out these fundamental functions that permit the processing of information.

One way in which a connectionist model functions is to place "weights" or degrees of "strength" on the connections among basic elements, such as the neurons in the case of the brain. When the relative strengths of the synaptic connections are altered, the information contained within the patterns of firing can be modified.[16] Subtle and rapid alterations in synaptic strengths are products of learning; the ability to have connection strengths in general is innate.[17] Some of these connection strengths may be predetermined by our genetic inheritance: Our brains may be preprogrammed to create systems that tend to process certain forms of input preferentially, such as the faces of attachment figures in the case of our attachment systems. These innate values are of evolutionary benefit and remain encoded in our genetic endowment.[18] But synaptic strengths are also determined by experience in a process that allows learning to occur. In this manner, as we've seen, *experience affects the brain by altering the strengths of synaptic connections.*[19]

Complex systems are also believed to have an innate property that creates a sense of order, cohesion, and stability across time. Again, this is called "self-organization."[20] Natural selection, connectionism, and information-processing views are all compatible with a complex systems or "dynamical" perspective on self-organization. Evolutionary theory helps us understand how systems evolved into adaptively complex forms designed to carry out specific problem-solving behaviors. Connectionist theory helps us understand how these skills in processing information can be carried out within the three-dimensional substance of interconnected neural tissue. Specialized information processing helps describe the fundamental components of the mind that reflect this evolutionary history and the physical reality of brain structure. Now we will add complexity theory to the conceptual mix in order to understand how the mind organizes its own functioning—and its states of mind.

The theory of nonlinear dynamics of complex systems, or complexity theory, provides several principles that will deepen our ability to understand many aspects of the mind, from emotions to human relationships. As Boldrini and colleagues have stated, "the spontaneity, unpredictability, and self-organizing properties of nonlinear dynamic systems are well suited to explain the notoriously spontaneous, unpredictable, and creative nature of human beings."[21] Dynamical systems have three major features: (1) They have self-organizational properties, (2) they are nonlinear, and (3) they have emergent patterns with recursive characteristics.[22] Let's take each of these abstract principles and try to make them clear and useful.

Self-Organization: The Movement toward Maximizing Complexity

Within an individual living being, *a driving force of development is the movement from simplicity toward complexity*. Esther Thelen has proposed that in child development, increasingly sophisticated abilities, such as reaching, crawling, and walking, can be viewed from this perspective as reflections of the increasingly complex patterns of the child's behavior.[23] The unfolding of the development of human beings throughout the lifespan from this point of view can be seen as governed by this movement toward increasing complexity. Rather than viewing children as having stepwise increments in their abilities, we can view development as the emergence of patterns of increasingly complex interactions between children and their environment. A child offers a variety of behavioral responses, such as trying to grasp a toy object, and then learns within a certain context that a particular movement is coupled with a specific outcome, such as finding the object. When the toy is then hidden under similar conditions, the child attempts to find it where it was before. If the effort is successful, the behavior is reinforced. From a dynamical viewpoint, the system is maximizing its complexity and therefore its stability by pushing behavior forward, applying old patterns in slightly new situations. Every moment, in fact, is the emergence of a unique pattern of activity in a world that is similar but never identical to a past moment in time.

Patterns emerge in interaction with the environment. Certain patterns of coordination become fairly stable under specific conditions or contexts. These reinforced patterns or states of activation are called "attractor states." A state consists of the activity of each component of the system at a given point in time; with unfolding experience, especially with the presence of the value systems of the living brain, certain states become more probable as they are engrained within the system. A "state of mind" as we have defined it earlier can therefore be seen as an "attractor state" of the system. *The probability of activation of a state is determined by both history and present context or environmental conditions.*

The ability to remember an event from a long time ago is an example of an attractor state. If you try to recall your tenth day in junior high school, you may be unable to remember anything. However, it you try to recall the most embarrassing day you experienced during junior high school, you may become flooded with visual images and bodily sensations of that day. This activation of various components of your brain, the heterogeneous elements of your dynamical system, assemble themselves in a pattern representing your recollection of that day long ago. As elements of your brain become active, they may recruit other neuronal groups to join in the pattern of activation. Your value systems including your appraisal centers, will have reinforced the strength of such an attractor state in the infinite range of possible patterns of neuronal activation. In this way, the self-organizational properties of the system create a sense of ordered complexity out of the trillions of synaptic connections that can be potentially fired.

In the brain, we can propose that emotional responses constitute a primary value system that engrains patterns of neuronal firing and shapes the emergent states of activation of the system. As states become engrained through repeated experience and emotional intensity, they become more likely to be activated. These attractor states help the system organize itself and achieve stability. Attractor states lend a degree of continuity to the infinitely possible options for activation profiles.

Repeated instantiation (activation) of a particular profile of activations, a state of mind, can make such a configuration a deeply engrained attractor state. What does this really mean? Think of this analogy. A hillside is filled with tall, flowing grass in the springtime. The snow has melted, and you seem to be the first person to take the trail to this spot. As you look out from the top of the hill, you notice that there are no paths toward the pond at the bottom. You wend your way down to the pond, spend a few hours there, and then walk back up the trail that you created earlier, so as to avoid stomping down any more grass. The next day, another hiker comes to the top of the hill, sees the pond, and without much thought follows your path down to the pond. He returns back up the hill the same way. Day after day, other travelers take the same path, carving into the vegetation on the hillside a path that did not exist before. The probability is high that other hikers will continue to take this pathway, further distinguishing it from other potential routes. As the feet keep pounding on the soil, any grass attempting to grow there will be flattened. The trail becomes this year's common pathway from the hill to the pond.

Such is the case for states of mind. With repeated activation, the state of mind becomes more deeply engrained, and the state is remembered. According to Hebb's axiom ("Neurons that fire together wire together"), the brain is more likely to activate this clustering of processes in the future as a cohesive state of mind. As we'll see, the mind also has a self-reinforcing quality to its organization, which serves as the mechanism for such reinforcement. Post and Weiss have provided a developmental perspective on Hebb's axiom: "Neurons which fire together, *survive together*, and wire together.[24] Thus repeated states of activation at critical early periods of development shape the structure of neuronal circuits, which then form the functional basis for enduring patterns of states of mind within the individual.

Stability of the system is achieved by the movement toward maximizing complexity. Complexity does not come from random activation, but instead is enhanced by a balance between the continuity and flexibility of the system. "Continuity" refers to the strength of previously achieved states, and therefore the probability of their repetition; it implies sameness, familiarity, and predictability. "Flexibility" indicates the system's degree of sensitivity to environmental conditions; it involves the capacity for variability, novelty, and uncertainty. The ability to produce new variations allows the system to adapt to the environment. However, excessive variation or flexibility leads toward random activation. On the other hand, rigid adherence to previously engrained states produces excessive continuity and minimizes the system's ability to adapt and change.[25]

Even pathological developmental pathways can move toward increasing complexity.[26] Complexity alone cannot be a criterion for defining mental health. Mental disorder can be envisioned in part as restricting the overall movement of the system in an adaptive manner toward complexity by an imbalance in continuity and flexibility. Pathological states may force the system into a range of excessive disorder or of rigidity; either one limits the movement of the system as a whole toward emerging complexity and adaptation to the environment. As we'll see in the next two chapters, examining the regulation of emotion and the flow of states of mind across time may serve as an important measure of the whole system's coherent functioning. An individual may experience relatively cohesive states that, in isolation, may function fairly well. However, the individual's ability to integrate states of mind across time into a coherent whole may be restricted if these cohesive states are themselves conflictual.

Nonlinearity

Dynamical systems are called "nonlinear," the second basic principle of complexity theory, because a small change in input can lead to huge and unpredictable changes in output. Part of this unpredictability is due to the context-dependent nature of the system's response. The unpredictability also stems in part from the fact that the system as a whole is inherently "noisy"; this means that there will be random activations that may or may not be reinforced by encounters with the environment. Systems have both determinate (predictable) and indeterminate features to their behavior.[27] Because of these features, *small changes in the microcomponents of the system can lead to large changes in the macro-behavior of the organism.*

In viewing the mind as a complex system, we can see that the "dysfunction" at one level of organization may produce large changes in the functioning of other levels and of the system as a whole. Within brain activity, one can envision these changes in the functioning of the mind as emanating, for example, from particular regions responsible for an emotion such as fear. In the case of obsessive–compulsive disorder, an excessive signal, coming from a limbic system that "checks" the environment for danger and finds evidence for fear when in fact there is none, can cause a cascade of responses from other systems in the brain: a sense of panic, with heart rate racing; obsessions composed of complex, abstract thoughts about death; and compulsive behaviors irrationally designed to avoid catastrophe.[28] Though the origin of a dysfunction may emanate from the abnormal messages sent from one component of the brain, the cascade of subsequent reactions can be unpredictable, can be huge, and can involve a widely distributed response from other components as well as from the brain and the mind as a whole. This is nonlinearity at its most painful, out-of-control worst.

On the more beneficial side of nonlinearity is the finding that small changes in a person's perspective, beliefs, or associations of particular forms of information processing can suddenly lead to large changes in state of mind and behavior. For example, the art of psychotherapy can be seen as finding a way to align oneself as a therapist with a patient in such a fashion as to know what sort of change is needed and what alterations in the constraints on the system might permit such changes to occur. Some of the most difficult kinds of ruts can be reinforced by deeply engrained, inflexible attractor states, including bad habits, intrusive memories, or isolation of information processing. For some people, a small change in behavior or memory processing can yield subsequent changes in mental set (or system state) that produce large changes in behavior and internal experience. The often challenging task is to figure out which system changes are needed in order to alter the constraints on rigidly engrained attractor states.

Emergent and Recursive Patterns

A third property of the nonlinear dynamics of complex systems is that of the emergent and recursive properties of the patterns of organization. "Emergent" means that each of us is filled with a flow of states that evolve across time. "Recursive" means that the effects of the elements of a given state return to further influence the emergence of the state of mind. We are always in a perpetual state of being created and creating ourselves. We will never be the same, and we have never been quite the way we are right at this moment. This emergence of being as we flow from state to state is characterized by an underlying sense that there is an incredible amount of both freedom and cohesion within the system in a given moment. As a person's states of mind emerge in ways determined by the system's own internal constraints and by the external constraints of interpersonal connections with others, the self is perpetually being created.

On a daily basis, we each experience this sense of emergence when we enter a "bottom-up" mode of perceiving reality. The sense of vitality in such living provides a window to the evolving quality of states of mind and human experience. In contrast, recursive or repeating patterns in these states can bring a sense of familiarity to these new encounters. This recursive quality reinforces patterns of representational response learned from earlier encounters with the world. This quality can be adaptive in allowing us to respond rapidly to our perceptions of the world. When engrained and restrictive patterns are taken to their extremes, however, the mind can become deadened to the vital and emergent uniqueness of lived experience.

The recursive nature of complex systems is revealed in the increasing specialization of a system's trajectory of states. Early on in development, for example, a wide array of states may be possible; as the system or organism evolves, it develops a more limited set of possible states. This increase in the system's differentiation, this specialization in the patterns of activation, is based on the coordination of basic elements into a more highly coupled, integrated system. Such differentiation may be a product of genetically encoded information and the unfolding of developmental processes in transaction with experience and the ongoing emergence of self-organizing brain states across time. Though at first glance such differentiation and the limitations in the flow of states with development may appear to limit the system's flow, such a differentiated system actually enables the states of activation to achieve more complexity. In this manner, the recursive, self-perpetuating nature of development moves the system toward increasingly differentiated and integrated states. As we'll see later in this and subsequent chapters, when differentiated subcomponent elements become functionally coupled into a larger system, such integration allows for continued movement toward maximizing complexity as the states of the system continually emerge.

Constraints

The system attains a balance between continuity and flexibility by having the ability to modify what are called the "constraints" on the system. These constraints are both internal, including the alteration of synaptic strengths (as described above as a part of connectionist theory and Hebbian associations) between neurons and neuronal groups, and external, governed by interactions with the environment. The modification of constraints is *not* performed by a hidden designer, a "homunculus," or a "ghost in the machine"—that is, some mind within the mind whose purpose is to help the organism adapt or organize its functioning. Constraints are modified by the mathematically predictable probabilities of the activities of the subcomponents of the system. *The mind organizes itself automatically, based on its ability to modify internal or external constraints.*

Adaptation occurs through modification of constraints. Self-organization is dependent upon the modification of constraints in an effort to achieve maximal complexity. Dysfunctions in self-organization can be conceptualized as due to any pattern of constraint modification that does not permit movement toward such complexity. As we'll see, patterns of modifying constraints can be effective in adapting to certain environmental conditions at one time, but can produce later limitations on the probabilistic movement toward maximal complexity. Such an adaptation may be the general process serving as the source of psychological dysfunction.[29]

Within given states of mind, dysfunction may be revealed as an incohesive clustering of mental processes. In posttraumatic stress disorder, for example, intrusions of memory, hypervigilance, and excessive arousal are experienced as fragmented mental states. In the states of mind characteristic of other disorders, such as personality disorders or chronic anxiety, there may be a semistable cohesiveness in which the isolated elements of the particular states of mind have a cohesive functional quality within themselves. The semistable or temporary quality of this cohesion is revealed when the whole system's constriction is examined. At the moment of activation of a semistable cohesive state, other elements (such as memories, other emotions, more flexible thought patterns, or responses to others) are strategically omitted from activation.

Attachment and Self-Organization

Attachment patterns illustrate how adaptation to the structure of parent–child communication can result in children's modification of constraints in characteristic ways to regulate their states of mind. For example, a securely attached infant uses both (external) communication with her mother and her own (internal) regulatory functions to help organize her self-system. During the first few years of life, this process involves a direct response of each partner to the signals of the other. As we've discussed in Chapter 3, Aitken and Trevarthen have defined this as "primary intersubjectivity."[30] As the child develops into the second half of the first year, her ability to have a representation of the mother, or a "virtual mother," allows for the interaction of the two to have a secondary intersubjectivity quality in which the child's perceptions of the mother are filtered through her expectations of the virtual, mentally constructed representation of the mother.

In the case of the securely attached infant, the perceptive, sensitive, responsive, and predictable communication from the parent allows a close correspondence between the infant's virtual parent and the actual parent. Cooperative communication involving the parent's capacity to perceive and respond to the mental state of the child is the hallmark of a securely attached dyad.[31] These mutually attuned experiences allow the infant to develop a reflective capacity that helps to create a sense of cohesion and interpersonal connection. The other's mental state is a positive element in the infant's life. The securely attached infant is able to use the communicative experiences with the parent to help regulate her internal state. Self-organization is thus achieved through a balance in the infant's use of external constraints (the attachment relationship) and internal constraints (the internal representations of the caregiver and of the attachment relationship itself).

An avoidantly attached infant, on the other hand, must rely primarily upon his own (internal) constraints to keep his system functioning. The emotionally barren and noncooperative nature of the patterns of communication lead to a nonresponsive virtual (representational) parent and to excessive reliance on internal constraints to achieve self-regulation. Reflective functioning is not developed well, in that the mental state of the parent is not available to the child. The actual mother provides little sense of mutual regulation; the acquired virtual mother offers little internal regulation. The learned autonomy keeps the individual's system isolated from that of others.

Ambivalently attached infants find themselves excessively responsive to their inconsistent attachment figures and unable to soothe themselves. Their virtual parents are unreliable; their internal working models of attachment are filled with uncertainty; and their capacity to self-regulate is compromised. Their distress becomes a dominant feature in their interactions with others. Though reflective functioning may be facilitated by the (inconsistently) available caregiving, mental states are often experienced as intrusive and not helpful in regulating the self. These children come to experience an approach–withdrawal cycle that leaves them in distress and yet clinging to others in attempts to achieve self-organization.

Infants with disorganized attachments are unable to use either internal or external means to regulate their internal states. They live in a chaotic internal world that reflects the external source of terror in the parents' behavior, which is incompatible with attachment and a sense of security. These infants are prone to have fragmented self-organizational patterns; achieving a cohesive state of mind is quite difficult under stressful situations, especially those involving separation and threat.[32] As noted in Chapter 3, these children are vulnerable to developing dissociative disorders and are more likely to develop clinical symptoms in response to overwhelming experiences. Reflective functioning may vary from state to state, as the parents may have been available in certain modes of being and quite threatening in other states. These children's fragmented internal worlds come to resemble the fragmenting interpersonal communication that shapes the development of their minds.

Beebe and Lachman's studies of communication patterns within various mother–child dyads have suggested the following findings. In avoidantly attached pairs, vocal rhythm matching (in which the response of one person corresponds to that of the partner) demonstrates a marked independence of communication signals. Each member communicates almost as if the other hasn't been heard. With ambivalently attached pairs, at the other extreme, there is an excessively matched pattern of response. Each individual acts as a tightly bound mirror of the other. Securely attached dyads have a midrange balance in which there is clearly a correspondence between signals, but each member has the freedom to vary responses, which in turn will be registered and contingently responded to by the partner.[33]

We can propose that complexity theory can be applied to view the midrange response in communicative contingency as the pattern allowing the maximal amount of complexity to be achieved. In this situation, we can suggest that two systems have become functionally linked or integrated in a manner that allows them to function as a single, complex system. *Maximal complexity* is achieved by the combination of individual differentiation and interpersonal integration. In contrast, being independent from one's partner (as avoidantly attached children are) is a situation in which the system of one individual acts as if alone, decreasing complexity by way of excessive internal continuity. Being tightly coupled with another, almost verging on intrusive matching or being paralyzed by being a mirror of the other, also decreases complexity by reducing any variability between the interacting systems.

People may find themselves experiencing this range in vocal rhythm matching with other individuals, often in nonverbal ways. Some people are exquisitely responsive to the most subtle nuances of others' signals—a yawn, a glance out the window, a concerned look. Others seem, at least to an observer, to be oblivious to the other persons' signals. This range of matching can be used to gain insight into people's present experience with others and reflections of past communication patterns. As a dynamical system, the mind may be restricted in its balanced movement toward complexity either by excessive responsiveness to others or by an intense autonomy and resistance to joining with others' states. Other people may tend toward dissociative states in which the overall state of mind can only be organized by dis-associations of the component parts of mental functioning.

STATES OF MIND ACROSS TIME

The activity of the brain creates the mind. We have reviewed how this activity is composed of the flow of neuronal activations, or energy, through a complex neural network that serves the purpose of carrying and transforming mental representations, or information. The processing of this information allows the mind to solve problems. The specific pattern of the flow of energy through the brain creates a particular neural net profile of activation, or state of mind. Emotion and its regulation play a central role in determining degrees and localization of neural activation. Emotion is fundamentally linked to the same circuitry that is responsible for creating meaning and value for mental representations. It is no surprise that particular emotions become associated with particular states of mind: Emotions, in fact, are a fundamental part of the process that creates a state of mind at a particular moment in time.

Marc Lewis has noted that the energy flow within states of mind can be seen as a flow of information through a self-organizing system.[34] Emotions reveal the way in which a system regulates its states of activation in processing information. This self-organization is dyadic—a part of the interaction between two people—and reflects the fundamental way in which the mind is created within interpersonal interactions and neurophysiological processes.[35] As Schore has commented, "These transactions represent a flow of interpersonal information accompanying emotion, and critical fluctuations, amplified by positive feedback, lead to disequilibrium and self-organization."[36] The state of the system is dependent upon the induction of alterations, or disequilibrium, in the movement toward self-organization.[37] These alterations are created by emotional transactions with others.

In clinical practice, therapists see a continuity of behavioral and emotional responses that can make people inflexible, nonproductive, dysfunctional, and unhappy. Their minds have lost the capacity for adaptive self-organization and have become stuck in inflexible patterns of activation. These are among the many reasons individuals may come to a psychotherapist for help. Certainly people show unpredictable, spontaneous behaviors that seem to "come out of nowhere." These are "predictable" from the nonlinearity of complex systems. As Boldrini and colleagues have stated, "In chaotic systems, several different patterns of movements are simultaneously present and very small changes in initial conditions can alter the system's trajectory. The system can itself give rise to turbulence and, under some circumstances, this leads to an evolutionary advantage, while, in other cases, it does not yield stability, but leads to intermittent chaos."[38] Often people seeking psychotherapeutic help feel stuck in patterns of response and internal experience that they are desperate to change but have been unable to alter. To help patients alter such an engrained and unhelpful pattern in the flow of states of mind, therapists need to consider how the brain establishes such a continuity across time and what interventions can be designed to change such a process.

Continuity in the flow of states across time is established in part by internal constraints—the neuronal connections that have been established by constitution and experience. In such a model of probabilities, the system moves toward increasing levels of complexity while maintaining elements of continuity, sameness, and familiarity in the face of new and unfamiliar activation patterns. The system by its very structure has a property that maintains some aspect of continuity. As the system produces outputs (behaviors in response to the environment), these too can produce a somewhat consistent pattern of reactions from the outside world, and thus can shape external constraints. For example, shy children may alter their responses to novelty slightly, but their hesitation may continue to irritate their parents, whose frustration continues to reinforce the children's anxiety. The result is that the seemingly "independent" variable of the external (parental) constraints is actually directly influenced by the children themselves. As discussed in Chapter 5, some studies suggest that behaviorally inhibited or shy children have a constitutionally active right hemisphere, which produces excessive withdrawal states. Negative responses from parents may reinforce such withdrawal reactions within their children. The system that began with a certain characteristic predisposition establishes continuity through both the internal and external constraints on its flow of states across time.

Information Processing

One way of viewing a state of mind is that the profile of activation includes *which* modules of information processing are active, as well as *what* they are processing. Of note is that certain circuits that function well in some states appear to be markedly impaired in depressed states, as evidenced, for example, by decreased ability to detect facial emotion and the corresponding brain imaging findings of decreased right hemisphere blood flow during these tasks. In depression, the module for processing facial affect is impaired.[39] The recursive (feedback-loop) nature of states of mind is such that the blockage of this module may reinforce the intensity of the very state of mind that produced the blockage. In other words, the depressed person loses the ability to utilize the facial expressions of others to help modulate his own emotional state. External constraints become unavailable, and the person must rely on the isolated and depressed functioning of the internal constraints alone. Such a person feels and is truly disconnected from others.

The selective activation or deactivation of information-processing modules of the mind creates its own continuity in the creation of a given state of mind. As Hofer has stated, "To accomplish various age-specific tasks, the brain must be able to shift from one state of functional organization to another and thus from one mode of information processing to others within an essential modular structure."[40] As clusters of neurons can become rapidly activated or deactivated in the creation of a state of mind, the pattern of neural firing can reflect abrupt shifts in self-organization. The complex system of the brain is inherently capable of abrupt transitions in states. One way of characterizing the nature of the brain's self-organizing properties is through its coordination of such transitions: When a brain remains stuck in a given state, such as depression, or exhibits dysregulated and abrupt shifts in state, such as in dissociation, this may be due to dysfunctional self-organization.

How does the encapsulated episode of experience, the state of mind, become reinforced by the process of self-organization? The characteristic flow of information within a given state helps to define its own boundaries. Being furious can lead to certain thoughts, images, and sensations that reinforce themselves in a rageful state. As this processing begins to become more flexible, the intensity of the state begins to subside, and the state dissolves into a more neutral flow of activations. In this manner, certain states have fairly definable boundaries and characteristics. Others are more adaptive and flexible in the patterns of activation that become clustered as a functional unit. In these more "fluid" and "neutral" states, there may be less easily defined beginnings and endings. Thus the *flexibility* in information-processing modules may help define the flow of states across time, rather than merely the processing by itself.

Continuity and Self-States

As we've seen in the case of disorganized attachment, unresolved trauma, and dissociation, the mind is capable of clustering its modules and the content of their information within fairly distinct states of mind. But is this the case only in those who have experienced disorganized attachments or childhood trauma? The answer appears to be no. Studies in child development suggest, in fact, that the idea of a unitary, continuous "self" is actually an illusion our minds attempt to create.[41] Childhood is filled with normal examples of the many ways in which a child must "be"—different roles to take, in order to adapt to different social contexts (with parents, siblings, peers, teachers). Adolescence is filled with new challenges to deal with the emergence of new "selves" with seemingly separate identities: a sexual self, a student self, a self independent of parents.[42] Even in cognitive science, the mind is considered as having many distinct "parts" responsible for a wide array of activities, from feeding and reproduction to affiliation and reading other people's minds. As intelligent beings with desires and beliefs, we attempt to achieve our goals by assessing our situations and applying our internal rules to interactions with the environment. Our many layers of information processing have unique sets of rules, as well as specialized problems they are attempting to solve. Dividing these information-processing modules is necessary to carry out efficient interactions with others in the world. We have multiple and varied "selves," which are needed to carry out the many and diverse activities of our lives.

Alan Sroufe has defined the "self" as an internally organized cluster of attitudes, expectations, meanings, and feelings.[43] In his view, the self emerges from an "organized caregiving matrix" that in part determines how the individual responds to and engages with or avoids the environment. Relationships also determine how children interpret experience.[44] An extension of this view, in combination with Susan Harter's research on the many "selves" of normal development, suggests that the "selves" in which we live are dependent upon relationship context.[45] Furthermore, our relationship histories may have shaped particular patterns of feelings, attitudes, and meanings that are more likely to become activated in the future. In these ways, history and present context shape whichever "self" is organized in the moment. As relationship experiences are repeated, these "self-states" become repeatedly engrained and develop their own histories and patterns of activity across time.

As we can see, both developmental studies and cognitive science appear to suggest that we have many selves. Within a specialized "self" or "self-state," as we are now defining it, there is cohesion in the moment and continuity across time. For example, a person's sexual self is made up of all of the states of mind that have been clustered over time to deal with sexual information: sexual arousal from within, sexual interaction with others. This sexual self then has a continuity by virtue of its connection strengths or internal system constraints, as discussed earlier. Within this continuity is a sense of cohesion. That is, the various modules of the mind cluster together in the service of specialized activity—processing information in order to achieve a particular goal. Within this cohesion of the specialized self emerges a continuity across time (in that self-state) of feelings, beliefs, intentions, memories, and so forth, which creates a qualitative sense of unity.

The mind as a whole, although it exists across time and is composed of many relatively distinct but interdependent modules, functions as a system itself. As a complex system, it is made up of subcomponent specialized self-states, as well as itself being a subcomponent of a larger interpersonal system. Let's continue to examine this issue of the continuity across states by looking at the selves of the mind.

Here's a bit of vocabulary clarification. We can use the term "state of mind" to refer to the cluster of brain activity (and mental modules) at a given moment in time. This "moment" can be brief or extended, and states of mind can have various degrees of sharpness or blurriness to their boundaries across time. The repeated activation of states of mind as time goes by—over weeks, months, and years—into a specialized, goal-directed set of cohesive functional units is what we are going to call a "specialized self" or "self-state."

The most basic division is that between a private, inner self and a public, outer self, which has been described in Chapter 4. Developmental studies have examined how individuals struggle with their various roles in life and how these may be composed of various degrees of "true" or "false" selfhood.[46] Other examples of specialized selves include sexual, affiliative, status-seeking, survival-oriented, and intellectual selves. Clearly the divisions could go on and on, until we get back to our basic unit of the state of mind in a given moment in time. And this is just the point: How does the mind create a sense of continuity across states of mind, if it does at all?

The proposal here is that *basic states of mind are clustered into specialized selves, which are enduring states of mind that have a repeating pattern of activity across time.* These specialized selves or self-states each have relatively specialized and somewhat independent modes of processing information and achieving goals. Each person has many such interdependent and yet distinct processes, which exist over time with a sense of continuity that creates the experience of mind.

Susan Harter and colleagues' developmental studies suggest that certain self-states may conflict with each other.[47] Such conflicts may be a central source of dysfunction, especially during adolescence. Also, the more extreme the degree of "false selfhood" within specialized selves, the more individuals may experience a sense of disconnection from others and from themselves. How a person resolves such conflicts may be an important determinant of future emotional resilience.[48] The question may not be whether there is a sense of unifying *continuity*, but how the mind integrates a sense of coherence—of effective functioning—across self-states through time.

If people become stuck and disabled, if they are filled with adaptive specialized selves without a sense of authenticity, or if they are filled with intense and unresolved conflicts across self-states, then the development of a specific process that integrates the selves across time may become important. Clinicians often encounter patients who face these dilemmas. Catalyzing the development of such an integrating process may be the central feature of psychotherapy for these individuals. The next chapters will examine how the mind achieves integration and self-regulation, and how interpersonal relationships can assist people in developing the vital capacity to transform their self-organization.

INTERPERSONAL SYSTEMS AND DYADIC STATES OF MIND

Our review of complex systems and the example of how attachment experiences shape patterns of self-regulation raises the issue of how two individuals come to function as a dyadic system.[49] Various theories of social psychology and psychodynamics suggest that learning, communication, role modeling, internalization, idealization, and identification may each play a role in how children develop.[50] From the point of view of the mind as emanating from the activity of the complex system of the brain, we can look at the question of development and interpersonal relationships from a different perspective.

Consider this view. The mind of one person, A, organizes itself on the basis of both internal and external constraints. Internal constraints are determined by constitutional features and experience. External constraints include the signals sent from others in the environment. Person B is in a relationship with A. A perceives the signals sent from B, and A's system responds by altering its state. Two immediate effects are (1) that A's state shifts as a function of B's state (or at least B's signals), and (2) that A sends signals back to B. B in turn responds to A's signals with at least these two alterations, and contingent communication is established. If A is an adult and B is a baby, then the pattern of responses will shape the function and the developing structure of B's immature brain, not merely B's present state of mind. So what's new about this view?

What's new is that the *patterns* of A's response to B and B's response to A can begin to shape the states that are created in both A and B. A and B come to function as a supersystem, AB. One can no longer reduce the interactions of A and B to the subcomponents A and B; AB is an irreducible system. Systems theory provides a hierarchical understanding of interpersonal relationships. For some people, sharing an "interpersonal state" is one of the most rewarding experiences in human life. For others, such dyadic states are occasionally welcome, but a hefty dose of isolation is preferred to the feeling of "disappearance" that such an AB state may create. Still others long for such a union, but feel they can never truly achieve it. Even when they are "almost in it," they fear it will disappear; that very fear can itself destroy the dyadic experience. Is this just another way of talking about the different attachment patterns? Certainly the attachment approaches may represent variations on the fundamental "I–thou" theme. There are selves, others, and their relationships together. But systems theory offers us a perspective and vocabulary on the constraints that help the system organize itself. These internal and external factors provide a new framework for understanding how one mind joins with others to form a larger functional system.

The imprint of a parent's patterns of self-organization is manifested within a child's own patterns of self-regulation. In this way, the joining of two systems into a single supersystem may continue to show its effects even when the child is away from the adult, or when the child has grown up. For example, in children with disorganized attachments and in dissociative adults, their chaotic and terrifying experiences with caregivers may have become not only a part of their memories, but a part of the very structure of their self-(dys)regulation. Such is the effect of early trauma on the developing mind.

Understanding the behavior of complex systems can provide insights into the sometimes automatic ways in which relationships with others seem to evolve. Looking toward the interpersonal state as the fundamental unit of "self-organization" for a relationship can be very helpful. For example, relationships that become stuck can be envisioned as unable to move in a balanced way toward increasing complexity in their interpersonal states. Rigid styles of communicating and unwillingness to enter into intense sharing of primary emotional states may lead to a sense of "deadness" in a relationship. The states of an emotional relationship may reflect both the elements of the here-and-now communication and remnants of past patterns of relating. Individuals join with each other in creating a system larger than the individual self.

Often the shift between states of mind within a dyadic relationship may be quite subtle. Context changes can be hidden—induced, for example, by alterations in a companion's tone of voice or facial expression. The ways we join with another person in forming an interpersonal system with its own emerging dyadic states can often be quite rapid and nonverbal.

Let's look at the example from earlier in this chapter of how an adult can experience a shift in her state of mind when she returns home for the holidays. If a family is viewed as a supersystem, a cluster of the smaller systems of its individual members, then we can begin to make sense of this common phenomenon. As we've seen, a state of mind includes the assembly of various processes via reentry loops, each of which may emanate from the activity of relatively distinct circuits in the brain. A state of mind involves the recruitment of these various subsystems into activity together—in other words, the coupling of disparate processes into a simultaneous set of reentrant, coassembled activating components. The adult child has her own developmental history in which her genetics and repeated encounters with the environment have reinforced her states of mind—specific patterns of clustered neuronal activations that are sensitive to initial, specific environmental conditions. Her parents also have their own developmental histories (part of which include having her as their child), which have created specific states and patterns of response. They may have been quite happy during the years since their daughter has moved away, but somehow on these holiday visits things for them, and for her, fall back into old patterns.

The context shift of the grown child's returning home—possibly sleeping in the same room, eating meals with her parents, having siblings present, and experiencing other old and familiar conditions— reestablishes a fertile setting in which each family member's mind can respond. The new contextual frame evokes old attractor states. Literally, what this means is that each of their brains is responding to this new setting with an alteration in its individual constraints to make old patterns of states of mind more likely to occur. The recruitment or coassembly of components of the individuals within the family allows us to see how the larger framework of a supersystem contains its own developmental history, with attractor states and coupling processes of its own. Recruitment is often automatic, without conscious awareness or intention. The family now functions as a whole system, reinstating its old attractor states. For the adult child, the experience may be one of being drawn back into old sensations and patterns of behavior without her initial awareness or sense of control.

Recall that states of mind contain the clustering of perceptual biasing, behavioral response patterns, emotional tone and regulation, memory processing, and mental models. For the adult child's parents, all of this may involve interpreting her behavior as oppositional, being harsh and critical in their own behavior, feeling scared and distrustful of her, recalling various conflicts she's had with them, and having a mental model of her as an impulsive, uncooperative teenager. Their shift in state probably occurs simultaneously with their daughter's. She may view their behavior as controlling and insensitive to her needs; she may find herself responding to them with impatience and disrespect; she may feel angry and disappointed, and challenged to keep these feelings from overwhelming her; she may have easier access to the memories of the painful years of her adolescence; and she may have a mental model of her parents as being unsupportive and of herself as a victim of their shortcomings.

The rapidity with which these virtually simultaneous and instantaneous shifts in state can occur once the daughter arrives back at her parents' home is astonishing. Neither part of this supersystem is to "blame" for such changes. Each subset of the larger system is taking part in a shift in state based on present context. Subsequent, often subtle, responses of one component to another reinforce the "appropriateness" of such shifts for adaptation. The daughter may find herself saying, "I knew I shouldn't have come home. They never change. This is hopeless." She may be right. Or she may be experiencing the tenacity of old attractor states, both within herself and within her parents, and especially within the relationship system. As her sense of helplessness continues, and the rapid interactions return to their old patterns, the old and painful mental state configurations are reinforced yet again. At this moment, she is in desperate need of a "change"—a way of healing old wounds and lifting herself out of engrained and dysfunctional patterns of dyadic self-organization.

Each of us needs periods in which our minds can focus inwardly. Solitude is an essential experience for the mind to organize its own processes and create an internal state of resonance. In such a state, the self is able to alter its constraints by directly reducing the input from interactions with others. As the mind goes through alternating phases of needing connection and needing solitude, the states of mind are cyclically influenced by combinations of external and internal processes. We can propose that such a shifting of focus allows the mind to achieve a balanced self-organizational flow in the states of mind across time. Respecting the need for solitude allows the mind to "heal" itself[51]—which in essence can be seen as releasing the natural self-organizational tendencies of the mind to create a balanced flow of states. Solitude permits the self to reflect on engrained patterns and intentionally alter reflexive responses to external events that have been maintaining the dyadic dysfunction.

We are all nonlinear dynamical systems. This means that small changes in input can lead to large, often unpredictable changes in output. It also means that a good portion of human behavior and the human mind are unpredictable in the long run. If this adult daughter becomes aware of these old patterns and decides, consciously, not to take part in them, she may find that they begin to change a bit. Solitude may permit the reflection necessary to enable her to initiate such changes. If she then makes a deliberate effort to alter her state—and especially her behavioral responses and patterns of communication—major changes in interpersonal interactions may occur. It takes diligence, but pulling out of the automatic reflexes of old family patterns for many people is often worth the effort. The daughter's changes in response, her internal awareness of her own and the family's processes, and her willingness to give up old beliefs that "I am right and they are wrong" can each bring about an alteration in system constraints, which can shift the patterns of the family system's trajectory, its pattern of state shifts, and subsequent behavioral patterns.

We have noted throughout this chapter that repeated activation of states, especially those involving significant emotional intensity during the early years of development, makes them more likely to be repeated in the future. In this manner, historical patterns of states of mind, both within an individual and within a family system, may become characteristic traits. It is in this way that attractor states become engrained within us and allow old interpersonal states to continue to influence our individual patterns of self-organization.

Rigidly engrained states produce reduced variability in the system, which diminishes its adaptability to the environment and its capacity to maximize the system's complexity. Self-organization, always attempting to move us toward increasing levels of complexity, is inhibited if flexibility is reduced. Individuals, families, or groups of people in whom states have become so engrained as to inhibit exploration of new possibilities can no longer grow and develop.[52] The subjective experience of such a condition is one of stagnation and malaise. Infusing energy into a system, destabilizing old states, and bringing new life to a stuck set of patterns mean establishing a new balance between continuity and flexibility—one that will allow for emergent states of increasing complexity. The dynamic experience of such emergent states of mind within responsive interpersonal relationships can create an electrifying sense of vitality.

REFLECTIONS: THE FLOW OF STATES

Emotional growth is based on the movement of dynamical systems toward a balance between continuity and flexibility in the flow of states across time. A balanced flow of energy within the system—without either rigid constraints on which neuronal groups will be recruited (excessive control) or a chaotic, random flow of activations (excessive disorganization), such as in "strange attractor states," which limit the complexity achieved by randomizing the recruitment process—is a goal of emotional development. In other words, past adaptations may have led to either excessively rigid or disorganized self-regulation. Either condition limits the stabilizing movement toward increasing levels of complexity of the system. These conditions reflect emotional dysregulation.

The attainment of maximum complexity is a function of the balance between flexibility and continuity of the system. Flexibility is based on the generation of diversity of responses and variation in the flow of states; it allows for the creation of a degree of uncertainty in the novel adaptations to changing environmental conditions. In contrast, continuity emerges from the system's learning processes, which establish a degree of certainty in response patterns as determined by an engrained set of constraints. This balance between flexibility and continuity, novelty and familiarity, uncertainty and certainty, allows a dynamical system to recruit increasingly complex layers of neuronal groups in maximizing its trajectory toward complexity.

Over time, cohesive states achieve enduring continuity within their organization as self-states. Each self-state is created and maintained in order to carry out specific information-processing tasks. As environmental conditions change, the context-dependent nature of states leads to the instantiation of a particular self-state required at the time. The healthy, adaptive mind is capable of entering a range of discontinuous (but minimally conflictual) self-states, each with its own cohesion and sense of continuity.

There are various ways in which cohesion and continuity may be impaired. Excessive rigidity in a state of mind leads to an inability to try new configurations and to adapt flexibly to changes in the environment. Such rigidity may be seen in those with avoidant attachment histories, in which input from other people is eventually adaptively blocked in order to maintain self-organization. Homeostasis is achieved at the expense of the connections with others and with primary emotional states of the self. In this manner, right-hemisphere information processing may be dis-associated from that of the left hemisphere in order to maintain functioning. Such a person faces the challenge of learning to create some tolerable level of disequilibrium, in order to allow the system to try new pathways toward balanced self-regulation. In such a case, we can envision strategies of moving toward growth and development as initially involving right-hemisphere-to-right-hemisphere communication between two people. Eventually, further internal change may be brought about by a process facilitating integration of the right and left hemispheres within the individual. Within a psychotherapy setting, such techniques as journal writing, guided imagery, and exercises for "drawing on the right side of the brain" have proven helpful to catalyze such a new form of bilateral resonance.

In ambivalently attached individuals, states may be somewhat fragile and easily disrupted. Cohesion may have a semistable quality that is particularly vulnerable to perturbation from social nuances. Some such individuals may be quite sensitive to subtle nonverbal cues and inadvertent misattunements; these disconnections may lead rapidly to states of shame from which it may be difficult to recover. For other people, past histories of parental intrusion make their semistable cohesion hypervigilant to the intrusion of others' internal experiences into their own. In this manner, they may defensively guard against the perception of others' minds, creating interpersonal disconnection.

In individuals with disorganized attachments, two major forms of dis-association can occur. One is within a state of mind at a given time, in which there is a "strange attractor" state of widely distributed activations. In the second form, cohesive states are dis-associated from one another across time; that is, there is a functional isolation of information transfer across states. Cohesion is achieved only through the restriction in complexity achievable by this particular configuration of self-states.

Complexity theory suggests that self-organization allows a system to adapt to environmental changes through the movement of its states toward increasingly complex configurations. Moving with a balance of flexibility and continuity, the system emerges within the internal and external constraints that define the trajectory of state changes. Internal constraints include the strength and distribution of synaptic connections within neural pathways; external constraints include social experiences and attuned emotional communication between people. By regulating these internal and external constraints, the self-system evolves through an emerging set of self-states that have cohesion and continuity within themselves. The mind as a nonlinear system is also quite capable of abrupt shifts in constraints, which lead to the instantiation of distinct, discontinuous self-states. The mind's creation of stable systemic coherence across these self-states is one of the central goals of emotional development and self-regulation.

CHAPTER 7

—

Self-Regulation

THE CENTRAL ROLE OF EMOTION
IN SELF-REGULATION

The self is created within the processes that organize the activity of the mind in its interactions with the world. As we've seen in Chapter 6, such self-organization is a part of the fundamental ways in which complex systems function. At a given moment in time, the array of possible mental activity becomes organized within a mental state that functions to create a cohesive set of goal-directed processes. Across time, we can understand how continuity is created within a given self-state through the various principles of complexity, connectionism, and information processing. Integrating these processes is emotion.

As Luc Ciompi has described, emotions function as "central organizers and integrators" in linking several domains: providing all incoming stimuli with a specific meaning and motivational direction; participating in state-dependent memory processes; connecting mental processes "synchronically" and "diachronically" (within one time and across time); creating more complex interconnections among abstract representational processes that share emotional meaning; and simultaneously attuning the whole organism to the current situational demands on the basis of past experience through neurophysiologically mediated peripheral effects.[1] Such organizing features intimately link what are traditionally considered the mental, social, and biological domains. As Alan Sroufe has pointed out, then, emotions are inherently integrative in their function.[2]

As we further explore the nature of the mind, we will find that understanding the creation of the self at the interface of brain and human relationships focuses our attention on the fundamental ways in which emotion is experienced and regulated. As many researchers have suggested, emotion is both regulated and regulatory. In its manifestations as neurophysiological events, subjective experiences, and interpersonal expressions, emotion interconnects various systems within the mind and between minds. Focusing on emotion regulation allows us to explore how the mind becomes organized and integrated.

In this chapter we'll explore some ways of viewing the regulatory processes that organize the mind. From a developmental perspective, the infant's first challenge is to achieve internal homeostasis via the activity of deep structures of the brainstem, which mediate sleep–wake cycles and other basic bodily functions (such as heart rate, respiration and digestion). Myron Hofer has described how even at this early stage, the parent provides "hidden regulators" that directly facilitate these basic functions in the infant.[3] As maturation unfolds, "dyadic regulation" becomes important in enabling the child to modulate more complex states of mind.[4] Attachment serves as a crucial way in which the self becomes regulated. As the child's evaluative mechanisms become more active, and memory processes enable the child to respond to discrepancies, subjective meaning is created in engaging with the social surround. Intimate attunements permit a resonance of states of mind that are mutually regulating. Misattunements lead to dysregulation, which requires "interactive repair" if the child is to regain equilibrium.[5] Achieving emotion regulation is dependent upon social interactions. At this early point, according to Sroufe, the child has become an emotional being—not merely a reactive one—in that arousal or tension is created via evaluative appraisals that create subjective meaning in engagements with the environment.[6] As infancy gives way to the toddler period, dyadic regulation is supplanted by "caregiver-guided self-regulation," in which the adult helps the child begin to regulate states of mind autonomously.[7] As the child's brain matures into the preschool years, the emergence of increasingly complex layers of self-regulation becomes possible.

As emotion continues throughout life to function in integrative ways, it reveals the continuing process by which our minds carry out intersystem integration: within our own modes of processing, across various modalities, and between our own minds and those of others.

As Antonio Damasio has noted, "Emotion, and the experience of emotion, are the highest-order direct expressions of bioregulation in complex organisms. Leave out emotion and you leave out the prospect of understanding bioregulation comprehensively, especially as it regards the relation between an organism and the most complex aspects of an environment: society and culture."[8] From our discussion of complexity, we can see that emotion and the development of emotion regulation move the self into more complex states of intra- and intersystem functioning. Emotion regulation that allows the mind a flexible manner in which to emerge in interaction with the environment reflects optimal state regulation. As we've discussed in earlier chapters, the prefrontally mediated capacity for response flexibility may be a central component to such a balanced capacity. Emotion "dysregulation" can be seen as impairments in this capacity to allow flexible and organized responses that are adaptive to the internal and external environment. As we'll discuss, such dysregulation can have its origins in constitutional elements, interactional experience, and the transaction between these two fundamental components of the mind.[9]

DYSFUNCTIONAL PATTERNS
OF SELF-REGULATION

The structure of the brain gives it an innate capacity to modulate emotion and to organize its states of activation. Sometimes referred to as "affect regulation," this capacity is crucial for the internal and interpersonal functioning of the individual.[10] Any of a number of psychiatric disturbances can be viewed as disorders of self-regulation.[11] Among these are the mood disorders, in which emotional state is massively dysregulated, producing states of depression or mania. Within these states of mind are characteristic dysfunctions in perception, memory, beliefs, and behaviors. These are disorders where the unique feature is a profound instability in mood. Anxiety disorders also reveal the flood of an emotion that evokes a dysfunctional state of mind. Individuals with these difficulties may be excessively sensitive to the environment and may also have autonomous signals of impending disaster, as in panic disorder and obsessive–compulsive disorder. Here, too, there is a marked incapacity to regulate one's state of mind. As individuals with these and other disorders (see below) develop, the instability of their states may become a characteristic feature, or trait, of their self-regulation. Indeed, in studies of patients with bipolar disorder, the untreated swings between mania and depression can begin to "kindle" the onset of more frequent, intense, and rapid cycling. In this way, the instability can become a repeated, "stable" feature of the individual's self-organizational dysfunction.[12]

In many of these disorders, a combination of pharmacological and psychotherapeutic interventions may be indicated. Even if the origin of the dysfunction is seen as the neural instability of some neuronal circuit in the deep or limbic regions of the brain, the mind of the individual is inextricably created by the brain's activity. As we've seen in Chapter 6, dysfunction of a subcomponent in a system can have profound and unpredictable effects on other subcomponents, as well as on the system as a whole. For this reason, interventions aimed at many layers of the functioning of the brain and the mind may be essential in helping the individual achieve a more balanced and functional form of self-organization. Within the clinical setting, the relationship of therapist and patient becomes the "external constraint" that can help produce changes in the individual's capacity for self-organization.

An example of the developmental origins of impaired self-organization can be seen within those with insecure attachments. With the experience of avoidant attachment, the mind learns to adapt to the barren psychological world by decreasing the awareness of socially generated emotional states. The rigidity of such a constrained pattern is revealed in the ways in which physiological responses continue to express the significance of social interactions, which are cognitively blocked from being processed. In disorganized attachment experiences, the child acquires the ability to respond to stress with a dis-association of processes leading to dissociative states. Whereas some of these states are quite disorganized and incohesive, others have the appearance of functional cohesion. Closer examination of even these dissociated states reveals a marked cognitive blockage restricting the overall processing of information and flow of energy through the mind as a whole. The apparently divergent avoidant and disorganized attachment patterns actually share the characteristic of restriction in the flow of states of mind. This convergence is supported by the finding in the Minnesota Parent–Child Project that during the early years of life, before adolescence, disorganized and avoidantly attached children have the greatest degree of dissociative symptoms.[13] This finding supports the proposal that impairments to mental well-being may be understood as adaptations that impair the balanced flow of energy and information in the formation of emerging states of mind.

As noted above, many psychiatric disturbances involve affect dysregulation. In addition to mood disorders (such as depression and bipolar illness) and the anxiety disorders (including panic disorder, phobias, obsessive–compulsive disorder, and posttraumatic stress disorder), these include dissociative disorders and certain personality disorders, such as borderline and narcissistic character structures.[14] However, rather than reviewing all of these disorders in detail, let us look at a single case example to gain additional insight into the nature of emotion dysregulation.

> "I couldn't help myself. He made me so furious with his mistakes that I told him to go jump in a lake. Not in those friendly words, of course. I was so angry. I wasn't going to let him get away with that kind of stuff again. Maybe for others it's OK, but not with me. Why is everyone in this world so stupid?"

This thirty-five-year-old attorney was fired by her client of ten years after screaming and apparently threatening a colleague at a meeting for missing a deadline in mailing a document she had given to him. This was not the first time her emotions had "taken over": she had lost several boyfriends in the past for her "instability" and was now at risk of being alone again, in addition to having lost her most important client. For this patient, the inability to regulate her emotions was a major problem in both her personal and professional lives.

Interactions with other people long before this episode of screaming at her colleague had historically evoked "sudden outbursts of intense emotion" in this woman. Within our framework for understanding emotional processes, let's examine what this phrase may have meant for her. "Sudden" refers to the notion that something seems to occur without a preparatory period giving some warning or clue that a process is even occurring. At a minimum, we can suggest that she was not consciously aware of the impending external expression of her emotional response. "Intense emotion" is a common term that we can now interpret in the language of the mind. "Intense" probably signifies a strong degree of activation or arousal, which became expressed in this woman's case as the categorical emotion of rage. So we have taken this a bit further, but not much. Is this just the use of new words to describe the familiar notion of an emotional "hijacking" or "outburst," in which rational thinking is suspended and anger or other emotions cloud perceptions and influence behavior?[15] It is much more than this, as we'll see later in the chapter when we review this attorney's childhood relationship history.

But, you may say, perhaps it was just this woman's "genetic legacy" to have uncontrolled outbursts of anger. Perhaps so. But in any psychiatric conditions that may have a large genetic component, understanding the mechanisms of the mind and the contributions of interactive experiences can help provide interventions that can alter the way the brain functions.[16] Recall that the reduction of human behavior into an "either–or" condition of "genetics versus learning" or "nature versus nurture" is unhelpful and clouds our thinking about the issues, especially when it comes to designing interventions. We will return to this example of the attorney toward the middle of this chapter, to examine ways of understanding how constitutional and experiential factors can lead to certain kinds of emotion dysregulation.

A CONCEPTUAL FRAMEWORK OF EMOTION REGULATION

The remainder of this chapter provides a conceptual framework for understanding some basic components of emotion regulation. These include regulation of intensity, sensitivity, specificity, windows of tolerance, recovery processes, access to consciousness, and external expression. This is not an exhaustive review of emotion regulation in its myriad manifestations, which can be found elsewhere in a number of useful texts.[17] Rather, this is a practical framework that draws on our study of the mind in order to illustrate how individuals achieve a flexible and adaptive capacity for the regulation of emotional processes.

The brain has developed a rich circuitry that helps regulate its states of arousal. The nature of this process of emotion regulation may vary quite a lot from individual to individual and may be influenced both by constitutional features and by adaptations to experience. "Temperament" describes some of the aspects of inborn characteristics, including sensitivity to the environment, intensity of emotional response, baseline global mood, regularity of biological cycles, and attraction to or withdrawal from novel situations. These inborn features of the nervous system, which are the results of both genetic and intrauterine factors, probably have powerful shaping effects throughout the lifespan. Temperament can evoke particular parenting responses and create its own self-fulfilling reinforcements, which further amplify the inborn trait. The example of a slow-to-warm up or shy child whose mother has little patience for his hesitancy illustrates how the response of others can engrain temperamental features.[18]

Attachment studies support the view that the pattern of communication with parents creates a cascade of adaptations that directly shape the development of the child's nervous system. Both longitudinal attachment studies and early intervention research support the idea that what parents do with their children makes a difference in the outcome of the children's development.[19] It is important to realize that both temperament and attachment history contribute to the marked differences we see between individuals in their ability to regulate their emotions.

If emotions influence the flow of states of mind that dominate so many of our mental processes, how do we keep them in some form of balance? The mind's ability to regulate emotional processes is essentially the ability of the brain to modulate the flow of arousal and activation throughout its circuits. Primary emotional processes, categorical emotions, affective expression, and mood can each be regulated by the brain. "Emotion regulation" refers to the general ability of the mind to alter the various components of emotional processing. The self-organization of the mind in many ways is determined by the self-regulation of emotional states. How we experience the world, relate to others, and find meaning in life are dependent upon how we have come to regulate our emotions.

Why should emotions and their regulation be considered so central to the organization of the self? As we've discussed in Chapter 4, emotion reflects the fundamental way in which the mind assigns value to external and internal events and then directs the allocation of attentional resources to further the processing of these representations. In this way, emotion reflects the way the mind directs the flow of information and of energy. The modulation of emotion is the way the mind regulates energy and information processing. With this perspective, emotional regulation can be seen at the center of the self-organization of the mind.

From the wide range of research on emotions, it is possible to propose here at least seven aspects of emotion regulation that can illustrate these ideas.[20] These divisions are derived from a synthesis of scientific concepts and clinical observations. Other aspects of regulation could also be proposed, but these seven areas provide a practical framework with which to begin to understand the various ways in which the mind regulates its own functioning.

Intensity

The foundation of emotional processing is the appraisal and arousal system, which can respond with various degrees of intensity. The brain appears to be able to modify the intensity of response by altering the numbers of neurons that fire and the amounts of neurotransmitters released in response to a stimulus. Degrees of arousal have a wide range. If initial appraisal and arousal mechanisms give a minimal activation of the body and brain, then the elaborating appraisal–arousal response will also be minimized. For example, studies have shown that subjects who are asked to meditate or who are given pills to reduce bodily responses and physiological arousal will interpret a stimulus as "not so important," and the primary emotion will not be as intense, as in subjects without such inhibitors of bodily reaction.[21] The body's state of arousal is mediated by the brain through the autonomic nervous system. As discussed in Chapter 6, the brain in turn monitors the state of the body and incorporates emotional meaning from the somatic markers that serve as representations of the body's change in physiological state.

The general pattern of high or low intensity of an individual's characteristic response may be a product of both constitutional and experiential factors. People with shy temperaments may have an inborn tendency to respond intensely to new situations and to withdraw when confronted with novelty. Geraldine Dawson has found that intensity of emotional response appears to be related to bilateral frontal activation, in contrast to the quality or valence of response, which is asymmetric (involving left activation for approach and right for withdrawal states).[22] Other individuals may experience milder degrees of intensity of emotion in response to novelty.

As noted in Chapter 5, Dawson has also found in studies of infants of clinically depressed mothers that the infant's capacity to experience joy and excitement is markedly reduced, especially if the maternal depression lasts beyond the first year.[23] Experience can thus directly shape the general intensity and valence of emotional activation in children. In particular, the sharing of positive emotional states may be missing from the experience of children with depressed parents. The sharing of such states under normal conditions permits an amplification of these pleasurable emotions, which sends both child and parent "into orbit" with waves of intensely engaged positive affect.[24] If such shared amplification of positive emotional states is missing, as in depressed dyads, then the capacity to tolerate (to emotionally regulate in a balanced manner) and to enjoy these intense states may be underdeveloped. Interactive experiences enable the child not only to experience high levels of "tension" or emotionally engaged arousal,[25] but to entrain the circuits of the brain to be able to manage such states.[26] Feeling comfortable with intense arousal and engagement with others may have its origins in both constitutional and experiential features of the individual.

As we'll see, intensity of arousal can be masked. It is often at the moments in which emotion becomes most intense that we seem to have the greatest need to be understood and the most intense feelings of vulnerability. This sense of exposure may make many individuals, especially those with unsatisfying past experiences with communication, reluctant to reveal openly what they are feeling. At a moment of intensity, a failure to be understood, to be connected with emotionally, can result in a profound feeling of shame.[27] The shame generated by missed opportunities for the alignment of states—for the feeling of emotional resonance, of "feeling felt"—can lead to withdrawal. Even with less intense states, not being understood may lead to a sense of isolation. Recognizing this vulnerability and the fact that moments of unintended disconnection are inevitable can allow us to repair such ruptures in alignment. Such interactive repair experiences allow us to learn to tolerate new levels of emotional intensity and the feeling of vulnerability that may accompany them.

Sensitivity

Each of us has a "threshold of response," or minimal amount of stimulation needed in order to activate our appraisal systems. Those with a hairtrigger response mechanism will find life filled with challenging situations by virtue of their brains' firing off messages of "This is important—pay attention!" frequently. Those with "tougher skins" will not respond with arousal and will be less emotionally sensitive to the same stimuli.

Sensitivity, like intensity, may be both constitutional and modified by experience. Both variables may also be dependent on an individual's state of mind at a particular moment in time. We can have times in our lives when our "nerves are raw" and we react quickly to previously innocuous events. We can also be not as sensitive as we might otherwise be when we are preoccupied by something else or emotionally defending ourselves. Alterations in our threshold of responding may be an important way our brains regulate emotional responses.

How can a mind alter sensitivity? Again, by turning to the foundation of emotions in appraisal, we can make some educated hypotheses. By increasing the amount of stimulation a value center needs to become activated, the brain can directly decrease its sensitivity to the environment. Later on, modifications in the appraisal system can decrease or increase sensitivity. For example, if you have recently seen a violent movie with gunshots and murders, your mind may be sensitized to loud sounds and dark alleys. If, upon returning to your car in a dark parking lot, you hear a sudden loud sound, you may be more likely to become aroused and to appraise such a situation as dangerous. If you had just been to a party with a lot of noise and fireworks, your mind would be less vigilant for signs of danger and would be less sensitive to those same sounds in the dark parking lot. Recent experience primes the mind for a context-specific change in sensitivity.[28]

Repeated patterns of intense emotional experiences may engrain chronic alterations in the degree of sensitivity. For example, overwhelming terror, especially early in life, may permanently alter the sensitivity of an individual to a particular stimulus related to the trauma. If a cat scratches and bites a young child, the sight of even a distant cat may evoke a strong emotional response of fear in this individual for years into the future. Furthermore, early trauma may be associated with an increase in release of stress hormones in response to daily life experiences.[29] Early alteration of the circuits of the brain involved in evaluative processes can deeply influence the appraisal mechanisms that directly influence the nature of emotional experience and emotion regulation.

One way of conceptualizing a therapeutic approach to excessive sensitivity involves the basic stages of emotional processes. Some early experiences that sensitize the arousal system to fire off may never be fully desensitized.[30] Patients may remain in a chronically hypersensitized state. However, specific appraisal of the excessively sensitive general arousal stage can be changed. Let us look at an example of this "cognitive override" mechanism.

As a young child, a forty-year-old man had been mauled by a dog; in the incident, he lost part of his left ear and sustained deep wounds to his arms and chest. Throughout his youth he naturally avoided dogs. As a young father, he dreaded the day when his own children would ask to have a dog as a pet. He came to therapy when that day indeed arrived. What could be done? Every time he saw a dog his heart would pound; he would sweat profusely, clutch his chest, and feel a sense of doom. This panic was once treated with medications, which were effective but excessively sedating for him. The man wanted to get a dog for his children but couldn't live with his fear.

Some might appropriately say that parents should let children know about the limits of what can or can't be done. They might feel in this case that the father's need to have a canine-free house should have been communicated and respected. Another possibility—the one that this man preferred—was to try to "deal" with his fears. The original accident had happened when he was two years old. He had little explicit recall of anything from that period. We know, of course, that this was a normal part of his childhood amnesia; that is, explicit auto-biographical encoding was not yet available to him, due to the immaturity of his orbitofrontal regions. And so his primary form of memory for this event was implicit: He exhibited emotional (fear and panic) and behavioral (avoidance) memories of the accident. Fortunately, he knew about the experience from the stories he had been told by his parents and from his own semantic memory. This knowledge was in a noetic form: He knew the facts, but did not have a sense of himself at this point in the past. Seeing his mauled ear in the mirror also reminded him each day that something terrifying had occurred.

This patient's amygdala was probably exquisitely sensitized to the sight of a dog. As we've discussed in Chapter 4, a preconscious feedback loop involving the perceptual system and the amygdala would have allowed for the fight–flight response to be initiated even before he became aware that he had seen a dog. These functional circuits have been evolutionarily helpful to us as human beings: Once we are hurt, our amygdalas will do everything they can to keep us from allowing it to happen again.

Teaching this man about the nature of the fear response and the neural circuits underlying it was relieving for him. Relaxation techniques and guided imagery with exposure to self-generated images of dogs were provided. Nevertheless, he still had an initial startle response to dogs. A "cognitive override" strategy was then tried. That is, this patient learned to acknowledge the relevance of his amygdala's response to the present dog and the past trauma (the initial arousal mechanism). He then would say to himself, "I know that you are trying to protect me, and that you think this is a dangerous thing" (the specific appraisal stage). What he would say next was what eventually allowed him to buy his children a (small) dog: "I do not need to see this sense of panic as something to fear or get agitated about." He would then imagine his amygdala sighing with relief, having discharged its duties to warn, and the sense of doom would dissipate. After several weeks of performing these internal override discussions, he felt ready to proceed with the purchase of the pet. Six months later, he and his family were doing well with the new addition to their household.

This example illustrates that even if the sensitivity to particular stimuli cannot be changed, a person's response to the initial arousal can be diverted in ways that lead to a more flexible life. This may have been made possible by the development and involvement of his prefrontally mediated response-flexibility process. In this case, this individual's past trauma had led to a rigid pattern in the flow of information processing and energy (the sight of a dog led to massive arousal and the sense of fear). By altering the engrained patterns of both the flow of information and energy, the patient became more flexible in his behavior and he was able to move forward more adaptively in his life. As we shall continue to explore, impediments to mental health may often be seen as blockages in information processing and energy flow. Experiences that allow for these fundamental elements to achieve a more flexible and adaptive flow or "circulation" through the mind can contribute greatly to emotional well-being.

Specificity

Emotion regulation can also determine which parts of the brain are activated by arousal. By determining the specificity of appraisal—the ways in which the value centers are establishing meaning of representations—the brain is able to regulate the flow of energy through the changing states of the system. For example, being awakened by a sound while taking a nap will probably lead your body to enter an aroused state of initial orientation. As your brain begins to process this stimulated state, it can assign meaning to various aspects of the sound. If you are expecting the arrival of your spouse while resting, the context of anticipating your spouse's return will be represented, and you may interpret the sound as a source of excitement. If instead you aren't expecting anyone, the sound may be interpreted as a possible intruder and a signal of danger, and you may feel fear. The representations activated at any particular moment, including the context of the situation, help shape the specific direction of stimulus appraisal elicited. The specificity of elaborated and differentiated appraisal directly shapes arousal and thus determines the specific type of emotional experience that unfolds.

Through its shaping of arousal, the specificity of appraisal directly influences the differentiation of primary emotions into categorical emotions. Characteristic differences among individuals in their appraisal mechanisms can directly determine the kinds of emotions generated and can influence the general "nature" of their moods and personality. Specificity of appraisal creates not only the meaning we attribute to stimulus events, but the meaning of the self–environment context and the form and meaning of the emerging emotional processes themselves. Specificity is thus a complex, recursive process of evaluation that appraises the meaning of events and the ongoing appraisal–arousal processes. The specificity of appraisal may be influenced by several elements of the evaluation of the stimulus, such as the individual's assessment of its relevance to the achievement of current or future goals, its threat to the capacity of the individual to cope and to maintain the self as the locus of control, and its meaning to global issues regarding the self and the self in relation to others.

As a child develops, the differentiation of primary emotions into categorical ones becomes more and more sophisticated. In this manner, there is a progression from the earliest states of pleasure or discomfort to the basic or categorical emotions, such as fear, anger, disgust, surprise, interest, shame, and joy. Sroufe has described the "precursor emotions" of pleasure, wariness, and frustration/distress as preceding the development of the more discrete emotional states of joy, fear, and anger, respectively.[31]

As the child continues to develop, more complex and "socially derived" emotions, such as nostalgia, jealousy, and pride, become differentiated. Linda Camras has suggested that dynamical systems theory may be useful in examining the development of emotional expression.[32] From this perspective, the infant's mind functions to incorporate internal processes with interactional responses from parents in the differentiation of the emotional processes within the interconnected domains of neurophysiology, subjective experience, and expression. The more differentiated, discrete emotions come to function as attractor states that have internally and externally determined constraints. As described by Carol Malatesta-Magai, such a process is a form of "emotion socialization," which reflects the fundamental way in which affect serves as a social signal and develops in part as a reflection of interpersonal history.[33] Such emotion socialization occurs both within the child–caregiver relationship and in peer–peer interactions.[34]

The specificity of emotional experience is determined by the specific complex layers of appraisal activated in response to a stimulus. These evaluative processes, mediated by our socially sensitive value centers in the brain, emerge within our individual constitutions and interactional histories. It is for this reason that in the same situation two people often have such qualitatively different reactions. Unique personal meaning is created by the specificity of our emotional responses.

Researchers have named a wide range of emotions in various categories.[35] Some of these include interest/excitement, enjoyment/joy, surprise/astonishment, sadness, anger, disgust, contempt, fear, anxiety, shyness, and love. Other types have also been described, such as the "self-conscious emotions" of embarrassment, pride, shame, and guilt, as well as a sense of exhilaration and humor. Individuals may have experienced many or all of these emotions at some point in their lives. They may also have noticed that each time they experienced a given categorical emotion (for example, sadness), it has both unique and universal aspects. As a state of the system is assembled, it has unique features of both inner processes and external contexts.

The differentiation of primary emotional states into categorical emotions is a rapid process illustrating how various layers of the brain are influenced by the unfolding state of mind. In its essence, emotion is a set of processes involving the recruitment of various circuits under the umbrella of one state of mind. Thus the appraisal and arousal processes create a neural net activation profile—a state of mind—whose characteristics in turn directly shape subsequent appraisal and arousal processes. This intricate feedback mechanism helps us to see why patterns of emotional response can be so tenacious in a given individual. The elements of continuity in specificity are self-reinforcing.

Creating change within rigid patterns of specific appraisals requires a fundamental change in the organization of information and energy flow. As we have seen in the example of the man who eventually bought the dog for his children, the alteration in sensitivity to the image of a dog took place at the level of altered specificity of appraisal: The specific appraisal response to both "dog" and "panic" needed to be revised before a new pattern of emotional reaction could be achieved.

Value circuits determine specific appraisal, creating the basic hedonic tone of "this is good" or "this is bad" and the behavioral set of "approach" or "withdraw." Value circuits also continue to assess the meaning of these initial activations as they are elaborated into more defined emotional states, including the categorical emotions. What determines the nature of the appraisal/value process itself? How does the mind "know" what should be paid attention to, what is good or bad, and how to respond with sadness or anger?

For human beings to have survived, this complex appraisal process had to be organized by at least two components. According to the fundamental principles of evolution, the characteristics of those individuals whose genes shaped the appraisal process in a direction that helped the individuals to survive and pass on their genes are more likely to be present today. This is one explanation, for example, of why some people are frightened of snakes though they may never have seen one before. This may also explain why infants have a "hard-wired," inborn system to appraise attachment experiences as important.

A second evolutionarily crucial influence on the appraisal mechanism is that it had to be able to learn from an individual's experience. Individuals who did not learn, for example, that touching a flame hurts would have been more likely to be repeatedly injured and unable to defend themselves, and therefore less likely to survive and pass on their genes. Those individuals whose brains could alter their evaluative mechanisms would have been more likely to survive. Hence, *the appraisal system is also responsive to experience; it learns. Emotional engagement enhances learning.*

Windows of Tolerance

Each of us has a "window of tolerance" in which various intensities of emotional arousal can be processed without disrupting the functioning of the system. For some people, high degrees of intensity feel comfortable and allow them to think, behave, and feel with balance and effectiveness. For others, certain emotions (such as anger or sadness), or all emotions, may be quite disruptive to functioning if they are active in even mild degrees. The intensity of a specific emotional state may involve arousal and appraisal mechanisms outside of awareness. As we've seen, these nonconscious activities of appraisal influence how the brain processes information. *One's thinking or behavior can become disrupted if arousal moves beyond the boundaries of the window of tolerance.* For some persons, this window may be quite narrow. For such individuals, emotional processes may only become conscious when their intensity nears the boundaries of the window and is on the verge of disorganizing the functioning of the system. For others, a wide range of emotion may be both tolerable and available to consciousness—from pleasant emotions including joy, excitement, or love, to unpleasant ones such as anger, sadness, or fear.

The width of the window of tolerance within a given individual may vary, depending upon the state of mind at a given time, the particular emotional valence, and the social context in which the emotion is being generated. For example, we may be more able to tolerate stressful situations when surrounded by loved ones with whom we feel secure and understood. Within the boundaries of the window, the mind continues to function well. Outside these boundaries, function becomes impaired.

At its most basic level this can be understood in terms of the activity of the autonomic nervous system's branches, which will be discussed in detail in the next chapter. Outside the window of tolerance, excessive sympathetic branch activity can lead to increased energy-consuming processes, manifested as increases in heart rate and respiration and as a "pounding" sensation in the head. At the other extreme, excessive parasympathetic branch activity leads to increased energy-conserving processes, manifested as decreases in heart rate and respiration and as a sense of "numbness" and "shutting down" within the mind. Other autonomic combinations are possible, with the most common being simultaneous activation of both branches; this creates the internal sensation of an "explosion" in the head and tension in the body, as if one were driving a car with both the brakes and the accelerator on at the same time. Some individuals refer to such a state as "explosive rage."

Under these conditions, the "higher" cognitive functions of abstract thinking and self-reflection are shut down. The circuits linking these cortical processes with the highly discharging limbic centers are functionally blocked, and rational thought becomes impossible. In states of mind beyond the window of tolerance, the prefrontally mediated capacity for response flexibility is temporarily shut down. The "higher mode" of integrative processing has been replaced by a "lower mode" of reflexive responding. The integrative function of emotion, in which self-regulation permits a flexibly adaptive interaction with the environment, is suspended. We can propose that under such conditions, the dynamical system appears to shift away from the movement toward maximizing complexity by entering into states characterized by either excessive rigidity or randomness. These states are inflexible or chaotic, and as such are not adaptive to the internal or external environment. The mind has entered a suboptimal organizational flow that may reinforce its own maladaptive pattern. This is now a state of emotion dysregulation.

A window of tolerance may be determined both by constitutional features (temperament) and by experiential learning. Present physiological conditions, such as hunger and exhaustion, may also markedly restrict individuals' windows of tolerance and make them more vulnerable to irritability and "emotional outbursts." The example of temperamental differences reveals how windows can be shaped by individuals' constitutional qualities. People with shy temperaments may find emotional intensity of many sorts very uncomfortable, and may seek environments that are familiar to them and that do not evoke such disturbing and disorganizing inner sensations. Within the social context of being with attachment figures with whom they have secure relationships, such individuals may feel safe enough to move toward novel situations. Without such a context, they may withdraw and become socially isolated. For others with more adaptive sensitivities, novelty may be quite pleasurable, evoking a feeling of excitement that is not disruptive to their sense of balance. Familiarity in these bolder individuals may sometimes become quite boring and create an internal sense of restlessness. Children with "easy" temperaments are characterized by such open approaches; on the whole, they make life for their parents less demanding. Those with the more irritable and unpredictable "difficult" temperaments are "moody" and have frequent bursts outside of their windows of tolerance, creating a challenge for many parents. As such children mature, many of them find more sophisticated ways to regulate their emotions, with a subsequent decline in the frequency and intensity with which they break through their windows of tolerance.

Windows of tolerance may also be directly influenced by experiential history. If children have been frightened repeatedly in their early history, fear may become associated with a sense of dread or terror that is disorganizing to their systems. Repeated senses of being out of control—experiencing emotions without a sense of others helping to calm them down—can lead such persons to be unable to soothe themselves as they develop. This lack of self-soothing can lead directly to a narrow window of tolerance. When such a person breaks through that window, the result is a very disorganizing, "out-of-control" sensation, which in itself creates a further state of distress.

A person's present state of mind can also narrow or widen the window of tolerance. Being emotionally worn, physically exhausted, or surprised by an interaction can each narrow the window of tolerance. In such cases, an individual may become "emotionally wrought up" or visibly upset by an encounter; under other conditions, the person's emotions might have merely indicated that something important was occurring.

Let's return to the example of the attorney offered earlier in this chapter. We cannot take the interaction with her colleague out of the temporal and social context in which it occurred. The document the attorney had given her colleague was addressed to one of her most important clients, a woman executive in her late sixties whom the attorney saw as a mother figure. She had always wanted to please this woman, because she felt (as she later revealed in therapy) that her actual mother had never been supportive of her or able to be pleased with her. The colleague's mistake (despite being reminded before the attorney left for a vacation, the colleague failed to mail the document on time, jeopardizing their legal case) created a sensation in the attorney that "yet again" she would be unable to please her mother. In this case, displeasing a mother figure gave the attorney an internal image, a cognitive representation, of herself in relationship to an angry mother. She had experienced as a child, and was now experiencing again as an adult, the state of mind that wanting to please but being unseen creates: shame. What was worse, the mother (and the business client's image, in the attorney's mind) had frequently expressed anger and hostility toward her, creating a sense of both shame and humiliation.

Some might ask how much of this patient's recollection was accurate, and, if it was accurate, how we can distinguish genetic from experiential effects. This patient's memories of these early events were independently supported after the patient entered therapy by the recollections of a cousin who had lived across the street and personally witnessed some of these humiliating interactions. In an even more uncommon type of corroboration, the therapist was able to interview the mother herself, at the request of the daughter.

The mother reflected on these incidents very much as the patient had reported them; she also stated that her own mother had "practiced" such a style of parenting, in order to "harden" her for the "real world." Her treatment of her own daughter, she said, was intentionally a "watered-down version" of the treatment she herself had received. Such single clinical case examples are not the same as research data, but they do offer us an in-depth example of how early experiences of dysregulated dyadic states can be associated with the development of individual dysfunction later in life. Still, "association" does not mean "causation." After all, the mother passed on her genes as well as providing a particular parental experience for her daughter. Having an explosive temper—a form of emotion dysregulation—can certainly be an inherited trait. The mixture of two individuals, mother and daughter, each with a constitutional tendency to break through windows of tolerance might help explain some of this patient's experience. The transgenerational passage of patterns of humiliating parenting could also explain such a finding. In any case, this woman found herself with the reality of dysregulation.

The repeated activation of these configurations of mental representations and a state of mind of shame/humiliation can be seen to have engrained this state as a repeating pattern of neural activation. We could almost say that the activation of this state had become a personality trait. The attorney was prone to entering this state of enraged humiliation at "inappropriate" times. In this manner, she entered an inflexible state that was no longer adaptive and inhibited new behavioral responses in interaction with the social environment. We can view this state as induced by the massive activation of the parasympathetic branch (the sense of not being understood or listened to when the colleague failed to mail the document on time despite a reminder) and the sympathetic branch (the internal state that she was being yelled at by her client and feeling anger toward her colleague) of the attorney's autonomic nervous system. The brakes and accelerator were being applied simultaneously. The car, her mind, could not be regulated. The cues that set her off were rationally related to the earlier states, but the logic of these reasons was of emotional and historical value only. Her colleague and her client couldn't care less about the "meaning" of her frightening rages. She was removed from all of the client's cases immediately after this last incident.

With intensive work during the months following this turning point in her life, the attorney began to become aware of the sadness and profound disappointment she had experienced as a child within her interactions with her mother. She also began to connect the meaning of her present interactions with others with what she (her value system) had learned through these repeated experiences of her childhood. Fortunately for her, this process apparently has allowed her to widen her window of tolerance for various disappointments she continues to encounter in life, as we all do. Her understanding of these layers of response and learning yielded a more flexible manner of relating to others and to herself as an adult.

Recovery Processes

When the intensity of an aroused state moves beyond the window of tolerance, a flood of emotion may bombard the mind and take over a number of processes, ranging from rational thinking to social behavior. At this point, emotions may flood conscious awareness. Some have called this an emotional "hijacking," "breakdown," or "flooding."[36] In such a situation, one's behavior may no longer feel volitional, and thoughts may feel out of control. Images may fill the mind's eye with visual representations symbolic of the emotional sensation. For example, when angry, some people may "see red" or visualize doing harm to the target of their rage. They may lose control of their behavior, performing destructive acts that would not be a part of their behavioral repertoire under "normal" conditions. In this "lower mode" of processing, the state of mind has pushed beyond the window of tolerance.

As we've seen, emotion, meaning, and social interactions are mediated via the same circuitry in the brain. Information in the brain is not handled independently of the biological reality of how the brain is in fact structured. For example, within the convergence zones of one of the central regions of emotional processing, the orbitofrontal cortex, we can see the way in which brain structure shapes mind function. In this neural region, inputs from anatomically distinct areas converge: Neural firing patterns transmitting the "information" from these regions are directly sent to the orbitofrontal cortex. This information includes social cognition, autonoetic consciousness, sensation, perception, various representations such as words and ideas, somatic markers representing the physiological state of the body, and the output of the autonomic nervous system (which allows for "affect regulation" via the balancing of sympathetic and parasympathetic branch activity).[37] As we've discussed earlier, the capacity to respond adaptively to the personal significance of an event, not merely with an automatic reflexive reaction, may require both the capacity for response flexibility as well as its integration with these other prefrontally mediated processes.

In states of excessive arousal, it has been suggested that the "higher" processing of the neocortical circuits is shut down, and that the direction of the energy flow within the brain and especially within the orbitofrontal regions is determined more by input from the "lower" processing centers of the brainstem, sensory circuits, and limbic structures than by input from the cortex. In this way, the beyond-the-window-of-tolerance state of hyperarousal leads, neurologically, to the inhibition of higher perceptions and thoughts in favor of the dominance of more basic somatic and sensory input. In this situation, we don't think; we feel something intensely and act impulsively. What this means is that an individual who enters a state outside the window of tolerance is potentially in a "lower mode" of processing, in which reflexive responses to bodily states and primitive sensory input are more likely to dominate processing.

In the attorney's interaction with her colleague, she went beyond the boundaries of her window and entered a state in which self-reflection, thinking about her emotions, achieving some distance from her reflexive reactions, and considering other options for behavior beyond her immediate impulses were not possible. All of these are thought to be cortical processes that are likely to shut down when a person is emotionally flooded in the state beyond the window. Having this patient learn the boundaries of her window of tolerance—that is, the points at which interactions with others began to generate intense responses in her mind that moved her to the edge of control—was a first step in helping her to try to avoid those "out-of-control" states. Becoming aware of the state of her body (tension in her muscles, tightness in her stomach and throat) and sensing images of anger in her mind were the first stages in her gaining some sense of control over her emotional outbursts. Prevention of the ruptures through the window was the most helpful for her. She also needed to learn techniques for increasing the speed at which she could recover, once she was out of the window.

How does the mind ever recover from this state of suspended cortical processing and thinking about thinking (metacognition)? The recovery process may vary from person to person, again depending on present context, constitution, and personal history. Certain states may be easier to recover from than others; specific contexts may activate a particular cluster of neural net profiles from which it is especially difficult to recover, whereas others may be more readily repaired. For example, if a person feels betrayed by a close friend who has never been suspected of being disloyal, then recovering from a flood of anger and sadness may be particularly difficult. On the other hand, being let down by an acquaintance of dubious reliability may create anger that is relatively easy to bring back into the window of tolerance.

Recovery means decreasing the disorganizing effects of a particular episode of emotional arousal. Recovery may be a primary physiological process in which appraisal mechanisms bring the degree of activation to tolerable levels. This modulation may involve a dampening in the intensity of arousal, as well as a restriction in the distribution of neuronal groups activated within the state of mind at that time. Recovery may also involve the reactivation of the more complex and abstract reasoning that the cortex mediates. This will then allow for the metacognitive processes of self-reflection and impulse control. The capacity to reflect on mental states and to integrate this knowledge about the mind of others and of the self may be important in enabling this aspect of emotion regulation. These reinstated cortical processes in part may help by altering the characteristics of the elaborated emotion and permitting an individual to begin to tolerate levels of arousal that previously would have been flooding. For example, the person engulfed in rage at a close friend may find that activating old memories of the friend and engendering a feeling of loss and sadness may allow the characteristics and intensity of this emotional experience to be transformed. For some, sadness is more easily tolerated than rage.

Some individuals have extreme difficulty recovering from emotional flooding of any sort. For these people, life may become a series of efforts to avoid situations that evoke strong emotional reactions. These avoidance maneuvers are defensive, in that they are attempts to keep the individuals' systems in balance. For those whose windows are quite narrow for certain emotions, such avoidance behaviors can shape the structure of their personalities and their ways of dealing with others and the world. If recovery processes are unavailable, then such individuals become prisoners of their own emotional instability.

Emotions are central in the self-regulation of the mind. It is inevitable that at times emotional arousal will be too much for any of us to tolerate. At these moments, the flood of emotions without an effective recovery process will result in prolonged states of disorganization that are ineffective and potentially harmful to ourselves or to others. Recovery allows us to move back within the boundaries of our windows of tolerance and to "push the envelope" but not to break it. In essence, recovery allows the self-organizational processes of the mind to return the flow of states toward a balance that maximizes complexity, moving the system between the extremes of rigidity on the one side and excessive randomness on the other. The system becomes more adaptive by tuning itself to both internal and external variables in a more flexible manner, thus enhancing complexity, which allows the mind to achieve stability.

How can recovery occur? Looking toward the two fundamental elements of the mind—energy and information—can help us to answer this question. Let's return to the example of the attorney. In her interaction with her colleague at the meeting, she remained in a state of hyperarousal, agitation, and rage, in which her cortical processing was surely suspended. The internal representations of the colleague's deadline error were probably linked, as we've discussed earlier, to the attorney's sense of shame and humiliation from interactions with her mother. "Linked" means that the error created within her a humiliated state of mind, with excessive arousal of both branches of the autonomic nervous system. This familiar state quickly flooded her beyond her window of tolerance. Her higher reflective processes were suspended. She began yelling at the top of her lungs, feeling misunderstood, demeaned, and enraged. Any attempts the colleague might have made to calm her down, she stated in retrospect, were interpreted as his being condescending (like her mother) and further irritated her. For hours after she had yelled at him she remained in a seething, agitated state.

Recovery from that episode was long in coming. As time wore on, she seemed to calm down, but was easily agitated by thoughts of the experience and of the eventual call from her client. As therapy progressed, the therapist and patient began to examine what had occurred in terms of these ideas about windows of tolerance, emotions, memory, and states of mind. She was very motivated at this point to understand how her own mind was "betraying" her. She was eager to change this pattern of emotional outbursts.

Within the sessions, she would again enter these hyperaroused, beyond-the-window states. Now entered the crucial elements of change. Within these states in the therapeutic session, her experience of being "out of control" was joined by the reflective and supportive dialogue with her therapist. She was able to listen in her agitation, but remained hyperaroused. However, she now had two objects for her attention—her internal state and the external dialogue. As time went on, she was able to begin to reflect on the nature of her own mental processes. She could picture her circuits with an excessive flooding of activity; she could notice her tense muscles contributing to the feedback to her mind that she was furious; and she could begin to see how the deadline error meant something to her and her past, beyond what the colleague and the mistake in reality were about.

This woman learned to enhance her recovery processes by learning to use the energy flow and information processing of her mind. Therapy allowed her to experience emotionally flooded states, and *within that state of mind,* she was then able to apply her newly acquired abilities. She could use relaxation and imagery to "lower the energy of her circuits" and the tension in her body. Her metacognitive cortical capacities were strengthened and made more accessible *during her rages* in ways that were not possible before. Such capacities allowed her to use previously inhibited pathways during this state of mind to alter the way she processed information. What had been a blockage in information processing and an inhibition in the flow of energy now became more adaptive states of mind. Her capacity for emotion regulation, and thus for self-regulation, became more flexible and more effective. She could say to herself, "This interaction is more about my feelings of shame than about my colleague," and focus her experience in a different way. The overall result, fortunately, was that in addition to entering these states less often, she learned that she was able to recover from them much more rapidly. The effect was to give her a deeper sense of stability and clarity than she had ever had before. This was just the beginning for this woman. Her next step, of course, was to work on getting new clients and establishing meaningful relationships with others in her life.

Access to Consciousness

As our appraisal mechanisms operate and as our primary emotions are differentiated into categorical ones, our minds are influenced by our value systems in every aspect of their functioning. These influences occur without the necessity of conscious awareness. The idea presented in this book is that emotion is a central set of processes directly related to meaning, social communication, attentional focus and perceptual processing. Emotion is not just some "primitive" remnant of an earlier reptilian evolutionary past. *Emotion directs the flow of activation (energy) and establishes the meaning of representations (information processing) for the individual.* It is not a single, isolated group of processes; it has a direct impact on the entire mind. By defining emotion in this way, we can begin to make sense of the wide range of interpretations of research findings on emotion, thinking, and social processes. Discussing the relationship of emotion to consciousness provides a useful opportunity to delineate our ideas about emotion further.

Huge amounts of evidence support the view that the "conscious self" is in fact a very small portion of the mind's activity.[38] Perception, abstract cognition, emotional processes, memory, and social interaction all appear to proceed to a great extent without the involvement of consciousness. Most of the mind is nonconscious. These "out-of-awareness" processes do not appear to be in opposition to consciousness or to anything else; they create the foundation for the mind in social interactions, internal processing, and even conscious awareness itself. Nonconscious processing influences our behaviors, feelings, and thoughts. Nonconscious processes impinge on our conscious minds: we experience sudden intrusions of elaborated thought processes (as in "Aha!" experiences) or emotional reactions (as in crying before we are aware that we are experiencing a sense of sadness). So we can say that for the most part, the self is not divided by some line between a conscious and a nonconscious self. Rather, the self is created by nonconscious processes, as well as by the selective associations of these processes into something we call "consciousness." To put it another way, we are much, much more than our conscious processes.

But then what do the "associations" of certain processes, such as perceptions or thoughts, with the phenomenon of consciousness do? What does it mean to have consciousness? Why do we even have consciousness at all? One answer to these questions, among many possibilities, is that *when processes become linked within consciousness, they can be more strategically and intentionally manipulated, and the outcome of their processing can be adaptively altered.* Consciousness may allow us to become free from reflexive processing and introduce some aspect of "choice" into our behavior. For example, by making a worry about who sits where at a wedding into a conscious concern rather than a nonconscious fret, a soon-to-be-married man can raise the issue with his fiancée, and then they can examine the options together; they can add new information and consider alternatives to decisions, which then can result in the selection of what may prove to be a more satisfactory seating arrangement. In this manner, a process made conscious can be directly shared across individuals, and the outcome can be strategically altered. The strategic manipulation, the introduction of choice, and the sharing of information are made possible by consciousness. If the groom is unable to be conscious of the meaning of his sensations of discomfort or thoughts about the wedding, it is likely that he will not bring up the issue for examination. What is a neuroscientific explanation for how this occurs?

Consciousness is important for focal attention and working memory, which allow information to be processed into long-term, explicit memory storage. As noted throughout this book, working memory is considered the "chalkboard of the mind"; it allows us the ability to reflect on several (seven, plus or minus two) items simultaneously. Such reflection allows us to manipulate these representations, to process them (for example, to note similarities and differences, create generalizations, and recognize patterns), and to create new associations among them. Working memory allows self-reflection and creates cognitive "choice." In other words, it introduces the possibility of personal intention and strategic, deliberate behaviors that are independent of automatic reflexes.

At the most fundamental level, we have discussed that consciousness involves the selective linkage or binding of representations, which then can be intentionally manipulated within working memory. The idea of intention is itself a philosophical puzzle. What we can say is that with consciousness, new information can be introduced or new manipulations can be attempted within the mind for a strategic purpose that is determined by the individual. Consciousness itself is not necessary for information processing, but it is necessary at times to achieve new outcomes in such processing.

From this vantage point, we can say that emotional processing—the initial orientation, appraisal, arousal, and differentiation mechanisms—usually occurs without consciousness. An individual's consciousness of these processes allows for the qualitative sensation of emotion, experienced as a sense of energy, meaning, and categorical emotion. Any and all of these sensations can be called a "feeling," which explains why people of many different ages respond with a range of reactions to the common query of "How are you feeling?" "I feel ... up ... down ... excited ... that this means the end of our relationship ... like I want to run and hide ... that he didn't understand my intentions ... that I am bad ... sad ... angry ... happy." "Feelings" can therefore involve energy, meaning, behavioral impulses, or the discrete categories of emotion. Why do emotional processes enter consciousness? What information processing does this permit?

The ability to involve conscious processing with something as fundamental as the creation of meaning, social relatedness and perceptual processing certainly does give the individual an increase in the flexibility of response to the environment. Having a consciousness of emotions is especially important in the social environment. Without it, we are likely not to be aware of our own or others' intentions and motives. Awareness of emotional processes has value for our survival as a social species: We can know our own minds as well as those of others, and can negotiate the complex interpersonal world with increased skill and effectiveness at meeting our needs.

Recall that consciousness may involve an integration of distributed neuronal activities that achieves a certain degree of complexity.[39] Effective processing within consciousness can thus be seen as the furthering of such an integrative process. Consciousness is more than the mere activation of representations in working memory that have become linked via the thalamocortical system and the lateral prefrontal cortex. Active, executive functions that direct the integrated flow of energy and information—possibly mediated also by nearby regions such as the orbitofrontal cortex and anterior cingulate—play an important role in the coordination of mental processes and response.[40] For example, Nobre and colleagues suggest that recent findings regarding the orbitofrontal cortex indicate that its activity may be important in "inhibiting prepared motor programs" and in "the tasks of motor selection and preparation requiring withholding of responses. The orbitofrontal cortex participates both in the redirection of the response based upon a violation in stimulus contingencies and in possible changes of emotional state. ... Activity in the orbitofrontal region is recruited as stimulus contingencies change, interacting dynamically with the basic neural–cognitive system that directs attention. The anatomical connections of the lateral orbitofrontal cortex support this ability."[41] Earlier we have called such a capacity "response flexibility" and have suggested that such a process may be an important element in self-regulation

and in the behavioral and attentional flexibility seen in the contingent, collaborative communication and coherent adult narratives
revealed in secure attachments.

What role does consciousness itself play in the regulation of
emotion? *Consciousness can influence the outcome of emotional processing.* Conscious awareness allows for self-reflection, which can
enable the mobilization of strategic thoughts and behaviors and can
therefore enhance the flexible achievement of goals. This can be seen
as the achievement of new levels of integration. For example, if a
person realizes that she is feeling sad about a friend who has left
town, she can then write or call that person and reestablish contact.
If, instead, her sadness remains nonconscious, she may never reach
out to her friend in this way. Given the fundamental role of the
appraisal system in distinguishing what is good and should be
approached from what is bad and should be avoided, emotions being
accessible to parts of cognition that can consciously mobilize behavior can be crucial in having emotion be effective in certain adaptive
ways as a value system. Consciousness allows emotion to play a
more adaptive role in the individual's behavior. But how does it help
regulate emotion?

Let's return to the example of the attorney in psychotherapy to
illustrate how consciousness can permit two fundamental elements of
emotion regulation: the modulation of the flow of activation or
energy through the brain, and the adaptive modification of information processing. After her "explosion" with her colleague and her
dismissal from the case, the attorney's motivation to understand her
social difficulties reached a peak. Though she had had a number of
brief encounters with therapists in the past, this was the first time she
felt driven to examine what role she was playing in these difficulties.
Earlier, she had focused on how troubled the world and other people
were. For the first time, she now became consciously aware of the
possibility that the source of her difficulties was within her own
mind.

Such a change in attitude was itself quite an accomplishment; in
this woman's case, it was brought about by "hitting bottom" with
her job. This new openness was a window of opportunity for therapy to provide her with some new tools. In the therapy sessions,
therapist and patient began a dialogue in which they examined the
patient's memories of experiences in both the recent and distant past.
The patient was also coached to reflect in the present on her own
internal processes—in other words, to begin the development of her

metacognitive abilities. The therapist strongly encouraged this self-reflection, knowing that it would be an essential tool for the patient to learn in order to regulate her emotions. Metacognition gives the developing minds of children (and adults) the ability to perform a number of unique processes: thinking about thinking itself; forming a representation of one's own mind; becoming aware of sensations, images, and beliefs about the self; and reflecting on the nature of emotion and perception.[42]

In formal terms, the mind develops the metacognitive capacity for the "appearance–reality distinction," which allows an individual to comprehend that what something looks like may be different from what it actually is in the world.[43] The notions that one's perceptions and ideas can change over time, and can be distinct from the equally valid ones of other people, are called "representational change" and "diversity," respectively. Metacognition also includes the awareness that emotion influences thought and perception, and that one may be able to experience two seemingly conflictual emotions about the same person or experience. Each of these areas became vital for this patient to develop a more adaptive capacity for emotion regulation.

These metacognitive abilities often, but not necessarily, involve consciousness. In this patient's case, her lack of metacognition required that it become a part of the focus of the therapeutic dialogue; its not being an innate ability at this point in her development also necessitated that she make it a conscious part of her processing of intense emotions. With time, these new capacities, which had to be initiated intentionally and with mental effort, might become more automatic for her and might not require as much exertion of conscious effort.

Before therapy, this patient's orientation, appraisal–arousal, and differentiation processes were often out of her conscious awareness. At some point, her rage became expressed externally as her screaming. Internally, she might first become aware of her emotional state through a burning sensation in her head and an intense focus of her attention on the "evil" of the person with whom she was interacting. Her consciousness was linked to the elements of emotional processing only when they burst through her window of tolerance in the form of uncontrolled fury and perceptual distortions filled with suspicion. In this state, she literally viewed others as "out to get her." Some might say that she was projecting her anger onto others. Another view might be that she was entering a state of shame and humiliation in which she was implicitly recalling an angry and

betraying mother. Whatever the explanation, her conscious awareness began at a time when self-reflection was impossible in such a
state of rage. Recall that in states of excessive arousal, higher cognitive functions, including metacognition, are shut down. The key to
this woman's development was to bring such "lower mode" states
into a more balanced modulation. Conscious awareness of emotional
processes is always a beginning; in this case, metacognitive reflection
on these processes was essential to enhance response flexibility and
self-regulation.

Therapy includes various aspects of an attachment relationship,
as well as the co-construction of stories, bearing witness, teaching,
and role modeling for patients. Each of these was essential in taking
the next step with this frightened individual. Giving her a conceptual
framework for how her emotions worked and influenced her experience of herself and interactions with others was vital in allowing her
not to feel "accused" of being defective. The shame state involves a
sense that something is wrong with the individual, and this emotion
is often at the root of why patients have not developed the ability to
reflect on their own contribution to their troubles. They may have an
inner belief that they are defective, and they seek to hide from revealing this "truth" to others.

As therapy permitted the patient to tell the story of her life, the
therapist could bear witness to the pain and vulnerability of her having been a child in a hostile family world. Making the link of these
emotional experiences to her present encounters, both with people in
her daily life and with the therapist himself, allowed the patient to
experience firsthand these emotional processes at work. She became
sensitive to the subtle sensations of primary emotions long before
they were elaborated into the categorical states that so often burst
through her window of tolerance. These primary sensations allowed
her to become aware of what was arousing to her ("This interaction
now has some meaning for me—watch out!"). They also permitted
her to reflect on how the specific meaning of an interaction had the
dual layers of her appraisal of its significance in the moment ("What
is happening now with this person?") and its parallel to historical
meanings for her ("How does this relate to my emotional issues from
the past?"). The important step for her was to associate primary
emotions with consciousness.

At first she continued to have outbursts, but these were less
intense and less frequent, and it seemed easier to recover from them.
Her feeling of success at actually stopping such an outburst was

exhilarating. This allowed her to consciously alter her bodily response by reducing the somatic marker feedback that was automatically reinforcing the cascading cycle of appraisal and arousal. This clearly allowed her to alter the flow of activation (energy) through her mind.

Simultaneously, she began a metacognitive analysis of the meaning of these interactions and emotional experiences. She could recognize that something "significant" was occurring, and was then able to connect (that is, to note similarities and to work with generalizations within working memory) the recurring themes of being ignored or misunderstood with her prior history of shaming and humiliating interactions with her mother. She was then able to examine the meaning of a representation (for example, the interaction with her colleague was associated with shame) and compare it to those from the past (her interactions with her mother had been humiliating and shameful). Such a nonconscious linkage in the past had created an explosion. Now, with conscious reflection, the same comparison permitted the outcome to be quite different: She altered the appraisal process to highlight a different aspect of the meaning of these representations. Previously, her mind would have nonconsciously noted the similarity in the interaction and created a state of humiliation and outburst. This was an automatic component of the Hebbian synaptic memory process, in which past states were reactivated by similar retrieval cues. Now, consciously, she was able to add the dimension of metacognition. This allowed her to state to herself, "I am becoming agitated because of the similarity of this interaction to my earlier ones, filled with feelings of shame. I am not a slave to the past, and I do not have to react in a similar way." Instead of the nonconscious, reflexive response, consciousness permitted response flexibility and a more adaptive reaction. By acquiring the ability to reflect on the relationships among past, present, and future, this patient was developing her capacity for autonoetic consciousness. She could choose not to become explosive. She could decide that what was best for her was to alter her initial impulses and try to achieve her professional goals in a more productive manner.

Appraisal processes, operating even without consciousness, recruit new neuronal groups into their active state of mind. The addition of consciousness to such a recruitment effort permits further mobilization of a new set of processes: Consciousness allows for the manipulation of representations in new combinations within working memory, the chalkboard of the mind. Consciousness involving the linguistic system and autonoesis allows for reflections on the past and future, moving us beyond the lived moment.[44] We are also able to be motivated by our awareness of emotions, which then facilitates more strategically focused achievements that are not likely without the involvement of consciousness.

External Expression

From the beginning of life, emotion constitutes both the process and the content of communication between infant and caregiver. Simply put, a baby's inner state is perceived by parents, who in turn feel in a parallel manner themselves. The baby perceives the parents' contingent response, and the affect is mutually attuned. Later, in addition, parents use words to talk about feelings and direct a shared attention to the infant's state of mind. The parents may state directly that the baby is feeling sad or happy or scared, giving the infant the interactive verbal experience of being able both to identify and to share an emotional experience. This earliest form of communication in a setting of safety and comfort provides the child with a sense that her emotional life can be shared and be a source of soothing from others.

By the second year of life, the infant has learned the adaptive behavior of not showing how she might be feeling. The social context in which an intense emotion is experienced may motivate the child to "hide" her inner experience. For example, if the toddler wants something but has learned that she will be yelled at if she shows an interest in that object, it will be best if she keeps a "poker face" and does not show an affect that reveals her true emotion. For us adults, complex social situations repeatedly teach us the essential ability to mask our inner states from the criticism and harsh reactions from others. Culture and family environments play a central role in a child's experiential acquisition of these often unspoken laws of emotional expression, called "display rules."[45]

Studies of children and adults of various cultures demonstrate that people may show emotions quite differently if they are with unfamiliar people or if they are by themselves. For example, one study showed that in the Japanese culture, facial expression showing emotional response to a stimulating film was quite evident if a subject believed that he was alone in the room. With the experimenter present, facial expression was quite flat.[46] If display rules tell people not to show emotion, does this affect how conscious they may become of their own emotional response? This may in fact be the case: We use our own facial responses to become aware of how we are feeling. This fits in with the general view that the brain has a representation of the body's state, including states of arousal, muscle tension, and facial expression, which it uses as information to register "how it feels."[47]

The self is capable of at least two contextual states: a private, inner, core self and a public, external, adaptive self.[48] Some authors have used the parallel notions of a "true" and a "false" self. This terminology, however, suggests that it is somehow false to adapt to social requirements; instead, it may be more useful to accept that different contexts evoke different states in each of us. Repeated patterns of social interactions can make a specific state, such as the masking of internal emotions from the outer world, an important adaptation. There is nothing "false" about a mechanism of survival. However, if the brain often relies on the expression of emotion as a signpost of what the individual truly feels, then this masking process certainly can create a challenge to knowing one's "true" response.

The regulation of emotional expression may assist the mind in modulating its states of arousal by social and intrapsychic mechanisms. Socially, masking internal states can permit the individual to avoid an experience of interpersonal resonance, in which the contingent response of the receiver can alter the initial state of the sender. Masking inner states can also enable an individual to avoid being misunderstood, in which case the painful state of shame would be induced. Within the individual, regulating affect can dampen the positive feedback loop in which an internal state is expressed externally as facial expressions and bodily responses, which then are perceived by the mind and heighten the initial emotional state. In both the individual and social feedback processes, regulating external expression of an internal state can help to keep the state of arousal from breaking through the window of tolerance.

A very difficult situation arises when an aspect of this form of emotional modulation, the inflexible and "nonexpressive" regulation of affect, is so engrained that it becomes a rigidly and repeatedly evoked state, or trait, of the individual. If there are no contexts available in a growing child's life when the inner, private self can be fully engaged in interactions with others, then the adaptive, external, public self may perpetually mask internal states even from the individual.

This condition may be experienced by the person as a sense of not knowing who she is. There may be a feeling that life is meaningless. In emotional terms, this person's access to awareness of her own emotions has been repeatedly blocked.

The danger of chronically blocking general affective expression is that it may also repeatedly inhibit the access of emotions to an individual's consciousness. The mechanism to block expression is unknown, but perhaps involves a temporary shutting down of the circuits that control affective expression. As we've seen, these appear to be primarily located in the right hemisphere, especially in the orbitofrontal cortex and the amygdala. Individuals with right-hemisphere lesions, for example, may have a reduced ability to perceive others' emotions, as well as to express and gain conscious access to their own. Furthermore, imaging studies of depressed individuals (who show reduced facial expression) have revealed a functional blockage in the activation of right-hemisphere facial perception centers.[49] The implication here is that the expression and perception of facial affect may be neurologically linked processes.

People vary widely in their ability to express affect. One way to can begin to make sense of these variations is to conceptualize nonverbal signals as the external expressions of internal states of mind. Primary emotions are expressed as the vitality affects described as the profiles of activation, including "crescendo" (increasing energy) and "decrescendo" (decreasing energy) states. A person reveals such vitality states in facial expression, tone of voice, activity of the limbs, gestures, and the timing and fluidity of these signals in interactions with another person. These signals may enter one's own awareness, and may also directly influence the adjustment of one's own state to that of the other person. Becoming aware of both the external signals from another person and those being given off by oneself can be crucial. Reflection on internal sensations may be an essential aid in knowing how another person may be feeling.

"Feeling felt" may be an essential ingredient in attachment relationships. Having the sense that someone else feels one's feelings and is able to respond contingently to one's communication may be vital to close relationships of all sorts throughout the lifespan. Such attachments foster the interactive sharing of states, which facilitates the amplification of positive, enjoyable emotions and the diminution of negative, uncomfortable emotions. The attuned communication within attachment relationships allows such interactive amplification and diminution to occur. The outcome is that each member of the pair may "feel felt" by the other. For the developing child, the secure attachment relationship provides the amplification that heightens pleasurable states and allows the child to engage in the self-regulation needed to diminish unpleasurable ones.

The challenge of communicating internal states may be a bit less demanding when it comes to the expression of categorical emotions. These more elaborated states of activation, with their cross-culturally similar patterns of expression that are probably embedded within the physiological response patterns of the brain, seem to involve a different form of communication. The studies cited above suggest that some aspects of categorical affect are mediated by social display rules. People sometimes mask certain intense feelings in the presence of strangers; in other situations, people only reveal certain responses (such as smiling or laughing) in the presence of others. These findings, combined with the developmental acquisition of masking categorical affects, support the social communication aspect of this form of emotion. The sharing of these states has a more "distant" quality and can involve more of the classic sense of empathy as a state of understanding another's experience rather than feeling another's feelings. We can feel sad when other persons feel sad, and we can rejoice in their excitement and joy. In this way, categorical affects can certainly be shared as well. But categorical emotions allow us to become more actively verbal within the communication with others. That is, we can use words with roughly shared definitions to encapsulate the shared experience: "It must have been so sad to have that happen," or "It is great to see you feel so excited about that event." In this way, the expression of a categorical emotion permits more linguistic distance from a shared moment in a relationship than the "feeling felt" of a primary emotional state alone.

Of course, categorical expressions are usually accompanied by all the undefinable nonverbal signals of vitality affects that are reflections of the ongoing primary emotional processes. But the point here is that the perception of a classic categorical affect, such as anger, sadness or fear, often overshadows the less classifiable and often more "subtle" aspects of vitality affects. The "risk" of a predominantly categorical emotional communication is that one may begin to use only one's intellect in classifying what this particular emotional experience means, rather than attending to the unique meaning of that moment, both for the other person and for the relationship itself.

REFLECTIONS: EMOTION REGULATION AND THE MIND

The capacity to regulate the appraisal and arousal processes of the mind is fundamental to self-organization; therefore, emotion regulation is at the core of the self. The acquisition of self-regulation emerges from dyadic relationships early in life. Attachment studies suggest that the type of interpersonal communication that facilitates autonomous self-regulation begins with healthy dependence. Such relationships involve sensitivity to the child's signals, contingent communication, and reflective dialogue that permits the child to develop coherence and mentalizing capacities. Achieving self-organization occurs within emotionally attuned interpersonal experiences. At the emotional core of attachment relationships are the amplification of shared positive states and the reduction of negative affective states. As these dyadic states are experienced, the child comes to tolerate wider bands of emotional intensity and shared affective communication.

A proposed model of emotion regulation includes seven elements: intensity, sensitivity, specificity, windows of tolerance, recovery processes, access to consciousness, and external expression. As we've seen, early attachment experiences and constitutional variables such as temperament help form these emotion regulation processes. "Epigenetic" factors—especially the social experiences that shape genetic expression and the experience-dependent maturation of the brain—directly influence how neuronal connections are established. In early childhood, such epigenetic attachment experiences create the neuronal pathways responsible for emotional modulation. Continuing emotional development within adult relationships can utilize the same attachment elements in helping to develop new paths to self-organization.

Lack of mental well-being may often be a result of emotion dysregulation. This may be experienced as abrupt ruptures of emotion through the window of tolerance, such as episodes of rage or sadness, from which it is difficult to recover. In these ruptured states, the mind loses its capacity for rational thinking, response flexibility, and self-reflection. Waves of intense arousal and sensations of "out-of-control" emotion such as anger or terror may flood the mind. In these states, the individual is both internally and interpersonally unable to function. Helping such an individual requires the development of a more effective self-organizational process. Metacognitive processes and mentalizing reflective functions may be important in the development of an integrative mode of processing, which is essential to achieve a more flexible and coherent experience.

If constitutional features, traumatic experiences, or severely suboptimal attachments have produced maladaptive emotion regulation, then individuals may be restricted in their ability to achieve emotional resilience and behavioral flexibility. In some situations, a form of "cortical override" mechanism may be useful. If there has been excessive parcellation (pruning) of corticolimbic structures, then the brain's ability to modulate states of arousal may be quite compromised. Learning to use neocortical reasoning abilities to observe and then intervene in reflexive initial dysregulatory responses is often a helpful approach. What does this mean? When people move beyond their windows of tolerance, they lose the capacity to think rationally. This initial response may be difficult to alter if it is engrained within deep circuits, such as those encoded early in life in the amygdala. However, the neocortex can override these responses and bring the deeper structures into a more tolerable level of arousal. This can be accomplished by any number of "self-talk" strategies in which imagery, internal dialogue and evocative memory (for example, evoking the soothing image of an attachment figure) can be activated. Over time and with continued practice, the frequency and intensity of breakthroughs into the "lower mode" of reflexive states beyond the window of tolerance can be significantly decreased, and the speed of recovery can be greatly enhanced.

Why is self-regulation seen as fundamentally emotion regulation? Emotion, as a series of integrating processes in the mind, links all layers of functioning. In fact, the study of emotion itself is essentially the study of emotion regulation. Though emotion can be defined as a subjective experience involving neurobiological, experiential, and behavioral components, it is "in fact" the essence of mind. "Emotional communication" is also the fundamental manner in which one mind connects with another. Early in life, the patterns of interpersonal communication we have with attachment figures directly influence the growth of the brain structures that mediate self-regulation.

CHAPTER 8

⌐⌐

Interpersonal Connection

This chapter explores more fully what is known about how the relationship between parent and child enables the child's brain to develop the circuits responsible for healthy emotion regulation. The intention here is not to imply that all or even most individuals' troubles with self-regulation stem from attachment difficulties. Instead, the aim is to review how what is known about the emotional communication inherent in attachment can guide us to understand the nature of emotion regulation within interpersonal relationships. Such an exploration allows us to look more deeply into the ways in which one mind directly shapes the development and function of another— the essence of interpersonal connection.

How can one mind influence another in this way? By viewing the substance of the mind as composed of the flow of information and energy, we can envision the complex neural systems from which it emanates as involving various dimensions: the parts of a single neuron, neurons in synaptic connections, groups of neurons organized within specific circuits, or systems such as the left or right hemisphere of the brain. The patterns of flow of information and energy through such systems allows them to form more and more complex layers of systems. But how can the system of one mind directly interface with that of another to create a "supersystem"? Just as we can receive information in various forms—from oral to written to digitally transmitted via facsimile or electronic mail—so too can the energy and information of the mind be relayed via means including the electric action potentials of single neuronal axons, the patterned release of neurotransmitters, the physiological neuroendocrine milieu, and the complex neuronal activation of a neural net profile.

The linking of minds occurs via different modalities of the transfer of energy and information. The physical proximity of one individual to another has direct effects that may serve as "hidden regulators" conveying, for example, warmth and tactile stimulation.[1] Touch may be an extremely important part of parent–child relationships.[2] Some studies suggest that close physical proximity also directly shapes the electrical activity of each individual's brain.[3] But even at a physical distance, one mind can directly influence the activity—and development—of another through the transfer of energy and information. This joining process occurs via both verbal and nonverbal behavioral responses, which function as signals sent from one mind to another. Both words and the prosodic, nonverbal components of speech contain information that creates representational processes within the mind of the receiver. Other nonverbal signals, including facial expression, tone of voice, gestures, and timing of response, have a direct impact on the socially sensitive value centers of the brain. The expression of these emotional elements of social signals serves to activate the very neuronal circuits that mediate the receiver's emotional response: orienting attention, appraising meaning, and creating arousal. This emotional engagement with another person creates a cascade of elaborated and differentiated appraisal–arousal processes, which serve to direct the flow of energy and information processing within one's own brain. It is in this manner that the emotional state of the sender directly shapes that of the receiver. In complexity terms, such "external constraints" as the signals sent from another person have a powerful and immediate effect on the trajectory or flow of one's own states of mind.

As we'll explore in this chapter, childhood patterns in the transfer of energy and information between minds can create organized strategies in relationships, which are revealed within characteristic behavioral responses in attachment-related situations. The minds of children learn to adapt specifically to the emotional communication they receive from their caregivers. Over time, such relationship-dependent patterns may become engrained as strategies that are employed in more general contexts. Aspects of children's emotion regulation (such as adaptation to stress), cognitive processes (as in memory and attention), and social competence (including peer interactions) have been related to attachment history.[4] In adults, one may see characteristic approaches to interpersonal intimacy and autobiographical narrative organization that reflect the development of this experiential learning into generalized states of mind with respect to attachment.

ATTACHMENT AND EMOTION REGULATION

Given the important role of emotions in creating meaning, it is understandable why the biological system that helps organize the self is so crucial in determining our subjective experiences in life. The view that has been proposed earlier, and that is explored further here, is that human emotions constitute the fundamental value system the brain uses to help organize its functioning. The regulation of emotions is thus the essence of self-organization. The communication with and about emotions between parent and infant directly shapes the child's ability to organize the self.

Allan Schore's work on affect regulation provides an extensive review of the neurobiology of emotional development.[5] This section highlights some of Schore's views and integrates them with the framework for emotion regulation proposed in Chapter 7. Children need to be able to regulate their bodily and mental states. They respond directly to their parents' neural activation patterns through the processes of emotional communication and the alignment of states of mind. A child's response to a parent's patterns can be described as the child's "internalization" of the parent. From a basic biological perspective, the child's neuronal system—the structure and function of the developing brain—is shaped by the parent's more mature brain. This occurs within emotional communication. The attunement of emotional states provides the joining that is essential for the developing brain to acquire the capacity to organize itself more autonomously as the child matures.

Reaching out from the brain to the body proper, the autonomic nervous system helps to control the body's state of arousal. This system can induce excitatory, arousing, energy-consuming bodily states, which are produced by the activation of one of its two branches, called the "sympathetic branch." Examples of physiological responses to the sympathetic branch are increases in heart rate, respiration, sweating, and states of alertness. The autonomic nervous system also includes an inhibitory, de-arousing, energy-conserving portion called the "parasympathetic branch." The parasympathetic branch mediates responses such as decreases in heart rate, respiration, and states of alertness to the outside world.[6]

The sympathetic branch's development predominates during the first year of life. The parasympathetic branch comes on-line during the second year. This timing is helpful because as the infant becomes ambulatory, it is important to have some way in which the primary emotional states mediated by the sympathetic branch—interest/ excitement and enjoyment/joy—can be modulated in order to inhibit potentially dangerous behaviors.[7] The sharing and amplification of these positive emotional states, so common during infancy, can be seen as a resonance of the sympathetic branch activity of the two individuals. These upbeat states are a major part of the emotional communication between infant and parent during the first year of life. By the second year, when a child becomes able to walk, prohibitions from the parent must be able to inhibit such activating emotional states in order for the child to remain safe. The baby must learn to stop moving in the face of danger. For example, if a child is climbing up the stairs, it is useful to have him learn what "No!" means: "Do not do that; stop what you are now doing." Before the first birthday, most parental communications are alignments with the aroused, positive emotional states. After that time, inhibitory comments from the parent become more prominent.

How does the need for contingent communication—for the alignment of states of mind between parent and child—influence the nature of parental behavior and prohibitions? How can these alignments occur if the child is learning that the parent may not share his excitement about doing something? Navigating this balance in needs between mental state alignment and parental prohibitions is one aspect of how the child acquires a healthy capacity for self-regulation. Let's look at one view of the biology of this process.

Schore has described shame as the emotion evoked when a child's aroused state is not attuned to by the parent.[8] Shame in certain degrees is actually an essential emotion for children to experience in order to begin to learn to self-regulate their state of mind and behavioral impulses. However, Alan Sroufe has noted that although this form of shame is inevitable and necessary, parents do not need to use shame intentionally as a strategic form of parenting.[9] Shame is thought to be based on the activation of the parasympathetic system (to an external "No!") in the face of a highly charged sympathetic system (an internal "Let's go!"). It's as if the accelerator pedal (the sympathetic branch) is pressed down and then the brake (the para-sympathetic branch) is applied.

Not connecting with a child's active bid for attunement has been proposed by Schore to lead to shame.[10] These types of transactions are necessary for a child to learn self-control and then to modulate both behavior and internal emotional states in prosocial ways. Shame, in this very specific sense, is not damaging. Emotional states emerge from the patterns of changes in states of activation. Parasympathetic states alone do not produce the feeling of shame. *Shame requires the dynamic profile of high sympathetic tone (a "crescendo" state) followed by onset of the parasympathetic system (a "decrescendo" state).* Shame is different from humiliation. Shame-inducing interactions coupled with sustained parental anger and/or lack of repair of the disconnection lead to humiliation, which Schore has proposed to be toxic to the developing child's brain.[11]

The orbitofrontal cortex—the part of the brain just behind the eyes and located at a strategic spot at the top of the emotional limbic system, next to the "higher" associational cortex responsible for various forms of thought and consciousness—plays an important role in affect regulation.[12] This area of the brain is especially sensitive to face-to-face communication and eye contact. Because it serves as an important center of appraisal, it has a direct influence on the elaboration of states of arousal into various types of emotional experience. Schore's detailed conceptualization of this region's role in attachment relationships helps describe the steps involved between emotional attunement and affect regulation.

A brief word on terms may be useful at this point. Researchers have used the term "affect attunement" to refer to the ways in which internal emotional states are brought into external communication with each other within infant–caregiver interactions.[13] Schore uses the term "attunement" in this manner, highlighting the importance of this communication in the interactive experiences upon which the brain's development depends. He and others have suggested that what are attuned are psychobiological states in both members of the interacting pair.[14] In this book, I am suggesting two related terms, "alignment" and "resonance." Alignment is one component of affect attunement, in which the state of one individual is altered to approximate that of the other member of the dyad. Alignment can be primarily a one-way process, in which one individual's state changes to match and anticipate that of the other; or it can be a bilateral process, involving movement by each member of the dyad. As an example of the former, imagine that a parent is preparing an excited child to get ready to go to sleep. The parent is likely to be more successful if he gets closer to the child's state and then brings the child "down" to a calmer state than if he simply expects the child to calm down suddenly on her own. Such an initial alignment allows the child to feel that she is being attuned to by the parent, and then the mutual change into a calmer state will be more readily achieved. Such alignments occur frequently, but of necessity they cannot occur all the time. Attunement requires times when individuals are in non-alignment—when they are not directly attempting to match or anticipate each other's states. In this way, attunement is a broader concept than alignment: It includes sensitivity to times when alignment should not occur.

The overall process of attunement leads to the mutual influence of each member upon the other—a characteristic described earlier in the book as "resonance." Emotional resonance, for example, involves more than the alignment of states; it also includes the ways in which the interaction affects the individuals in other aspects of their minds. Resonance also continues after alignment has stopped. The mutual influence of the alignment of states persists within the mind of each member after direct interaction no longer occurs. Attunement yields moments of both alignment and nonalignment, and it also permits emotional resonance to occur between two people even after they are no longer in direct communication.

The effects of attachment relationships and the process of attunement on the mind have been postulated by Schore to have direct impacts upon the orbitofrontal cortex.[15] The orbitofrontal cortex can facilitate the regulation of bodily arousal by pushing down a kind of emotional "clutch" that disengages the sympathetic "accelerator" and activates the parasympathetic "brakes." The parasympathetic system is later deactivated with realignment, and the proper adjusted or regulated level of arousal is established through reactivation of the sympathetic system. In other words, the brakes are applied with the disconnection; the repair process allows the child's energies to be redirected, and then the accelerator is applied again with resumption of the emotional connection during the repair process. The child essentially learns this: "My parents may not like what I am doing, but if I change my activities they will then connect with me; things in the end will be OK." There is a balance between the accelerator and the brakes. This is the essence of affect regulation.

The band of tolerable levels of activation of the autonomic

nervous system—of either the sympathetic or parasympathetic branches—may vary widely among individuals. Movements beyond this window of tolerance, in either the sympathetic or parasympathetic branch direction, may be accompanied by diminished ability to function in an adaptive and flexible manner. Neither excessive, nonregulated arousal (sympathetic activity) nor excessive inhibition (parasympathetic activation) is healthy for the development or the ongoing functioning of the brain.

Parenting Approaches

Children challenge parents continually. How parents respond will set the tone of their interactions and will shape the development of their children's capacity to regulate their states of mind and shifts in emotions. Take, for example, a fourteen-month-old boy who wants to climb onto a table with a lamp on it. One possible parental response would be to yell "No!" and then take the boy outside, where his drive to climb can be "attuned to." Another response would be not to notice the attempt to climb, to hear the lamp come crashing down, to pick it up, and either to tell the boy quietly not to do it again or just to ignore him the rest of the evening. A third response would be for the parent to yell "No!" and reprimand the boy, hug him out of guilt, then distance herself from him because he has disappointed her. A fourth approach would be to become enraged and throw the lamp to the floor next to the boy, to teach him never to do that again. Which attachment pattern would be associated with each form of prohibition/disconnection and repair? Think of how the child over time would learn to regulate his baseline emotional state as well as his aroused state in each case, if each pattern of interaction were to be repeated many times. These four parental responses would be associated with the attachment patterns of security, avoidance, ambivalence, and disorganization, respectively.

Security

The first year of life is filled with the attunement of infant and attachment figure, which often centers around the upbeat, high-vitality affects of interest/excitement and enjoyment/joy. The sympathetic system is being activated and developed at a high level during this period. Children who become securely attached to their parents are likely to have a good baseline autonomic tone. They are capable of tolerating high-intensity emotional states. Specifically, if a pattern of attunement like the first one described above is chronically repeated, the securely attached child will experience an aroused state (excited about climbing) that is responded to by the parent with a prohibition (inducing parasympathetic activation and a sense of shame), rapidly followed by a repair (attuning to the gist of the initial aroused state and redirecting it in socially acceptable ways). This child's orbitofrontal cortex "learns" that even high-arousal states (in need of connection) can be modified, and *then* connection will be reestablished. We can propose that such connection–disconnection–repair transactions are one means by which patterns of parent–child communication promote the prefrontally mediated capacity for response flexibility.

Avoidance

The avoidantly attached child is not so fortunate and learns little about the emotional state of the parent, with no warning about the parental response, which in fact may be quite uninvolved (neglectful) or severe and misattuned (rejecting). In such a dyad, it is likely that the general level of shared emotion is quite low, possibly resulting in an underdevelopment of the child's capacity for normal levels of interest/excitement and enjoyment/joy. Prohibitions may be behaviorally severe and emotionally disconnected. This, coupled with the generally low levels of attunement and sensitivity to the child's signals, may produce an excess in overall parasympathetic tone. The child's early experience may have a significant impact on the expression of affect and access to conscious awareness of emotion. The child learns to minimize the expression of attachment-related emotion, which may serve to reduce the disabling effects of overwhelming frustration in the face of continuing interactions with the caregiver.[16]

Ambivalence

In the third approach, parental facial expressions of continued disapproval, eye gaze aversion, and body language of disconnection or anger are all perceived by the child. The child's high-arousal states may be attuned to sometimes, but if they are not, disconnection and shame may be associated with humiliation and may thus become toxic, especially if disconnection is prolonged or associated with parental anger. The child's range of tolerable emotional arousal may be broad, but uncontrollable swings beyond the window of tolerance may occur. Inconsistent attunements and repair may lead to excessive arousal, so that the sympathetic system may often be unchecked because of a diminished parasympathetic system response. Alternatively, prolonged despair may result if the parasympathetic system is excessively activated. Anticipatory anxiety and fear of separation may be evident. Separation in the ambivalently attached child means having to rely on the self for ineffective emotion regulation. Repeated experiences of going beyond tolerable levels with excessive arousal or despair teaches these children that they themselves are unreliable affect modulators; this is the reason for their paradoxical excessive reliance on the inconsistent attachment figures. Such experiences may produce an apparent increase in a child's sensitivity, especially in relationship to interactions with others and to situations of loss and separation. Overall, there is a maximizing of the expression of attachment-related emotions, which some authors suggest may serve to attempt to enhance the chances that the inconsistent parent will pay attention to the child.[17]

Disorganization

In the fourth pattern, the child's behavior elicits a rageful parental response, producing terror in the child. This is not simply the child's fear of consequences, but a fear for safety induced by the attachment figure. The child's adaptation to this suddenly induced fear state (high levels of both sympathetic and parasympathetic discharge) is a conflictual one: The accelerator and the brakes are being applied simultaneously. This is an example of a disorganized form of attachment. The parent, often with unresolved trauma or loss as described in Chapter 3, may unintentionally and unknowingly be providing the child with a set of responses that are disorienting and disorganizing. As an attachment figure, such a parent has become a source of fear and confusion, not of safety and security. The intense and frightening moments of disconnection with the parent remain unrepaired. As the parent disappears into rage, the child becomes lost in terror. These disorganizing and disorienting experiences become an essential part of how the child learns to self-regulate behavior and emotional states. The child has the double insult of becoming engulfed in confusion and terror induced by the parent, and of losing the relationship with an attachment figure that might have provided a safe haven and sense of security.

RELATIONSHIPS AND AFFECT REGULATION

The lessons from attachment research can guide our understanding of the powerful effect interpersonal relationships can have on the development and ongoing functioning of self-regulation. Studies suggest that the orbitofrontal cortex remains plastic throughout life; that is, it is able to develop beyond childhood.[18] The orbitofrontal cortex mediates neurophysiological mechanisms integrating several domains of human experience: social relationships, the evaluation of meaning, autonoetic consciousness, response flexibility, and emotion regulation. The nonverbal social signals of eye contact, facial expression, tone of voice, and body gestures communicate the state of mind of each member of a dyad. The interactions that occur have direct effects on the emotional experience *in that moment*. Within the context of an attachment relationship, the child's developing mind and the structure of the child's brain will be shaped in such a way that the ability to regulate emotion *in the future* is affected.

The proposal being made here is that interpersonal relationships can provide attachment experiences that can allow similar neurophysiological changes to occur throughout life. In extreme cases of trauma, such as neglect or abuse, the deeper structures of the brain may be impaired to such a degree that improvement may be difficult to achieve. Even in these situations, however, the principles learned from attachment research may perhaps still prove useful in organizing an approach to helping people adapt to life's stresses. In many cases of disorganized attachment and clinical dissociation, for example, therapeutic relationships can facilitate effective movement toward well-being and adaptive self-regulation.[19] In less extreme cases, the deeper structures of the brain may have developed well, but the states of mind that have been engrained may be maladaptive. For these people, therapy may help to move the systems of their minds toward more adaptive modes of processing information and regulating the flow of information. Sometimes specific techniques within a psychotherapy relationship are needed to alter engrained patterns of emotion dysregulation. The patient–psychotherapist relationship may provide a sense of proximity, a safe haven, and an internal model of security. These elements of an attachment relationship, within therapy or other emotionally engaging relationships such as romance and friendship, may possibly facilitate new orbitofrontal development and enhance the regulation of emotion throughout the lifespan.

An example of a five-year-old girl seen for "impulse control" problems in school illustrates the use of psychotherapy to enable the mind to develop flexible self-regulation. A review of the child's history revealed that she had severe visual problems, which had remained undetected until she was three and a half years of age. Even after she received proper glasses and could see objects in focus, however, she continued to have "outbursts of emotion" and impulsivity at school. In the therapist's office, it was clear that she did not look to other people's faces to "check in" with how they might be responding to her. She seemed to have an impairment in the normal process of social referencing, which is usually evident during the first year of life.[20] At school, she seemed oblivious to the reactions of her teachers and her classmates. This social disconnection gave her the outward appearance of being oppositional and perhaps of having a basic deficit in social cognition—the ability to perceive and process social signals. Face-to-face communication is one route by which attunement and social referencing enable the emotional state of one individual to be perceived by another. Such abilities allow for emotionally contingent communication, which is at the developmental heart of emotion regulation.

In therapy, the child was encouraged to look at the therapist's face. Her parents and teachers were counseled about the nature of attachment, social referencing, and the use of face-to-face communication in the development of emotion regulation. The impairment in her vision, now corrected, was offered as a working hypothesis for why this girl exhibited such social difficulties. Over a period of several months of intervention, she began to look more frequently at others when she spoke. In play, she engaged more in identifying dolls' internal states, and their emotions became a more active part of the stories that unfolded in therapy. With the development of these capacities for facial perception, "theory of mind," and social referencing, she began to engage more appropriately in social interactions. The use of reflective dialogue—talking about feelings, thoughts, memories, beliefs, and perceptions—in conjunction with the nonverbal face-to-face communication enabled her to develop previously unstimulated abilities in her mind. Her ability to regulate her emotions seemed to improve: Her explosions became less frequent and less intense, and her impulsive behavior diminished significantly. One could hypothesize that each of these developmental accomplishments was mediated by the interactive maturation of her orbitofrontal cortex.

In theory, this therapeutic approach enabled this young girl to use the nonverbal signals that she had generally missed because of her visual difficulties. Other modalities that can allow two individuals to communicate their states of mind, such as hearing and touch, are also important in communication during childhood. The use of this approach allowed this child to take in the vital information of other people's minds instead of living in isolation, where her frustration level was high and her behaviors appeared "impulsive" because they were so independent of the signals and needs of others.

PATHWAYS OF EMOTIONAL GROWTH

This section integrates many ideas about memory, attachment, and emotion in exploring some insights gleaned from therapeutic work with adults and children. These illustrations are offered not as scientific data, but as clinical impressions that can serve to further our discussion of the ways in which interpersonal experiences may shape the developing mind across the lifespan.

Avoidance and Dismissing States of Mind

Although emotional relationships of all sorts can be healing and promote healthy maturation, facilitating a movement toward an "earned" secure/autonomous adult attachment status,[21] at times the unique configuration of psychotherapy is needed to catalyze this growth. For Main and Goldwyn's dismissing adult,[22] without awareness of "what life could be like," promoting this growth may be quite a challenge for his therapist and his partner alike. On the one hand, the individual has the right to remain as he is; there are no definitions of absolutely "normal" ways of relating that some "objective" therapist can push onto others. However, isolation and emotional distance take their toll—within the person's romantic relationship; within relationships with others, including children; and within the self. His intense emotions and enjoyment in life may be severely muted. Part of this neutral emotionality may be attributable to the proposed parcellation of the sympathetic (accelerator) branch of the autonomic nervous system, which is responsible for heightened states of arousal. His mindsight—the ability to sense the subjective mental life of others, or of himself—may also be severely restricted. The result is that his basic emotional needs are not met by anyone. However, the avoidantly attached individual does not believe this, because it appears to his adaptive self that his approach to survival has been successful thus far. His private self remains highly underdeveloped and consciously unaware.

The avoidantly attached (dismissing) adult often comes to therapy at the insistence of his securely or ambivalently attached romantic partner. The partner feels that the relationship is too distant, too emotionally barren, to tolerate. Ironically, the partner may have been initially attracted to the patient because of his "independence and autonomy—he didn't have to rely on anyone." This autonomy gives the ambivalently attached mate a feeling at first that intrusion (the dreaded experience of the mate's own childhood) need not be feared. As adult development progresses, however, the ambivalently attached partner may change and come to feel the need for more emotional intimacy. The avoidantly attached partner is less likely to develop as quickly toward models of security, because he often lacks awareness of internal pain or dissatisfaction with the relationship, which might otherwise serve to motivate change.

Logical discussions, which are so natural for avoidantly attached individuals, only go so far. Gentle and unintrusive attunements to their shifts in states begin to open up new possibilities. These are right-hemisphere-to-right-hemisphere connections between a therapist and a patient. In addition to these affect attunements, activation of right-hemisphere processes can be helpful. For example, by encouraging imagery and other nonverbal processes (such as "drawing on the right side of the brain" art techniques,[23] awareness of bodily sensations, dance, and music), psychotherapy can facilitate the emergence of new ways of experiencing the self. Such self-awareness often facilitates the development of new ways of seeing the world, especially the subjective mental lives of others. This process may be helpful for many other individuals besides those who have a history of avoidant attachment.

Guided imagery provides direct access to prelinguistic symbolic imagination and processes driven by implicit memory. The results can be deeply moving, though often initially logically derided by some avoidant/dismissing patients as "weird" and useless. As time goes on, emotional states become accessible to these patients in the form of images that they can come to respect. These nonverbal, nonrational, right-sided processes begin to influence the patients' behavior and make them more aware of similar states in others around them. In some cases, psychotherapy can catalyze the development of new conscious awareness of the self's and others' emotional processes. As the attuned and resonating emotional communication within psychotherapy continues, new models of the self and of the self with others can gradually begin to develop. These right-hemisphere models facilitate the promotion of emotional connections with others. As such resonant experiences unfold, an integrating process emerges and a more coherent narrative evolves, coupled with a more complex and enriching sense of meaning in life. The nature of such an integration will be explored in depth in the next chapter.

In one case, a man who had a dismissing state of mind with respect to attachment was introduced over time to the techniques of guided imagery and asked to do the drawing exercises outlined in Betty Edwards's art book.[24] At first, this man seemed very reluctant to consider these new experiences as important in any way. He had come to therapy at the insistence of his wife, who stated that he was "too cold and intellectual." As the imagery continued over several sessions, however, the emerging stories became more and more complex and compelling to him.

For the therapist, this imagery process revealed a previously quiet, nonconscious, and dormant right hemisphere's construction of reality. It was filled with sensations, intense emotions, visual scenes, thematic struggles, and new perspectives on dilemmas of which the left-sided individual was quite unaware. For example, he experienced the notion that he had better let his "wilting" marriage "blossom" by buying her roses when she didn't expect them. He had never done such a thing as buying flowers for her without a particular "reason," such as a birthday or anniversary. He got the roses simply because it "felt" right. He couldn't explain it at the time, but he just followed his gut instinct. His right hemisphere took his wife's internal world into account, provided him with a metaphor for her needs, and enabled him to feel her feelings. Though there was no logic to the act, this man learned—from his own gut (literally, represented in the right orbitofrontal region)—the importance of letting another person fill him.

Over many months of therapy as he continued to allow his innate right-hemisphere processes to "blossom," he found himself slowly becoming aware of new types of internal sensations. He would feel his body more in response to interactions with his wife; he also began to become aware of shifts in her facial expressions, and found himself responding more to these internal and external emotional cues. What was particularly striking to him was that his internal experiences seemed to shift. He stopped being so concerned about goals and outcomes, and became more focused on the process of things, both at home and at work. These changes at first were quite subtle. Though this man would not openly admit it, he seemed to feel very vulnerable experiencing and expressing these new sensations. His life seemed to be opening up to a new mode of experiencing both himself and his wife.

Ambivalence and Preoccupied States of Mind

For an individual with a history of ambivalent attachments, the intrusion of parental emotional states onto those of the child has led to an intense sense of vulnerability and loss of the self. As this individual struggles to connect, she feels perpetually at risk of losing her connections to others, or to herself. Retreating into chameleon-like imitations of meeting others' expectations is a learned, reflexive public adaptation to these intrusive assaults. In psychotherapy, this may lead to an attempt to be the "perfect patient." As this individual tries to define herself, there may be patterns of withdrawal and approach similar to those in her childhood history of attachment, which lead to fluctuations in openness to being understood in psychotherapy.

As this person's inner, private states of mind become slowly accessible, the therapist must be ever vigilant to the critical micromoments of interaction, where attunement is crucial. Responding to the patient's nonverbal signals, including tone of voice, facial expressions, eye gaze, and bodily motion, can reveal the otherwise hidden shifts in states of mind. Resonating with these expressions of primary emotions requires that the therapist feel the feelings, not merely understand them conceptually. Resonance involves the alignment of psychobiological states between patient and therapist.

One aspect of this attunement is the recognition that everyone seems to go through naturally oscillating cycles of internal versus external focus of connection. There are times when an individual needs to have self-focus, perhaps reflecting the internal self-regulation of emotional states. Within moments, however, there may be a noticeable shift to an other-focus, in which external connections are used for dyadic self-regulation. These natural oscillations suggest the use of modifications of the internal versus external constraints of the individual's system, in order to regulate the flow of states and self-organization. These ideas also remind us of the important concept that self-organization is a result of both internal individual processes and dyadic processes. Another implication of such oscillations comes from the findings on hemispheric specialization discussed in earlier chapters, in which the left hemisphere mediates approach states and the right hemisphere facilitates states of withdrawal. The changing focus of processing, mediated via a cycling of left- versus right-hemisphere dominance and of external versus internal focus, may be a part of what we sense when others have a cycling need for external versus internal connection.

Missed opportunities for attunement and misattunements, whether these occur in psychotherapy, parenting, or other emotional relationships, are unavoidable. Unless repair of these disruptions in attunement is undertaken, toxic senses of shame and humiliation can become serious blocks to interpersonal communication. These dreaded states are not merely uncomfortable and disliked; they can feel like a black hole, a bottomless pit of despair, in which the self is lost for what seems to be forever. Repair requires the recognition that a rupture has occurred in the attunement process, and then the realignment of states between the two individuals involved. The repair process is an interactive one, requiring the openness of both people in attempts to reconnect after a rupture.

The public self strives to avoid the dreaded states of shame and humiliation; it scans the social environment for clues of connection, but is often unable to prevent the activation of these states. The anxiety accompanying the emergence of these dreaded states into one's consciousness can induce defensive adaptations. Fears of annihilation and of abandonment are the origins of the desperate withdrawal and anxious approach common in ambivalently attached individuals. The excessive parcellation of the parasympathetic "brakes," proposed to be one adaptation to inconsistent and intrusive parenting, may make these states especially vulnerable to dysregulation. An adaptive, public self may emerge at these times to avoid the dreaded state by meeting the needs of others. The adaptive defenses of such a public self vary greatly and can include primitive modes, such as denial and the projection of the sense of disconnection onto other people or life events. In contrast, some individuals may utilize more mature approaches, such as seeking emotional connection with others or sublimating their painful experiences into efforts to help others through professional work (for example, teaching with an emphasis on supporting others' self-esteem, working in the government to establish laws protecting the rights of children, or becoming a therapist and emphasizing the importance of understanding others and respecting their individuality).

From primitive, "nonproductive" defenses to mature, "socially helpful" ones, an ambivalently attached (preoccupied) individual may experience any of a wide range of adaptive modes within differing emotional and social contexts. The relative distance of a work setting may permit sublimation to flourish; the close quarters of a romantic relationship or a parent–child relationship may periodically activate an intense sense of intrusion or other forms of misattunement, and yield a sudden emergence of the dreaded states of shame and humiliation. In an effort to avoid these painful states, activation of more primitive modes of defense filled with fear, anger, and associated distortions of perceptions and misinterpretations of other's behavior may occur. These are moments of intense vulnerability and risk for dyadic dysregulation.

Romantic Attachments and Interlocking States

Knowing the attachment histories of each member of a couple can be essential in clarifying how micromoments of misattunement can be blown up into major battles and interlocking, dysregulated dyadic states of despair and distancing. Small changes in input, such as subtle shifts in the emotional expression of one member of the pair, can produce large and rapid alterations in output in the nonlinear complex systems of each individual and of the dyad. These interlocking states often have their origins in the attachment models of each member of the pair. In these situations, a historical rut has created the opposite of resonance of states of mind: a cascade of emotional reflexes and defensive distortions, locking a romantic pair into a series of mutually induced misunderstandings and misattunements. These repeated ruptures in connection are rarely repaired.

"Interlocking" in this context means that the separate states of mind activated by these repeated patterns of induction reinforce the historical mental models of relationships and keep the partners continually reexperiencing lack of attunement, misattunements, and repeated verification of the lessons learned from their own individual attachment histories. Interlocking states strengthen earlier maladaptive self-organizational pathways. They create a rigidity that prevents the partners from joining together as a larger system capable of moving toward dyadic states of increasing complexity. At one extreme, these ruts can be experienced as a sense of malaise or deadness, which each member of the pair may feel but may be unable to articulate; at the other extreme, these ruts may be filled with anxiety and a sense of intrusiveness and uncertainty. To remain healthy, a dyadic system, like an individual, must find a balance between flexibility and continuity in its perpetual move toward increasingly complex states of existence. Couple therapy may sometimes be necessary for the partners to recognize and then to alter these profoundly frustrating and deadening interlocking states.

In a dynamical sense, an ambivalent attachment can be seen as a system that cannot dyadically regulate itself in a way allowing for a healthy resonance between two individuals. The state of the child is intruded upon by that of the parent. There is often an inability to sense and respect the child's oscillating need for internal versus external connection. In this way, maximal complexity cannot be achieved by the two as a dyadic system. Instead, a lesser degree of complexity must be settled for, because the parent rigidly defines the nature of the interaction. There is no true collaborative communication. The dance of attunement is severely constrained by the parent's entangled preoccupations with the past and inability to align states with the child.

In an avoidant attachment, maximal complexity is also not attained because the states of the two individuals are so independent of each other. The parent's dismissing approach leads to an emotionally disconnected form of communication, which minimizes the resonance between the parent and child. In this sense, the two systems act independently of each other, and the dyad remains in a segmented and noncomplex mode of existence.

As these early models of attachment are later activated within a couple's relationship, the opportunity emerges to learn about how early experiences shaped implicit reality. Both partners' private selves are hungry and in pain, fearing annihilation or abandonment by the narcissistic intrusion of parental states that have historically obliterated their own (as in ambivalent attachments) or having adapted to an emotional distance and sense of rejection (as in avoidant attachments). Nurturing their private selves requires that the members of the couple join together in supportively reflecting on how their public selves have struggled to adapt to these intrusions, inconsistencies, and experiences of disconnection without repair. Growth emerges as reflective and resonant dyadic states become achieved within the attuned relationship. Such a process can then allow the couple to achieve more fulfilling and adaptive levels of dyadic self-organization.

Disorganization and Unresolved States of Mind

Unresolved parental trauma or loss can lead to disorganized/disoriented attachment, which is a much more chaotic form of dyadic system than either avoidant or ambivalent attachment.[25] For the person who has experienced disorganized attachment, the experience of parental fear or fear-inducing behavior has often been associated with the parent's lack of resolution of trauma or loss. That is, the incoherence of the parent's life narrative has been behaviorally injected into the child's experience by way of the parent's own disturbance in self-organization and the resultant dysregulated states and disorienting actions. These parental behaviors, which are incompatible with providing a sense of safety and cohesion, are "biological paradoxes" and directly impair the developing child's affect regulation, shifts in states of mind, and integrative and narrative functions. The result is that the child enters repeated chaotic states of mind. From a dynamical point of view, these can be considered "strange attractor states"—neural net configurations that are widely distributed throughout the system and that have become engrained, repeated states of dissociated and dysfunctional activation.

When a patient has a history of disorganized attachment, the therapist is faced with the especially crucial challenge of providing the essence of a secure attachment: a predictable emotional environment in which the patient can learn to depend upon the therapist for regulating state shifts. The therapeutic relationship and the dyadic self-regulation subsequently become "internalized" through the development of a mental model of the self with the therapist and through the acquisition of new capacities for autonomous emotion regulation. As we'll discuss in the next chapter, achieving this new level of self-organization is often facilitated by an integrating narrative process which facilitates a deep sense of internal coherence.[26]

TRAUMA AND GRIEF

In addition to the influence of repeated patterns of communication within attachment relationships, specific overwhelming events may produce marked effects on the developing mind. Psychological trauma can overwhelm affect regulation mechanisms, and various forms of adaptation may be required to maintain equilibrium. The flood of stress hormones can produce toxic effects on the development of brain systems responsible for self-regulation. In this way, early, severe, and chronic trauma may create impairments in a child's ability to adapt to future stress.[27] The individual's developmental stage at the time of a trauma—be it loss of a loved one, an abusive experience (especially those involving a sense of betrayal), or the witnessing of a violent event—markedly influences the adaptive responses available. In general, loss or trauma can have a negative impact on a child's expectations for the future, directly shape his anticipational models and prospective memory, and disrupt his narrative process. These influences produce impairments to achieving self-regulation and integration of self-states, and in these ways damage the individual's deepest sense of the self and the ability to regulate the flow of internal states.

In some cases of engrained patterns of dysregulation—due to a number of combinations of constitutional and experiential factors—psychiatric medications may be needed to help the brain achieve the capacity to regulate the flow of states of mind, through direct biochemical effects that alter the synaptic strengths determining the internal constraints of the system. A positive response to medications does not confirm some "genetic disorder." For example, some of the symptoms of posttraumatic stress disorder respond well to medications. Furthermore, studies of laboratory animals that have experienced maternal deprivation and reveal subsequent behavioral disturbances find that these animals respond well to selective serotonin reuptake inhibitors, but relapse when these medications are removed.[28] It may be the case that certain individuals—whether because of genetic factors, early traumatic experiences, or some combination of inherited vulnerability and stressful environmental conditions—have developed such maladaptive brain structures and self-organizational capacities that intensive psychotherapy and/or medications are essential. It is important to keep in mind, however, that the limbic regions of the brain (especially the orbitofrontal cortex) may continue to be open to further development throughout the lifespan, and thus remain open to experience-dependent maturational processes. Psychotherapy can utilize this potential in helping facilitate the further development of the mind.

If severe trauma occurs early in life, or if a form of divided attention (such as entering a state of intense imagination or trance) is utilized during an overwhelming experience, explicit memory for the traumatic experience(s) may be impaired. Intense and frightening elements of implicit memory will be encoded and may later be automatically reactivated, intruding on the traumatized individual's internal experience and external behaviors without the person's conscious sense of recollection or knowledge of the source of these intrusions.

In the case of loss of a loved one, especially an attachment figure, the mind is forced to alter the structure of its internal working models to adjust to the painful reality that the self can no longer seek proximity and gain comfort from the caregiver. Loss, especially early in childhood, can have a deep impact on the growing mind. The degree of impact may be related in part to how well the family can meet the child's ongoing attachment needs. The child's developmental stage at the time of the loss will also influence the nature of the grieving process. As the child continues to develop, grieving may need to be revisited so that the new developmental capacities can process the loss. For both a child and an adult, dealing with loss takes time and a nurturing environment. John Bowlby's view of the grieving process is that the attachment models must be deeply altered to take the loss into account.[29]

Delayed or pathological grief can be seen as the impairment in the ability to make such alterations within the attachment system. States of mind continue to be activated in which connection to the actual attachment figure is expected. Prohibitions to sharing the grieving process may result in impaired grief, as can be seen in families whose members are unable to communicate about painful issues or to recognize the different emotional needs of individuals within the family. If conflictual feelings toward and mental models of a deceased attachment figure were present, then grieving may also be difficult.

The effects of unresolved loss or trauma in relation to specific overwhelming events can be powerfully disorganizing and often hidden from conscious awareness. At the most fundamental level, such a lack of resolution involves disturbances in the flow of energy and information in the mind. As the mind emerges at the interface of neurophysiological processes and interpersonal relationships, such disturbances can be seen within neural pathways and within dyadic communication. Knowledge of impaired resolution of grief or trauma is crucial, given its devastating effects on the individual and its potential to impair attachment with future offspring. Attachment disturbances in the children of parents with lack of resolution result directly from the impairments to contingent, collaborative communication. As suggested above, the flow of energy and information between parent and child—the essence of attuned relationships—is disturbed in cases of parental unresolved trauma or loss.

Prospective memory allows us to "remember the future." In memory-related terms, lack of resolution means that the mind has a tendency to create repeated patterns of disorganizing states, often without conscious awareness of their origin. These states may be created by sudden and unwanted activations of implicit elements of memory, such as flashbacks of traumatic events or mental models of a deceased attachment figure as if the figure were still alive. These activations can seriously impair functioning, especially in the realms of response flexibility, emotional modulation, and contingent communication with others. Unresolved trauma or loss leaves the individual with a deep sense of incoherence in autonoetic consciousness, which tries to make sense of the past, organize the present, and chart out the future. This lack of resolution can produce lasting effects throughout the lifespan and influence self-organization across the generations.

Making the connection within psychotherapy between these aspects of memory and past experiences allows patients to understand the origins of their disturbances. Such reflections must take place within the therapeutic attachment setting, which allows the mind to experience intensely dysregulated states and learn—dyadically at first—how to tolerate them, then to reflect on their nature, and eventually to regulate them in a more adaptive manner. Much of this emotional processing is in its essence nonverbal and is probably mediated via right-hemisphere processes (both those within the patient and those between patient and therapist).

Bringing conscious reflection to such unresolved reactivations permits the consolidation process of explicit memory to become involved and traumatic experiences to be integrated within autobiographical narrative. As we'll explore in the next chapter, this process may allow for cooperative processing in both hemispheres of what may have been only unilateral representations. The attuned resonant relationship with the therapist allows patients to make left-hemisphere, verbally mediated, interpreter-driven sense out of their right-hemisphere autobiographical representations. This integrative process probably has direct effects on the right hemisphere's capacity to regulate primary emotional states. The patient's mind is prepared for such a process by the development of a secure attachment with the therapist. Furthermore, the elaboration of autonoetic consciousness permits patients to reflect on the past, understand the present, and help actively shape the future. Such mentalizing reflective dialogue is also a fundamental component of secure attachments. Individuals with histories of disorganized attachments can thus become freed from the "prison of the present," in which they were repeatedly trapped when they had no words to reflect on their rapidly enveloping and terrifying states of mind.

REFLECTIONS: EMOTIONAL RELATIONSHIPS AND THE JOINING OF MINDS

We all need contingent communication. Our history of being close with others, having affective attunements and resonating states of mind, allows us to connect with others and to have a sense of coherence within our own internal processes. Adaptations to patterns of misattunements without repair, and to the subsequent dreaded states of shame and humiliation, shape our subjective experience of self, others, and the world. These patterns of relationships can lead to a large disparity between our adaptive, public selves and our inner, private selves. The attachment models that reflect these early, pre-explicit-memory experiences influence our emotions and their regulation, response flexibility, consciousness, self-knowledge, narrative, and openness to and drive toward interpersonal intimacy.

At times, engrained dysfunctional patterns of self-organization may require the specialized interpersonal relationship of psychotherapy to alter the emotion dysregulation that has come to be the source of pain in some individuals' lives. Psychotherapy establishes a safe environment in which present and past experiences can be explored. A therapist and a patient enter into a resonance of states of mind, which allows for the creation of a co-regulating dyadic system. This system is able to emerge in increasingly complex dyadic states by means of the attunement between the two individuals. The patient's subtle nonverbal expressions of her state of mind are perceived by the therapist and responded to with a shift in the therapist's own state, not just with words. In this way, there is a direct resonance between the primary emotional, psychobiological state of the patient and that of the therapist. These nonverbal expressions are mediated by the right hemisphere of one person and then perceived by the right hemisphere of the other. In this way, the essential nonverbal aspect of psychotherapy, and perhaps all emotional relationships, can be conceived as a right-hemisphere-to-right-hemisphere resonance between two individuals.

The left hemispheres of both members of the dyad are also

important and active in the verbal exchanges and logical reflections on the patient's present life, past history, and the therapy experience itself. The left hemisphere's interpreter function attempts to "make sense" of experiences and therefore can be seen as a motivational force in the narrative process. As we'll explore more fully in the next chapter, coherent autobiographical narratives—a primary focus of therapy of all sorts—probably involve a resonance of left- and right-hemisphere processes in both the teller and the listener. In this way, the joint construction of narratives reflects the interhemispheric resonance within both members of the therapeutic relationship.

The flow of states within the dyadic system is allowed to achieve increasing degrees of complexity as the individuals themselves achieve increasingly coherent states of interhemispheric resonance. Such a state is achieved via the right-to-right and left-to-left attunements that emerge from the nonverbal and verbal communication between patient and therapist. The emergent sense of flow, of connection, between two individuals in such a state of resonance is deeply compelling.

As self-states emerge over time, the mind has the challenge of integrating these relatively autonomous processes into a coherent whole. Psychotherapy can catalyze the development of such a core integrative process by facilitating dyadic states of resonance: right hemisphere to right hemisphere, left hemisphere to left hemisphere. In such a process, the mind of the patient (and that of the therapist) can become immersed in primary emotional states while simultaneously focusing on reflective narrative explorations. Such affect attunement and reflective dialogue catalyze an internal, bilateral form of resonance within each member of the dyad. As will be explored in the next chapter, this form of resonance may be at the core of an integrating process that permits emotion regulation across time and across self-states. It is from this state of cooperative activation that coherent narratives emerge, and through this process that the mind is able to achieve maximal complexity and thus stable self-organization.

Psychotherapy is a complex process. The brain can be ravaged by interactions between genetically influenced mental storms and experiential histories of family strife. Both inherited disturbances and adaptations to traumatic experiences can have complex effects on the neurophysiologically constructed reality of our subjective lives. Our minds are complex systems constrained in their activity by neuronal connections, which are determined by both constitution and experience. Different therapeutic tools, including medications and specific psychotherapeutic techniques, may be useful at various times in helping patients achieve self-organization and live balanced and enriching lives. Whatever tools or techniques are used, the relationship between patient and therapist requires a deep commitment on the therapist's part to understanding and resonating with the patient's experience. The therapist must always keep in mind that interpersonal experience shapes brain structure and function, from which the mind emerges.

It is a challenge, and a profound privilege, to keep an objective focus on a patient's emotional needs while at the same time allowing oneself as the therapist to join with the patient's evolving states of mind. This resonance of states bonds patient and therapist. By joining, they become part of a larger system that develops its own self-organizational processes and coherent life history. In many ways, therapy reflects the challenge of all human relationships: understanding and accepting people as they are, and yet nurturing further integration and growth. These connections within ourselves and with others are the essence of living vital lives and remaining open to all layers of our own emerging experiences.

CHAPTER 9

Integration

One of the mind's most robust features is its capacity to interconnect a range of processes within its present activity, as well as its functioning across time. Researchers studying diverse aspects of mental life—from social psychology to the neurosciences—have used the term "integration" to refer to the collaborative, linking functions that coordinate various levels of processes within the mind and between people. This chapter explores various ways in which integration can be understood as a fundamental aspect of interpersonal experience and the developing mind.

NEURAL INTEGRATION

Within the brain itself, complex functions emerge from the coordination of neural activity in a range of circuits. Those regions that receive input and send output to widely distributed areas of the brain play an important role in neural integration. The limbic regions and associational circuits, especially the prefrontal areas such as the orbitofrontal cortex, serve such a coordinating function. From this neurobiological perspective, Tucker, Luu, and Pribram have stated that

> the theoretical challenge at the neural level is to go beyond labeling the functions of the frontal lobe to formulate the key neurophysiological mechanisms. These mechanisms link the operations of frontal cortex to the multiple systems of the brain's control hier-

archy, ranging from the control of arousal by brain-stem projection systems to the control of memory by reentrant corticolimbic interactions. When sufficiently understood, these mechanisms must be found to regulate not only physiology of neural tissue, but the representation and maintenance of the self."[1]

In this manner, neural integration is fundamental to self-organization, and indeed to the capacity of the brain to create a sense of self. Tucker and colleagues further suggest that integration within the brain may consist of at least three forms, which focus on particular aspects of anatomic circuits: "vertical," "dorsal–ventral," and "lateral."[2] Vertical integration is the integration of the "lower" functions of the brainstem and limbic regions with the "higher" operations of the frontal neocortex such as cognitive and motor planning. In vertical integration, somewhat isolated processes at various layers of complexity or "order" are coordinated into a functional system. This vertical process is common throughout the brain.

Dorsal–ventral integration focuses on the dual origins of the frontal cortex from the archicortical and paleocortical regions of the paralimbic cortex. As we've seen in Chapter 5, these differences begin in the embryo and may stem from the asymmetry in what Trevarthen has called the "intrinsic motive formation."[3] Each hemisphere has a dominant pathway: right with dorsal and left with ventral. Each circuit or "stream" mediates differential forms of motivational processes and motor control, and creates different representational processes on either side of the brain. As suggested earlier, the finding of less hemispheric specialization in women may be proposed to be partly due to the participation of both dorsal and ventral circuits in each hemisphere. Dorsal–ventral integration would allow for less lateralization of the more complex representational processes originating from each side of the brain.

Lateral integration is the coordination of functions of the circuits at a similar level of complexity or order. Coordinating perceptual processes across sensory modalities, such as bringing together vision with tactile and auditory perceptions, to create a "whole picture" of an experience is an example of lateral integration. This integration may be mediated by associational neurons, which link distinct systems. When lateral integration connects the complex representational processes of one hemisphere to another, the term "bilateral" or "interhemispheric" integration can be used. The associational neurons that link various anatomically and functionally distinct regions on either side of the brain may be the means by which the coordination of interhemispheric information processing occurs. According to Trevarthen, the cerebral commissures (the corpus callosum and the anterior commissures) are "the only pathway through which the higher functions of perception and cognition, learning and voluntary motor coordination can be unified"; this is achieved through a sorting process, which he proposes "creates complementary sets of associative links between the cortical maps of various sensory and motor functions."[4] In this form of lateral integration, the isolated functions of each hemisphere can be coordinated into a functionally linked system.

The fact that the "greatest integration of sensory, motor, and evaluative information may occur in the primitive paralimbic cortex" has led Tucker and colleagues to suggest that these three forms of integration, each of which involves aspects of this region, may actually be interdependent.[5] For example, vertical integration is revealed in the capacity of the right hemisphere (especially the paralimbic orbitofrontal cortex) to have predominant control over certain "lower" functions, such as the regulation and representation of bodily function as mediated via the autonomic nervous system. Lateral integration is revealed within REM sleep and encoding–retrieval processes, in which left and right orbitofrontal cortices are involved in representational integration in dreams and the consolidation of memory. At a minimum, then, the orbitofrontal cortex coordinates vertical and lateral integration. Future studies will need to explore whether and how these coordinating regions play a role in dorsal–ventral integration on one or both sides of the brain.

Another illustration of how distinct regions of the brain may be coordinated into integrated circuits is in the connections of frontal cortex to the basal ganglia. As outlined by Steven Wise and colleagues, this integrated system functions to guide behavior by assessing a variety of inputs.[6] In their view, the basal ganglia mediate rule-guided behavior, whereas the frontal cortex provides alternatives that incorporate context-dependent processing. This can also be seen as an example of the integration of implicit encoding in the basal ganglia and explicit processing in the frontal cortex. This frontal cortex–basal ganglia system serves to allow the individual to reject maladaptive rules that are no longer useful in the currently assessed situation. The integrated functioning of such a system has powerful implications for the acquisition and application of new behavioral responses. This integration of "motor" areas (basal ganglia) with those thought of as responsible for more abstract "planning" (frontal lobes) may be an adaptive way through evolution that our brains have come to integrate a wide array of systems.[7] This view is consistent with our earlier discussions of the orbitofrontal cortex's role in mediating response flexibility, the altering of responses based on unexpected or changing conditions.[8]

At an even more basic level of neurobiology, we can examine the notion of how neurons integrate their functioning within neural networks to produce neural net activation profiles. As we've seen, the brain learns from experience through the shaping of patterns of neuronal firing that create these networks. van Ooyen and van Pelt have stated,

> As a result of these activity-dependent processes, a reciprocal influence exists between the formation of neuronal form and synaptic connectivity on the one hand, and neuronal and network activity on the other hand. A given network may generate activity patterns which modify the organization of the network, leading to altered activity patterns which further modify structural or functional characteristics, and so on . . . the realization is growing that electrical activity and neurotransmitters are not only involved in information coding, but also play an important role in shaping neuronal networks in which they operate.[9]

In this manner, basic neuronal connectivity creates representational abilities and also directly influences the nature of the network activity itself. What this means is that a process that links distinct circuits not only creates a new form of information processing, but also establishes a more complex, integrated network that influences its own capacities. Integrated systems, by virtue of their coordinated activities, establish their own characteristic features; the whole is greater than merely the sum of the individual parts. As we'll see, such neural integration becomes a central process that is directly related to self-regulation.

The fundamental role of complexity has helped to clarify the development and functioning of neural networks and has pointed to the central role of "spatiotemporal integration."[10] Various levels of hierarchical systems—from sets of neurons to the interaction of complex circuits—involve space–time patterns of neuronal activity. What this suggests is that the brain is capable of representing, in the moment, patterns of activity in which direct influences from the past are encoded. As we've discussed, the organization of memory and the brain's function as an anticipation machine enable it to "represent the future." Such anticipatory mechanisms directly shape the ways in which linkages may be made across various processes and across time.

For example, the ways in which neural circuits anticipate experience may help us understand how the mind develops through a recursive set of interactions. As representational processes anticipate experience, they also seek particular forms of interactions to match their expectations. In this way, the "bias" of a system leads it to perceive, process, and act in a particular manner. The outcome of this bias is to reinforce the very features creating the system's bias. As development evolves, the circuits involved become more differentiated and more elaborately engrained in an integrated system that continues to support its own characteristics. These recursive and anticipatory features of development may be at the core of how the dorsal and ventral circuits influence the unfolding of the lateralization in hemispheric functioning. Infant studies suggest that traditional theories attempting to understand hemispheric lateralization and brain asymmetry may be looking at the problem from a limited end-product perspective. According to Trevarthen, a clearer understanding of the developmental origins of these different systems may be achieved by examining how the anticipation of encounters with the world influences each hemisphere in quite distinct ways. As Trevarthen explains, "With a change of theory that recognizes the priority of intrinsic motor planning and prospective motor imagery in cognition, and that also takes into account the expression of emotional states related to anticipatory self-regulation and the subject's evaluation of the consequences of intended action, a different perspective on cerebral asymmetry of awareness and memory can be proposed, one that seeks the origins in cerebral activities that *anticipate* experience."[11] This anticipation can be seen as emanating from a form of spatiotemporal integration: The mind creates complex representations as a process between perception (input) and action (output) in an effort to interact with an environment that changes across time and space. The value of such a representational process is that it allows the individual to anticipate the next moment in time and in this way to act in a more adaptive manner, enhancing the chance for survival. Spatiotemporal integration may therefore be a fundamental feature of how the human mind has evolved.

DEVELOPMENT AND
INTEGRATIVE PROCESSES

How do integrative processes develop within the individual? What are the neural mechanisms that allow integration to occur? How do experiential and genetic factors transact in the development of integrative processes? One approach to answering these questions may be to view the foundation of the mind as emanating from patterns in the flow of energy and information. Experience, as we've discussed repeatedly, activates neurons in such a manner that genes may become expressed and may produce alterations in neuronal connectivity. Information is transferred by the assembly of neural circuits into recruited clusters of activation that become functionally linked. This information transfer itself creates new representations and mental states. When new elements of informational processing are recruited into a new state of the system, this linkage of differentiated elements into a functional whole occurs and is the essence of integration. Such a flexible process, as we've seen, becomes disrupted in childhood trauma and in suboptimal attachment experiences. But normal development appears to move in the direction of more differentiated and integrated states. How does this integration happen in the brain?

The capacity to link a widely distributed array of neural processes can be proposed to be mediated by neuronal fibers that serve to interconnect anatomically and functionally distributed regions of the brain. In this manner, differentiated information processing modes, such as different sensory modalities, can become functionally linked.[12] This basic neuronal process may also help us to understand, for example, how highly engrained mental states, such as those of fear and shame, may become, or fail to become, integrated within the flow of the system's complex states. For example, we've seen that certain suboptimal attachment experiences produce multiple, incoherent working models of attachment and engrained and inflexible states of mind that remain unintegrated across time within specialized and potentially dysfunctional self-states. We can propose that the creation of new neuronal linkages, then, allows the internal constraints of the dynamical system of the brain to change. New interconnecting neuronal linkages may thus serve to integrate not only anatomically independent processes, but functionally isolated ones such as engrained mental states that have produced inflexibility and impairments in the system's capacity to adapt.

Central to this integration is emotion. As we've discussed earlier, emotion is inherently an integrative function that links internal processes and individuals together. This view reinforces the central role of emotion in self-regulation and in communication within interpersonal relationships. As the neurologist Antonio Damasio notes:

> It would not be possible to discuss the integrative aspects of brain function without considering the operations that arise in large-scale neural systems; and it would be unreasonable not to single out emotion among the critical integrative components arising in that level. Yet, throughout the twentieth century, the integrated brain and mind have often been discussed with hardly any acknowledgment that emotion does exist, let alone that it is an important function and that understanding its neural underpinnings is of great advantage.[13]

Fortunately, we are in a time of great strides in examining the neurobiology and interpersonal nature of emotion.

Emotionally meaningful events can enable continued learning from experience throughout the lifespan. Such learning may be seen as, in effect, the ongoing development of the brain. Experience plays a primary role in stimulating new neuronal connections in both memory and developmental processes. Findings from neurobiology suggest that such development may continue to some degree throughout the lifespan.[14] In particular, the neural circuitry facilitating integration may also continue to develop throughout life. Those neurons that serve to coordinate information from distributed regions may continue to develop perhaps with genetic programming, with the inherent mechanisms of aging, and with specific forms of experience. For example, in studying the progressively increasing myelination across the lifespan in the hippocampal pathways that interconnect widely distributed regions, Francine Benes has indicated:

> Growth and development of regions in the human brain occur not only in childhood but also much later during adolescent and adult years. ... Myelination represents one of the final stages in neuronal maturation where cells acquire a fatty lipid sheath around their axons, a change that increases the propagation of electrical signals from the neuronal cell body to terminal areas. ... These axons might well play a role in the integration of emotional behaviors with cognitive processes, a putative function of the limbic cortex. ... Therefore the functions influenced by this ongoing myelination may themselves "grow" and mature throughout adult life.[15]

In this manner, experiences and innate developmental processes may allow our neural capacity to integrate an array of processes to continue to develop throughout our lives. The mechanism of this differentiation of circuits, as we've discussed earlier, may involve a range of processes from the growth of axons into widely distributed regions of the brain, the establishment of new synaptic connections, and the increased conductance of nerve fibers via their increased myelination. These mechanisms may be at work in the dramatic maturation of the corpus callosum during the first decade of life, and perhaps, we can propose, in its possible ongoing development throughout life. Future studies may enable us to investigate how experience enhances or hinders the development of these integrating neural processes.

The movement toward such integrating neural connections is consistent with complexity theory: highly differentiated and functionally linked subsystems maximize the complexity achievable by the system. In this manner, it may be a natural developmental outcome for increasing levels of differentiation and integration to occur across the lifespan. One outcome of such a process for some individuals, we can imagine, might be the development of wisdom with age: The capacity to "see the forest for the trees" may emerge from an integrative capacity to focus on patterns over time and across situations rather than on the details of particular events. Disturbances in mental health, as we've discussed, may emanate from recursive processes that impair this natural movement toward integration by fixing the system's flow in the maladaptive direction of excessive rigidity or chaos. Fixed constraints to the system, either internal or external, may create an inflexible state for the individual. Normal development may thus continue to promote integration throughout life if it is unimpaired by elements of our constitution, experiential history, or ongoing interpersonal relationships.

Internal processes and interpersonal relationships that entail subcomponent differentiation and intercomponent integration can be proposed as those that promote healthy, ongoing development within and between individuals. Consider the musical analogy of a choir. At one extreme each individual sings his or her own song totally independently of the others. The ensuing cacophony occurs as a result of the lack of clustering of the individuals into a functional whole. There would be no cohesion, and the resultant sounds over time would be incoherent. Such a random set of isolated, though differentiated, interactions does little to move the system toward complexity.

But at the other extreme, the matching of each singer's voice to those of the others produces an amplification of the mirrored sounds. While the tune may be pleasing (and loud), it does little to maximize the complexity possible, if differentiated singers were to join together in a resonant integrational process. Neither independence nor mimicry creates complexity. With each singer having well-developed individual skills, integration allows them to contribute to a functional whole that has continuity and regularity on the one hand, and yet flexibility and spontaneity on the other. As we've seen, such a blend allows for the movement toward maximal complexity within the individual mind and between minds. At the heart of such integration is emotion and the flow of energy and information through the system. Such a dynamic condition achieves stability as the system moves forward in time through the various states of activity. These reciprocal and cooperative processes may characterize the healthy ongoing development of the individual mind, dyadic relationships, and nurturing communities. The blend of individual differentiation and interpersonal integration allow each of us to move forward in life with our minds forever developing in a complex biological interdependence of our social and inner worlds.

INTEGRATION OF MINDS

The concept of integration has also been applied to mental activity at a more macroscopic level, in both the intraindividual and interindividual domains. For example, several authors use the concept of intraindividual integration to refer to various ways in which developmental achievements and processes interrelate at one time or across the lifespan.[16] Interindividual integration focuses on the relationships between children and their caregivers and peers. From this psychological perspective, various layers of integration can be seen as interdependent, influencing one another in the moment and affecting the developmental trajectory of the child within a social world.

Integration can also help us understand the notion of "selves" within a given individual. For some adults, their developmental path has led to a coherent set of interactions with the world—interactions that have enabled the emergence of various self-states, which perform their functions with relatively minimal conflict among themselves. Such individuals may live a comparatively carefree existence, without internal tumult or impairment in functioning. Part of the developmental challenge of normal adolescence, as identified by Susan Harter and her colleagues, is the resolution of potential conflicts among various adaptive "selves" defined by specific social relationship role contexts.[17] The teen years bring a significant change in metacognitive capacity, with the new ability to reflect on one's own existence in more complex and integrative ways than were possible at earlier stages of life. Adolescents become aware of conflictual role patterns in their early teens, but often only develop the capacity to resolve tensions about these roles in later adolescence. This lag time between the onset of awareness and the capacity for resolution may be a characteristic feature of normal adolescent development. As the need for various roles is accepted and teenagers find ways to resolve potential conflicts within their experiences with peers and parents, an integration of selves across time and role relationships becomes possible. This is the essence of the integrative capacity to achieve coherence of the self.

Not all individuals are able to find emotional well-being in integrating multiple self-states into a coherent experience of the self. From early in development, the resolution of multiple models of attachment may be one of the determinants of later developmental outcome. Particular forms of self-states may have been constructed in relationship to different caregivers, resulting in potentially conflictual conditions. Within a given state, there may be cohesive functioning; across these self-states, however, spatiotemporal integration may not be possible, given the inherent incompatibility of mental models, drives, and modes of emotion regulation. Experiences within relationships and the ways in which the mind comes to create a coherent perspective, access to information, and models of such experiences are important variables in determining emotional resilience or vulnerability. In other words, an integrative process across self-states may be essential in the acquisition of well-being. The capacity for such internal integration may be intimately related to interpersonal experience—derived initially from attachment relationships, and later shaped by individuals' ongoing involvement with parents, teachers, and peers.

We can study various layers of integration, such as the coordination of elements of a given perceptual process into a hierarchy of functioning: sensory input, pattern analysis, and the creation of complex visual representations. We can also study the ways in which more widely distributed neural circuits interact to form a coherent process of increasingly complex processing, such as in the creation of multimodal representations that include perceptual and linguistic components. Such processes may involve the vertical, dorsal–ventral, and lateral domains of integration discussed above. For example, the combination of linguistic and nonverbal prosodic elements of speech requires the bilateral integration of representational processes.[18] The brain is normally integrating information processing across widely distributed circuits at any given moment in time, or in a "synchronic" fashion. As Ciompi has suggested, emotion may be essential in such an integrative process at a given time ("synchronic"), as well as across time ("diachronic").[19]

What does integration at a given time or across time look like? We can propose the following possibilities. Synchronic integration involves the elements discussed in Chapter 6, which create a cohesive mental state. Various aspects of neural activity are clustered together within a functional state of mind as a part of vertical, dorsal–ventral, and lateral integration in a given moment in time. At another level, we can suggest that as the individual's states of mind flow across time, diachronic integration somehow "links" these together in a manner that facilitates flexible and adaptive functioning. This is an example of spatiotemporal integration. Such cross-time integration serves as a mechanism of self-regulation, in that it serves to organize the flow of states. In Chapter 6, we have focused primarily on how complex systems can function as a cohesive state—a form of synchronic integration as we are defining it here. In this chapter, we will explore ways in which the mind may create coherence across time through diachronic integration. As time itself flows, it is in fact difficult to distinguish between cohesion in the moment and coherence across time. In the physical world, when does a "moment" actually end? The complex system of the brain, however, has the capacity for abrupt shifts in state that more clearly define the neural edges of time. Though time itself may have no clear boundaries, these neural shifts give a functional reality to the temporal contrasts between states. In this manner, cohesion exists within a given state of mind as a form of synchronic integration. The recursive nature of systems establishes a continuity in a given self-state across time. As a given state changes, it goes through a phase transition involving the temporary disorganization and then reorganization of the system's state. In contrast to cohesion of a given self-state, coherence is created across states of mind as a form of diachronic integration. As we'll discuss, such abilities to create coherence can be proposed to be a function of the individual's experiential history, which enables the acquisition of a core integrative process.

ATTACHMENT AND INTEGRATION

Main and Goldwyn have suggested that the way adults can flexibly access information about childhood and reflect upon such information in a coherent manner determines their likelihood of raising securely attached children.[20] The abilities to reflect upon one's own childhood history, to conceptualize the mental states of one's parents, and to describe the impact of these experiences on personal development are the essential elements of coherent adult attachment narratives. Moreover, the capacity to reflect on the role of mental states in determining human behavior is associated with the capacity to provide sensitive and nurturing parenting. Fonagy and Target have suggested that this reflective function is more than the ability to introspect; it directly influences a self-organizational process within the individual.[21] We can extend this idea to suggest that the reflective function also enables the parent to facilitate the self-organizational development of the child. We will explore how the coherent organization of the mind depends upon an integrative process that enables such reflective processes to occur. As we'll see, integrative coherence within the individual may early in life depend upon, and later facilitate, interpersonal connections that foster the development of emotional well-being.

The coherence of one's own states of mind permits a form of relationship with others—especially one's own children, friends, or intimate partners—that fosters integration, reflective processes, and emotional well-being within the relationship and within the emerging minds of each person. In other words, internal integration allows for vital interpersonal connections.

Attachment studies suggest that coherence can be observed and measured within autobiographical narrative reflections. As Pearson and colleagues have stated, "congruity, unity and free-flowing connections" in such narratives are central features revealing what is thought to be "coherence of mind" in the AAI studies.[22] The intergenerational transmission of suboptimal parenting within insecure attachments is thought to be due to the persistence of incoherent adult stances toward attachment. Given the view that insecure attachment can be considered a risk factor for future difficulties, understanding the nature of coherence becomes a pressing concern for parents and mental health professionals interested in early intervention and preventative measures.

What is incoherence of mind, and how can it be transformed

into coherence? Incongruity, fragmentation, and restricted flow of information are the elements of such incoherence, as seen within the AAI narratives of individuals who are classified as dismissing, preoccupied, and unresolved/disoriented. Studies of those individuals who appear to have had suboptimal attachment histories but receive "earned" secure/autonomous AAI classifications in the Main and Goldwyn system[23] reveal that their parenting, even under stressful conditions, is sensitive and nurturing.[24] "Earned" secure/ autonomous status is most often achieved through supportive personal or therapeutic relationships (for example, marriage or psychotherapy). The implication of these findings is that even with difficult past childhood experiences, the mind is capable of achieving an integrated perspective—one that is coherent and that permits parenting behavior to be sensitive and empathic. If integration is achieved, the trend toward transmission of insecure forms of attachment to the next generation can be prevented. Achieving coherence of mind thus becomes a central goal for creating emotional well-being in both oneself and one's offspring. As we'll see, such integration involves internal processes and their facilitation by interpersonal interactions.

Integration can be proposed to be a key process that influences the trajectory of developmental pathways toward resilience or toward vulnerability. For example, one factor in the adolescent onset of certain psychiatric disturbances, such as mood, eating, or identity disorders, may be the challenge of the need for integration.[25] Those who are not fortunate enough to achieve this sense of coherence may live with adaptive selves whose goals are incompatible with each other; in such individuals, mental modules and the information they process create anxiety and conflict if shared across modalities. For these people, emotional imbalance may be due to the inability to integrate the self diachronically into a coherent whole. For example, an individual who has been humiliated repeatedly as a child may find rejection as an adolescent or adult extremely disorganizing. The self-state that needs affiliation and acceptance from others is in direct opposition to the need to gain status and rise, say, in the school setting or the corporate world, where being in a position of authority inevitably involves evoking the displeasure of others. Such an individual may find her career hampered by such a conflict in needs. Most people experience some degree of conflict between inner desires and outer realities. But at times these desires are a part of fairly distinct states of mind, which can remain out of the awareness of many individuals. Even without awareness, the mind may experience the emotional imbalance of such conflicts as the onset of depression, anxiety, uncontrolled rage, a feeling of meaninglessness and disconnection (as in a "false self"), loss of motivation, and interpersonal difficulties. Harter and coworkers' studies suggest that the more adolescents experience their roles as "false" and not "authentic," the more turmoil they feel.[26] Social contexts that force individuals to adapt via self-states that are not reflective of their own experiences, mental states, and needs may place these persons at higher risk of developing emotional disorders.

Attachment relationships may therefore serve as catalysts of risk or resilience, to the extent that they facilitate the flow of inauthentic versus authentic states within interactions with others. We can propose that *insecure attachments confer vulnerability because they fail to offer children interpersonal experiences that foster an integrative self-organizational process.* Later relationships with peers and teachers can also make a difference; interpersonal influences on the self-states that emerge to adapt to social contexts directly shape mental health. Though early attachment experiences have been shown to have a direct influence on social competence, sense of autonomy, ego resilience, and peer acceptance, it seems clear that dyadic relationships beyond those with early caregivers may continue to influence the development of regulatory capacities.[27] As Cicchetti and Rogosch have noted, resilience is not a trait or some fixed achievement, but is an emergent state function dependent upon self-organizational processes and continued interdependence within social connections.[28]

The capacity for self-integration, like the processes of the mind itself, is continually created by an interaction of internal neurophysiological processes and interpersonal relationships. Resilience and emotional well-being are fundamental mental processes that emerge as the mind integrates the flow of energy and information across time and between minds.

As Ogawa and colleagues have paraphrased the work of Loevinger, "Integration is not a function of the self, it is what the self is."[29] They go on to state, "Therefore, the failure to integrate salient experience represents profound distortion in the self system. When salient experience must be unnoticed, disallowed, unacknowledged, or forgotten, the result is incoherence in the self structure. Interconnections among experiences cannot be made, and the resulting gaps in personal history compromise both the complexity and the integrity of the self."[30]

THE INTEGRATING SELF
Creating Coherence

The integrating mind attempts to create a sense of coherence among multiple selves across time and across contexts. We have discussed in Chapter 6 how the inherent features of computation, complexity, and connectionism create a property of cohesion within a state of mind in a given slice of time. Self-states have a repeating pattern of cohesive activity, which lends a sense of historical continuity to their existence. If each of us existed as a continuous flow of states, this might be the end of the story. But as we've discussed, the complex systems of our minds are capable of abrupt transitions into markedly different states. These state transitions lack cohesion and continuity. How, then, does the mind achieve coherence across self-states?

The struggle to satisfy needs and desires within a complex social world is often filled with conflict. Examples can be found in many periods of life: a married adult's desire to explore his sexuality with other adults, but also to maintain affiliation with spouse and family; a young professional's struggle to balance her drive to achieve on a personal level with her need to be a part of a group process; an adolescent's need to have an identity as a member of his peer group, while at the same time seeking a sense of individuality and autonomy; a child's drive to master new situations and yet her desire to feel safe in a familiar environment. Each of these individuals can be seen as experiencing "conflictual needs," which are a part of the experience of segmented self-states. The properties we've seen in states of mind, the research on normal child and adolescent development, and the findings of cognitive neuroscience all suggest that in fact the normal functioning of the mind consists of many processes that can indeed function fairly autonomously. Just as the body is made up of its component parts, the mind as a whole system is made up of the activity of these multiple self-states.

At the transition between self-states, there may be a temporary disorganization or incohesion and discontinuity in the activity of the brain; however, once a new state of mind is instantiated, cohesion is reestablished. How can a four-dimensional sense of coherence be created with such discontinuous transitions across states? Why can't the mind merely function as independent sets of self-states? Answering these questions is facilitated by reviewing the way the mind functions as a self-organizational system.

Self-organization at the level of the mind must involve the integrative processing of these self-states across time and context. It is at the moments of transition that new self-organizational forms can be constructed. Indeed, integrating coherence of the mind is about state *shifts*. Congruity and unity emerge at the interface of how information and energy—the defining elements of the mind—flow across states. As Allan Schore has stated,

> The term "self-organization" can be imprecise and misleading, because first, despite the implications of the two words used to describe the process, self-organization occurs in interaction with another self—it is not monadic but dyadic. And second, the organization of brain systems does not involve a simple pattern of increments but rather large changes in organization. Development, the process of self-assembly, thus involves both progressive and regressive phenomena, and is best characterized as a sequence of processes of organization, disorganization, and reorganization.[31]

Integration is about how the mind creates a coherent self-assembly of information and energy flow across time and context. Integration creates the subjective experience of self.

Some people, then, can spend the vast majority of their time in cohesive, albeit relatively independent, self-states. If these states are not conflictual with one another—if the desires, beliefs, goals, and behaviors of one state are not in destructive competition with another—then what is the problem? Perhaps there is none. For these individuals, a coherent mind may be a natural developmental outcome of authentic nurturing relationships, supportive experiences with teachers in school, meaningful friendships, and identification with peer groups, which have all contributed to the development of a capacity for self-organization in a wide variety of contexts. *Integration establishes a sense of congruity and unity of the mind as it emerges within the flexible patterns in the flow of information and energy processes of the brain, both within itself and in interaction with others. This is coherence.*

For other people, *conflicts among different needs, mental models, and self-states may lead to internal distress or external difficulties that create dysfunction. Such a conflict among self-states within an individual can create incoherence.* Incoherence may develop from insecure or conflictual attachments, difficulties in meeting school or job expectations, or significant trouble with finding companions in friendships or peer groups. Incoherence may be revealed in various ways, such as impairments in affect regulation, insecurity, unresolved trauma or loss, and dysfunctional social relationships. Whether with professionals or in intimate relationships, an active approach to creating coherence may become necessary.

The Adapting Mind: Disorganized Attachment as an Example of Impaired Integration

As noted in earlier chapters, the parents of children with disorganized attachments have provided frightened, frightening, or disorienting shifts in their own behavior, which create conflictual experiences leading to incoherent mental models.[32] Such a child may develop an internal mental model for each aspect of the parent's behavior. Abrupt shifts in parental state force the child to adapt with suddenly shifting states of his own. Such state shifts may occur if the nature of these experiences is profoundly incompatible with attachment and/or if the child is neurobiologically capable of intense dissociative processes. With frequent experiences, the child can rapidly enter "altered states" to meet the interactive demands of the parent's sudden shifts in behavior. When such shifts are early, severe, and repeated, these states can become engrained in the child as self-states. The child both learns the processes of abrupt, dissociative state shifting and develops specific self-states that can be activated in response to specific external context cues. The result of these internal state shifts can be that the child may come to develop several forms of attachment with the parent: some avoidant, some ambivalent, some disorganized, and perhaps even some secure. These can be considered nonintegrated working models of attachment.

The quality of the relationship between the parent and child may thus vary significantly across repeated clusters of interactive experiences. Parent and child may enter various forms of "dyadic states" characterized by unique communication styles. A parent who disavows the existence of certain dyadic states (such as during periods of terrifying a child), without later repairing and reconnecting after such ruptured connections, will promote dissociative adaptations. A parent with unresolved trauma or loss may enter trance-like states that are frightening to a child but are unrecognized and unacknowledged by the parent. Such state shifts lead to disconnections in attunement, which, if left unrepaired, can lead the child to have profoundly disturbing underlying feelings of shame and humiliation.[33]

Some individuals have experienced secure attachments with certain caregivers and disorganized ones with others. In such cases, isolation of the attuned dyadic states may maintain high functioning within self-systems that have reflective functioning, as well as the capacity to integrate a coherent sense of self *across the self-states within that securely attached clustered system.* The AAI narratives of such persons may reveal an integrated coherence that on the surface appears to be highly functional. This is revealed in coherent stories about limited parts of the persons' lives. When certain psychosocial contexts, moments of stress, or less integrated subsystems emerge, then integration, reflective functioning, and narrative coherence may become impaired. In the narratives and lives of less well-functioning individuals, there may be a more generalized absence of any such reflective or integrative capacity, as a result of their more pervasive insecure attachment histories. These individuals may have had no developmental experience of interactive communication, which would have promoted such abilities. These individuals may have more difficulty utilizing internal or interpersonal resources, and thus have more marked impairments in their ability to cope with stress and to self-organize.

Giovanni Liotti has proposed that several different trajectories are possible in the setting of disorganized attachment.[34] If parental behavior becomes more predictable later in a child's life, even in the non-nurturing direction, then the child may minimize the conflict among the mental models of attachment that have been developed in the context of the abrupt and confusing shifts in the parent's behavior. In the case of a parent's becoming more predictable, then, the child may "settle" on one model or another. If the parent continues to exhibit disorienting behaviors, but these are not overly traumatizing, the child may develop the potential for future dissociation, especially under conditions of stress. A third pathway suggested by Liotti is that if the parent's behavior remains severely traumatizing and chronic, then the disorganized attachment may evolve into a dissociative disorder. At the extreme of this spectrum is dissociative identity disorder (formerly known as multiple personality disorder).

Elizabeth Carlson, working with the Minnesota Parent–Child Project, has provided longitudinal support for Liotti's proposal that children with disorganized attachments are predisposed to develop clinical symptoms of dissociation later in life.[35] This, combined with the finding that dissociation itself puts those who experience stressful events at risk of developing clinical posttraumatic stress disorder,[36] suggests that disorganized attachment experiences early in life may lead to inadequate coping mechanisms and impaired interactive capacities. This vulnerability, in turn, makes these individuals less likely to be able to resolve trauma or grief, if such stressors are encountered later in life. In disorganized attachments, the core of the self remains fractured. As Ogawa and colleagues have stated,

> Self, in fact, refers to the integration and organization of diverse aspects of experience, and dissociation can be defined as the failure to integrate experience. . . . When experience is acknowledged and accepted, integration inevitably follows, because the self cannot help seeking meaning and coherence from experience. When experience is dissociated, however, integration is not possible, and to the extent that dissociation prevails, there is fragmentation of the self. A coherent, well-organized self depends on integration, and thus psychopathological dissociation represents a threat to optimal development of the self.[37]

For the child with disorganized attachment, in other words, relationship experiences have severely hampered the developmental acquisition of the capacity to achieve coherence. The segmentation of mental processes becomes an engrained process itself: dissociation.

What is dissociation? Numerous books have been written about the conceptualization, history, genesis, evaluation, psychopathology, and treatment of dissociative disorders. For the purposes of this chapter, let us look briefly at the self-organizational aspects of dissociative states of mind, and see how such states involve an impairment in the ability to achieve coherence of the self. The reader is referred to other sources for a more comprehensive review of this important area.[38]

"Dissociation" is a term with many meanings. Clinicians use the term to refer to a discontinuity in mental functioning that is a part of a number of disorders, such as panic, borderline personality, and posttraumatic stress disorders. Dissociation includes the phenomena of depersonalization, derealization, and psychogenic amnesia. The term is also used to refer to a specific group of clinical disorders, including dissociative identity disorder, dissociative fugue, dissociative amnesia, and depersonalization disorder. In any of these latter conditions, there is a disruption in the integration of various processes, including memory, identity, perception, and consciousness.[39]

Clinical dissociation can be viewed as a dis-association in the usually integrative functioning of the mind. How does this happen? Mental functioning emanates from anatomically distinct and fairly autonomous circuits, each of which can be dis-associated from the function of the others. Studies of a drug called ketamine demonstrate that administering it to normal subjects leads to dissociative symptoms, such as depersonalization and derealization.[40] Subjects with prior histories of trauma experience the additional symptoms of terror and panic. Ketamine blocks the transmission of signals across the synapses of large neurons, which are especially plentiful in the associational regions of the cortex. This finding suggests that the disassociation of functions in dissociation may be mediated by a blockage in the integrative capacity of associational regions, which coordinate an array of neural pathways.

As an information-processing system, the mind has layers of representational processes that are created by various inputs from more and more complex representational levels. Studies of brain function reveal that neural pathways have such layers of input, in which secondary and tertiary association areas link streams of neural activity into more and more complex networks of activation.[41] These processes in turn influence a widely distributed set of neural processes responsible for our emotional states, bodily response, reasoning, memory retrieval, and perceptual biases.[42] Regions of the brain such as the orbitofrontal cortex, which function to coordinate these disparate functions across time, may be proposed to play a crucial role in the integrative process. Various mental processes may thus be functionally isolated from one another with the blockage of integrative circuits. As we've seen, these associational functions include social cognition, autonoetic consciousness, response flexibility, stimulus appraisal, and affect regulation.[43] Isolation of these functions may be at the core of incoherence during dissociative experiences.

OBSERVING INTEGRATION

Coherence and Complexity

We can propose that integration creates coherence by enabling the mind's flow of information and energy to achieve a balance in its movement toward maximizing complexity. This movement of the flow of states of mind can involve activity both within the mind itself and in interactions with other minds. This balance means that the system moves between sameness and rigidity on the one hand, and novelty and chaos on the other. As we've seen, systems achieve stability as they flow between these extremes in their movement toward maximal complexity. Within this optimal flow are connections of the processes both within a single mind and between minds. Integration involves the recruitment of internal and interpersonal processes into a mutually activating co-regulation, which we have earlier defined as "resonance." We can thus look at resonance within both internal processes and interpersonal relationships to understand how the mind's attempts at integration bring about coherence.

Resonance, as we've discussed earlier, is the property of interacting systems that defines the influence of each system's activity on the other. Between two individuals, for example, emotionally attuned and contingent communication creates interpersonal resonance; each member of the dyad is influenced by the other. Within the brain, the neural process of reentry can help us to understand how distinct circuits can become involved in a resonating state. Circuit A sends signals to B, which in turn sends signals back to A, and so on. The reentrant activity of such a circuit links A and B as an integrated system at that moment. In this manner, A and B are part of a state-dependent process. In a different state, the activity of A may have little influence on that of B. Resonance is a term that can thus be used to describe the nature of a system's contingent, reentrant, co-regulating influences of the interacting elements—whether these are clusters of neurons, circuits, systems, hemispheres, or entire brains (as in interpersonal communication). In resonance, the subcomponent parts become functionally linked in an integrated system.

Let's try to define the relationships among the terms "integration," "coherence," "cohesion," and "resonance." We've defined "integration" as the process that creates coherence in the mind. "Coherence" is the state of the system in which many layers of neural functioning become activated and "cohere" to each other over time. Complexity theory gives us some insight into why this linking process may occur: States of the system that maximize complexity achieve stability. In this way, integration defines the self. As the mind moves toward complexity, it recruits various layers of processes into a cohesive state of mind. "Cohesion" is thus a state in which subcomponents become linked together at a given moment in time. As the mind emerges across time, cohesive states become a part of a coherent flow. The linkages of subcomponents—whether in a given moment (cohesion) or across time (coherence)—are achieved by the process of integration. Integration recruits differentiated subcomponent circuits into a larger functional system through a fundamental reentry process. The co-regulating, mutually influencing state of reentrant connections is called "resonance." In other words, *integra-*

tion utilizes the resonance of different subsystems to achieve cohesive states and a coherent flow of states across time. Such a process creates a more complex, functionally linked system, which itself can become a subcomponent of even larger and more complex systems.

Translating this often nonconscious process into words is quite a challenge. Within particular sensory modalities, for example, there may be a feeling of "connection" with the object in the focus of conscious attention. Looking at a flower can become a dynamic, consuming process in which the self and the flower lose their boundaries within conscious experience. The act of creation in many activities can feel as if some powerful flow of energy and information within the mind is occurring without intention and with a life of its own. Within interpersonal relationships, integration may be experienced as fullness of communication and spontaneity, in which the self is both fully present and lost within the flow of a vibrant, unpredictable, and yet reliable dyadic connection.

These experiences have the quality of "joining," in which the individual becomes a part of a process larger than the self. As integration occurs, the creation of coherence represents the flow of states of the system on the "fertile ground between order and chaos"[44]—a path of resonance with a balanced trajectory between rigidity and randomness. The particular "system" whose states are flowing may involve any level of functioning: localized circuits in the brain, larger neuronal systems, both hemispheres, or two or more minds. The subjective experience of coherence will depend on the nature of the elements of the system activated in the resonance created by the integrative process.

Is there empirical support for the relationship between integration and the creation of such joining experiences? One possible source of corroboration may come from the studies of "optimal experiences" by Mihaly Csikszentmihalyi.[45] In these investigations, subjects who had the experience of "flow"—a process in which one creatively loses oneself in an activity—often seemed to have well-developed skills at becoming highly focused and fully immersed in an activity, such as athletics, playing music, or writing. Csikszentmihalyi has suggested that such flow experiences involve the individual's moving between the boundaries of boredom on the one hand and anxiety on the other. We can propose that these experiences maximize the complexity of an individual's states in their movement between rigidity/order (boredom) and randomness/chaos (anxiety). We can also suggest that such experiences actually become self-reinforcing, as they facilitate the development of integrative processes within the individual that enhance the capacity for joining in a variety of contexts. The capacity for such a joining process might be revealed in an individual's immersion within an activity ("flow"), as well as within the collaborative communication of interpersonal relationships. This possibility is supported by Csikszentmihalyi's finding that individuals who experienced flow tended to have a combination of highly specialized individual skills and a capacity for being socially integrated with others. Future studies may be helpful in exploring the possible ways in which the capacities for joining within activities and within interpersonal relationships are related to each other as well as to the development of integrative processes, and perhaps emotional well-being, across the lifespan.

The Narrative Process

What evidence is available to help us understand the integrative process and to support the notion that it actually exists? There are several sources of data. The first we will examine is the integrative function of narratives. Studies of child development reveal that by the third year of life, a "narrative" function emerges in children and allows them to create stories about the events they encounter during their lives.[46] These narratives are sequential descriptions of people and events that condense numerous experiences into generalizing and contrasting stories. New experiences are compared to old ones. Similarities are noted in creating generalized rules, and differences are highlighted as memorable exceptions to these rules. The stories are about making sense of events and the mental experiences of the characters. Filled with the elements of the characters' internal experience in the context of interactions with others in the world, these stories appear to be functioning to create a sense of coherent comprehension of the individual in the world across time.

Is this related to a drive to create coherence among the disparate aspects of one's own mind? We could argue that it is, but this is not necessarily the case. Narratives may at times selectively focus on the minds of others and on external contexts, not on one's own internal experience. Children begin as biographers and emerge into autobiographers. As Dennie Wolf has discussed, a child begins to develop an "authorial self" by two years of age. In her view, "authorship is the ability to act independent[ly] of the impinging facts of a situation." Such a process requires the ability to "uncouple" various versions of experience, as well as the "emergence of explicit forms of representation to mark the nature of and movement among the stances of the self."[47] This view is based on the notion that the child can adopt different perspectives on or versions of the experience of self. As Wolf states, "Our most immediate definition of self is that of a coherent and distinctive center: a bodily container, an anchor point for our sense of agency, a single source for our emotions (no matter how chaotic), or a kind of volume where the chapters of a very personal history accumulate."[48] As the child experiences different domains of self-experience (or "self-states," as we have defined them), the authorial self is challenged to incorporate these different "versions of the self" into an autobiographical narrative process. The development of such a personal process, as we've seen in other domains, is extremely dependent upon social experience.[49]

The narrative process in this way attempts to make sense of the world and of one's own mind and its various states. In some individuals, however, one sees narratives that reflect upon a particular self-state without creating a more global coherence of the mind as a whole. The narrative process is thus a fundamental building block of an integrative mode, but insufficient by itself to create coherence across self-states through time. Let's look at three other sources of data that can help us explore the nature of integration and its potential relationship to the narrative process.

Hidden Observers

A second source of information regarding an integrative mode of processing consists of studies of normal subjects in hypnotic or trance-like states. In this condition, the vast majority of the population appears to have a third-party observing capacity, which has been called a "hidden observer," "observing ego," "internal self-helper," or "inner guide."[50] The hidden observer reveals itself under hypnosis or guided imagery as a form of mental output that makes comments about the person: "Dan is working too much; he should slow down and relax more," or "Her need to get this project done is interfering with her ability to exercise. She should stop being so busy with the project." This function reveals the mind's capacity for processing mindsight, representing states of mind, and processing the context of an experience over time. Comments such as these, made under the hypnotic condition of focused internal concentration, are intended to *alter the functioning* of the individual as a whole. This appears to be not just an observing function (information representation), but also an effort to use this information to change other aspects of behavior (processing the information and causing further effects). We can therefore view the hidden observer as an integrative attempt of the mind to create a sense of coherence across its own states through time and contexts.

Does the hidden observer exist beyond the conditions of hypnosis? Several sources of information suggest that it does. First of all, as we've just seen, children develop the capacity at an early age to narrate their own lives from multiple perspectives, including the third-person, observer perspective. Second, studies of memory reveal that people have the capacity for observer recollections in which they recall themselves from a distant perspective, seeing themselves in a scene from the past as if they were watching themselves from afar.[51] Furthermore, clinical studies of patients with a variety of disorders reveal an internal process that comments on ongoing experience. In patients with dissociative disorders, an "internal self-helper" that attempts to coordinate some of the disparate activities of the mind is quite a common self-state.[52] Individuals with depression may experience an "internal voice" that is demeaning and pessimistic, and that further entrenches the negative, depressed mood.

What does the hidden observer tell us about interpersonal experience? In examining the relationship between hypnosis and developmental processes, Brian Vandenberg states, first, that hypnosis reveals how "social exchange and intrapsychic functioning interpenetrate, that self and other, cognitive and social, individual and culture are intimately enmeshed"; second, that it suggests that "thought and experience are not always continuous, seamless, autonomous, and internal but involve discontinuities, dislocations, and alterations that are structured by contextual factors"; and, third, that hypnotic states reflect "the childhood experience of lability of grounding, and of 're-ceiving speech' from an authoritative other who provides stability in an uncertain world."[53] Communication with a parent, in other words, can enable a child to achieve a sense of coherence in the face of confusing shifts in the internal and external worlds. Could it be that children's early relationship experiences with contingent communication and reflective dialogue facilitate the development of an "internal voice" that addresses the self from a third-person perspective and helps integrate a sense of coherence? Could this form of thought be the internalization of interpersonal dialogue, as Lev Vygotsky has suggested?[54] Future studies examining the relationships among parent–child attachment, discourse, narrative, and the hidden observer will help elucidate these processes.

Hemispheric Laterality

A third source of information supporting the existence of an integrative mode of processing consists of research on the specialized functions of the brain's two hemispheres. The following findings (many of which have been reviewed earlier) have been consistently obtained in investigations ranging from studies of "split-brain" patients to studies involving brain function imaging. When information is presented to only the left hemisphere, verbal output reflects an effort to create a story or make sense of what it sees or hears. Michael Gazzaniga and colleagues have called this the "interpreter" function of the left hemisphere.[55] For the isolated left hemisphere, these words are confabulations—made-up stories that fit with the data, but are unrelated to the gist or context of the situation. In these studies, the left hemisphere appears to lack the contextual representations of the right hemisphere, but nevertheless creates a story to explain the limited information at its disposal. The left hemisphere uses syllogistic reasoning, stating major and minor premises and deducing logical conclusions from a limited set of data in an attempt to clarify cause–effect relationships. For example, if a subject with an isolated left hemisphere is asked about a picture showing a boy and his father, the left hemisphere will take the details of the scene and create a fabricated explanation of what the two people are doing. Surrounding elements, such as the fact that the other parts of the picture reveal a baseball game or the facial expressions of the pair, are ignored. These contextual elements do not appear to be perceived by the left hemisphere, or at least they are ignored when it comes to explaining what the scene is about. The left hemisphere's interpreter function seems to be driven primarily by a need to reason about cause–effect relationships, rather than to establish some coordinated or coherent view of "truth." In this manner, some authors have suggested that the left hemisphere may be primarily responsible for the creation of distorted and "false" memories of past experiences.[56]

  In contrast to the left, the right hemisphere appears to be able to make sense of the essential meaning of the input it is able to perceive: Contextual information is perceived and processed, and the gist of a situation is sized up and understood. The right hemisphere does not use syllogistic logic to deduce conclusions about cause–

effect relationships, but rather represents information about the environment. Such information includes the relationships of various components of experience, including elements of mental processes and spatial relationships. Since the right hemisphere is nonverbal, the output of its processing must be expressed in non-word-based ways, such as drawing a picture or pointing to a pictorial set of options to make its output known to the external world.

As discussed at length in prior chapters, these hemispheric differences have embryological origins and reflect a dominance of processing in the dorsal or ventral circuits on each side of the brain. Numerous studies support the view that the capacity for mindsight is right-hemisphere-mediated. The registration and regulation of bodily state, the perception and expression of nonverbal signals of affective state, the coordination of social and emotional input with the appraisal centers of the brain, and the retrieval of autobiographical memory all appear to be predominantly mediated by the right hemisphere. The capacity to represent states of mind within the mind is probably mediated within the right-hemisphere's domains of processing. We have thus proposed that reflective function, which permits mentalizing, is likely to be mediated primarily by the right hemisphere.

These laterality studies suggest several relevant aspects of the mind's functioning. The left hemisphere tries to create explanations for the information it receives, but it lacks the ability to process the context of this information, and so its conclusions are based on selected details without relational meaning. The left hemisphere's interpreter deduces an explanation that is superficially logical but is often without contextual substance if this hemisphere is acting in isolation from information from the right hemisphere. The right hemisphere processes the overall gist of a scene and creates a context-rich representational "understanding." The right hemisphere specializes in the ability to perceive the mental states of others and to represent others' minds. Although it may not use syllogistic reasoning to interpret and deduce cause–effect relationships, it has a reflective understanding of the social world of other minds.

Making Sense of Minds

Another important implication of the three sets of studies reviewed to this point is that people are constantly trying to "make sense" of what they experience. On one level, making sense means trying to understand cause–effect relationships—what is happening and why it happened. Why does the mind try to do this? (Even the asking of this question reflects the human mind's need to make sense of things, including the mind itself!) A straightforward answer comes from the reverse-engineering approach of evolutionary thinking: Individuals whose brains were able to understand cause–effect relationships were more likely to survive and to pass on their genetic material. Why? Because if the mind can perceive the events of the world, remember them, extract cause–effect relationships (understanding, making sense), and use these processes to influence the outcome of future behavior in the world, then it will be more likely to survive. As we have noted throughout this book, the brain functions as an anticipation machine; it takes data from the perceived world and prepares itself for the next event. Individuals whose brains were good at anticipating did better than those whose brains merely lived in the here-and-now. For instance, it was easier to avoid a lion if people figured out that a growl (cause) could indicate the presence of a lion who would eat them (effect). Such is the basis for learning. Such is the basis for making sense of the world.

Making sense of the social world of minds is a bit more complicated, but it involves the same basic problem of cause–effect relationships. What does the scowl of another person "mean"? How do the subtle and rapid signals, both verbal and nonverbal, from other people reveal what is happening and what may happen next? Knowing whom to trust and whom to be wary of is essential in negotiating one's way through the human world of social interactions. The states of mind of others—their intentions, beliefs, attitudes, and emotions—predispose an individual to behave in a certain way. *The ability to anticipate the behavior of others is dependent upon the ability to understand other minds.*

Functioning in a complex social network enhances people's capacity to survive as individuals, reproduce, and create a group of like-minded individuals who share such a capacity. This can be seen as a form of interindividual integration, in which an individual becomes a member of a community beyond the dyadic relationships of attachment and friendship. The potential for such a group to become a functionally cohesive system of individuals will enhance the chances of that group's surviving in competition with isolated humans or with groups that cannot process such social communication signals as well. Such shared mentalizing abilities permit the group to function as a cohesive system composed of connected individuals. This allows for a "group state" to be achieved, which can facilitate the development of a highly effective problem-solving system to meet challenges in a world filled with competition. Being a member of a group in this way confers a sense of safety, security, and stability on an individual. A number of studies suggest complex relationships among early attachment history, experiences with teachers, relationships with friends, and social competence in peer groups.[57] One of these studies has shown, for example, that peer acceptance and leadership abilities are associated with a history of secure attachments.[58] Relationships, both early and later in life, clearly make a difference as our lives evolve. Overall, these findings support the notion that the individual continues to develop in interaction with an evolving set of internal processes as well as social experiences within interpersonal and group relationships.

Through the life course, the individual mind attempts to create a coherent internal, interpersonal, and group experience. Such an integrative process places the system of the individual mind within the context of complex social forces, which directly shape the life course in often unpredictable ways. As Glenn Elder has described, "life course theory and research alert us to this real world, a world in which lives are lived and where people work out paths of development as best they can. It tells us how lives are socially organized in biological and historical time, and how the resulting social pattern affects the way we think, feel and act."[59] Our minds are in this manner continually processing both internal and social experiences as we develop through time.

The finding that our minds appear to have "cheater detectors," which identify misleading social communications intended to mask the true inner states and intentions of others, supports this idea that group functioning has been a central shaping force in the evolution of the human mind.[60] Natural selection has thus enabled our minds to evolve mindsight capacities. Being able to navigate our way through such an intense social world requires the ability to make sense of other minds. Communicating the more elaborate and intricate learned aspects of this mentalizing knowledge to others allows the benefits of one individual's wisdom and experience to be shared with others in the group. This knowledge is transmitted from one individual to others in the group by means of storytelling. *Making sense of other minds is the essential stuff of narratives.* This means that the mentalizing representations of the right hemisphere may need to be integrated with the interpreting ones of the left in both the expression and reception of such information. What can stories tell us about such an integrative process?

AN INTERPERSONAL NEUROBIOLOGY
OF STORIES

Narrative and Neural Integration

Narrative may have originated as a fundamental part of social discourse. Recall that stories are created within a social context between human minds. The process of narrative is thus inherently social. The contents of stories are human lives and mental experiences. Describing an interpersonal neurobiology of stories may be helpful in elucidating the fundamental processes involved in how narrative facilitates the integration of coherence within the mind. Let's first review some aspects of the neural integration involved in stories.

The hippocampus is considered a "cognitive mapper": It gives the brain a sense of the self in space and in time, regulates the order of perceptual categorizations, and links mental representations to emotional appraisal centers.[61] These are multiple layers of integration.

A number of authors propose that the associational areas of the neocortex, such as the prefrontal regions (including the orbitofrontal cortex) that link various widely distributed representational processes together, form dynamic global maps or complex representations from the input of widely distributed regions in order to establish a sensorimotor integration of the self across space and time.[62] This capacity allows for the anticipation of and planning for future events as they are created from the integrated representation of the experiences of the self. This is autonoetic consciousness. Such a spatiotemporal integrating process can be proposed to be fundamental to the narrative mode of cognition. This mapping process may be at the heart of autobiographical narrative and the way the mind attempts to achieve a sense of coherence among its various states: trying to make sense of the self in the past, the present and the anticipated future. We can propose that the capacity of the mind to create such a global map of the self across time and various contexts—to have autonoetic consciousness—is an essential feature of integration that may continue to develop throughout life.

Narrative can also be viewed as requiring both right- and left-hemisphere modes of processing information. The right brain's perceptually rich, analogic, context-dependent, autonoetic, mentalizing representations create much of the imagery and many of the themes of the narrative process. The logical, linear, "making sense" interpretations of these representations and the communication of narrative details stem from the left hemisphere's interpretive and linguistic processing of digital representations. On each side of the brain, these processes may reflect a vertical integration of various representational processes. As the dorsal tract processes (dominant in the right hemisphere) interconnect with those of the ventral tract (dominant in the left hemisphere), dorsal–ventral integration begins to occur. Within these forms of integration, processes on the right begin to be integrated with those on the left. We can propose the following bilateral integration process for narratives: *The left hemisphere's drive to understand cause–effect relationships is a primary motivation of the narrative process. Coherent narratives, however, require participation of both the interpreting left hemisphere and the mentalizing right hemisphere. Coherent narratives are created through interhemispheric integration.*

Integration that recruits multiple layers of circuits may create the most complex states as it links various forms of representation throughout the brain (and, as we'll see, between brains). Vertical, dorsal–ventral, lateral, interhemispheric, and spatiotemporal forms of integration are all present within the narrative process. The "drive to make sense of the mind," drawing on these multidimensional layers of integration, may in part be seen as a way the brain achieves a more stable (complex) connection among its various representational processes. The left hemisphere's effort to find cause–effect relationships draws upon the right hemisphere's retrieval of autobiographical and mentalizing representations. Such multilayered integration may exist independently of narration. In other words, the mind may be internally driven to link these layers of representational processes as a function of achieving coherence within the mind itself. Such internal coherence may be revealed within the orbitofrontal cortex's capacity for response flexibility and may reflect the integration of a range of prefrontally mediated processes. As we attempt to communicate a shareable set of representations within autobiographical stories, we must use the linguistic translations and interpretations of the left hemisphere in order to express the narrative of our lives. Such a communication process lets us see for ourselves, and share with others, the fundamental way in which our minds come to integrate experience.

As we've discussed in Chapter 2, Endel Tulving and colleagues have postulated a dual role for the frontal lobes on each side of the brain. In their "hemispheric encoding–retrieval asymmetry" hypothesis, the left hemisphere is seen as the primary mediator of autobiographical encoding, whereas the right is responsible for retrieval.[63] Autonoetic consciousness gives us the ability to perform "mental time travel," in which we can represent the self in the past, present, and future.[64] We have also discussed the possibility that the consolidation of memory into permanent storage may require REM sleep and thus depend on the synchronous activation of both hemispheres. We have proposed that this bilateral activation of the brain may permit a rhythmic process in which right frontal activation retrieves autobiographical representations from more posterior regions of the right brain. The transfer of this information to the left orbitofrontal regions may then allow encoding to occur. In essence, this may be the encoding of the newly assembled representations created from retrieved memory. Items in long-term (nonpermanent) storage in this way may be retrieved (right side) and encoded (left side) in a process that integrates information from recent and more distant past experiences as well as from imagination, current perception, and random activations. As Winson has suggested, the electrical activity and neuroendocrine milieu of the REM stage of sleep may allow for the consolidation of memory via the induction of the long-term potentiation of synaptic connections.[65] This bilateral encoding–retrieval process may facilitate the creation of new and strengthened associational links. This process may also reveal how memory retrieval acts as a "memory modifier" in this setting of bilateral activation, permitting recent recollections of the day's experiences to be synthesized with prior elements of memory within a constructive and thematic narrative process.

In this proposal, interhemispheric integration is essential for memory consolidation. Dreaming, REM sleep, and cortical consolidation become the integrating processes that mediate autobiographical narrative. Blockage of these integrating processes may be seen as the core of unresolved trauma and may be revealed as one form of incoherence in autobiographical narratives. Autonoetic consciousness may thus be impaired as the ability to integrate representations of the self across past, present, and future is disrupted in lack of resolution. This proposal regarding narrative, consolidation, and bilateral integration is a hypothesis in need of validation. As Milner, Squire, and Kandel have noted, we are still far from understanding the exact mechanisms behind the consolidation process.[66] Future research will need to clarify exactly how this consolidation process occurs.

The ways in which interpersonal experience shapes both implicit memory and explicit memory directly affect our life stories. Narratives, though they draw on consciously accessible explicit memory, are also influenced by implicit recollections. Our dreams and stories may contain implicit aspects of our lives even without our awareness. In fact, storytelling may be a primary way in which we can linguistically communicate to others—as well as to ourselves—the sometimes hidden contents of our implicitly remembering minds. Stories make available perspectives on the emotional themes of our implicit memory that may otherwise be consciously unavailable to us. This may be one reason why journal writing and intimate communication with others, which are so often narrative processes, have such powerful organizing effects on the mind: They allow us to modulate our emotions and make sense of the world. Integration, as observed in coherent narratives, directly shapes self-regulation.

Narrative and Interpersonal Integration

The narrative process also enables a form of interpersonal integration. The external expression of narrative through storytelling is a form of discourse inherently influenced by listeners' expectations. Early attachment experiences in this way have a direct effect on how children learn to narrate their lives and perhaps to develop autonoetic consciousness. Patterns of collaborative communication allow children to develop what Trevarthen has called "narratives of cooperative awareness."[67] As parents reflect with their securely attached children on the mental states that create their shared subjective experience, they are joining with them in an important co-constructive process of understanding how the mind functions. The inherent feature of secure attachment—contingent, collaborative communication—is also a fundamental component in how interpersonal relationships facilitate internal integration in a child. We can propose that a parent's engaging in what we have called reflective dialogue (focusing on the central importance of mental states in human behavior and their manifestations as feelings, perceptions, intentions, goals, beliefs, and desires) is also central to both secure attachment and the integrative process of co-construction of narratives. Social competence and a sense of autonomy, mastery, and self-determination are aspects of resilience that secure attachment fosters.[68] We can propose that integration also becomes a developmental capacity within the foundation of nurturing and reflective early relationships.

Secure attachment facilitates integration in the developing child by allowing for different forms of interpersonal resonance to occur. Left-hemisphere-to-left-hemisphere resonance takes the form of verbal communication within a linear, logical mode of discourse. Right-hemisphere-to-right-hemisphere resonance involves the nonverbal components of communication, such as tone of voice, gestures, and facial expressions. *In the co-construction of stories, parent and child enter into a dyadic form of bilateral resonance: Each person enters a state of interhemispheric integration, which is facilitated by interpersonal communication.* In this manner, secure attachment involves an intimate dance of resonant processes involving left-to-left, right-to-right, and bilateral-to-bilateral communication. This highly complex form of collaborative communication allows the dyad to move into highly resonant states, and also enables the child's mind to develop its own capacity for integration. Such a capacity may be at the heart of self-regulation.

In insecure attachments, such contingent, resonant communication often does not occur. For example, the avoidantly attached child's and dismissing adult's experience can be understood in part as dominated by a primarily left-hemisphere form of communication. These interactions may stem from the parent's tendency to access primarily the nonmentalizing representations of a dominant left-hemisphere interpreter. In fact, studies of the correspondence between affective expression (right hemisphere) and verbal communication (left hemisphere) reveal such a dis-association in these dyads.[69] The capacity to blend the nonverbal/prosodic elements of dialogue with those of semantic/linguistic meaning requires the harmonious collaboration between the hemispheres.[70] As Sroufe has noted, "shared emotion is the fabric of social relationships" and "provides the rhythm or punctuation in human interaction and communication."[71] Thus avoidant attachment reveals an emotional impairment in the ability of two minds to communicate fully. Resonance and the capacity to integrate experience in a complex and interhemispheric way are significantly restricted. This absence of emotion produces a severe restriction in the level of interpersonal connection that parent and child are able to achieve. Such a condition reflects the central role emotion plays as an integrating process, both within the mind and between minds.

Within the individual mind, bilateral integration may occur in creative processes of many forms. My clinical work with insecurely attached individuals who experience a transformation in their "state of mind with respect to attachment" within psychotherapy or other emotionally involving relationships suggests that their new experience of interpersonal connection allows them to achieve new levels of mental coherence. This new capacity for integration—both interpersonal and internal—may create a sense of vitality and a release of creative energy and ideas, leading to an invigorating sense of personal expression. Such spontaneous and energized processes can give rise to participation in various activities, such as painting, music, dance, poetry, creative writing, or sculpture. It can also yield a deeper sense of creativity and appreciation within the "everyday" experience of life: communication with others, walks down the street, new appreciation of the richness of perceptions, feelings of being connected to the flow of the moment. Life becomes a process, not merely a focus on products. Part of this experience of creativity may be derived from the way in which activated elements in one modality freely recruit those in another. Much of this is nonconscious, but the new resonance among processes can give rise to an awareness of the activated flow of an emerging, coherent mind. Many people find this sense of vitality, intensity, and clarity to be quite exhilarating.

The integrating experience of resonance also gives rise to a sense of spontaneity and creativity when it occurs between two people. Such vibrant connections between minds can be seen within various kinds of emotional relationships, such as those of romantic partners, friends, colleagues, teachers and students, therapists and patients, and parents and children. Two people become companions on a mutually created journey through time. Interpersonal integration can be seen in spontaneous, resonant communication that flows freely and is balanced between continuity, familiarity, and predictability on one side and flexibility, novelty, and uncertainty on the other. Neither partner of a dyad is fully predictable, yet each is quite familiar. The collaborative communication between the two is not merely a reflective mirror, but a reciprocal, contingent process that moves the pair into vibrant states neither alone could achieve. The resultant evolving process creates a sense of the emerging complexity and coherence of integrating minds.

REFLECTIONS: INTEGRATING MINDS

As the mind emerges within the flow of self-states, it creates coherence across these states by a process we have defined as "integration." Integration allows the mind to experience the mutual co-regulation of energy flow and information processing, which permits adaptive, coordinated functioning. Incoherence derives from the inflexible, maladaptive, and restricted flow of energy and information within the mind across time. Interpersonal processes can facilitate integration by altering the restrictive ways in which the mind may have come to organize itself.

Creating coherence is a lifetime project. Integration is thus a process, not a final accomplishment. It is a verb, not a noun. This process perhaps is best seen as a form of "resonance," defined as the mutually influencing interactions between two or more relatively independent and differentiated entities. This resonance allows two systems to amplify and co-regulate each other's activity. In the case of one mind, integration allows for the spontaneous flow of energy and information within the whole brain. This spontaneity does not mean random activation, but the flexible influence of layers of processes upon each other. By contrast, insecure attachment patterns produce incoherence, in that individuals' adaptations to suboptimal parenting experiences have placed marked restrictions on their capacity for resonance—both within their own minds and with other minds.

Autobiographical narratives can reveal integration or incoherence. A coherent narrative reveals a blending of left- and right-hemisphere processes. The interpreting left hemisphere is driven to weave a tale of what it knows. When access to the right hemisphere's representational processes is limited, such a tale is incoherent. When the mentalizing, primary emotional, somatosensory, and autobiographical processes of the right hemisphere can be drawn upon, the left brain is able to "make sense" by integrating a coherent life story. Bilateral integration promotes coherent narratives.

The multilayered resonance of contingently communicating dyadic states allows each individual to acquire new integrative capacities. Two people connect across space by means of the flow of energy and information from both sides of each brain. This flow is contained within patterns of communication. As seen in attachment relationships, the development of the mind depends upon the basics of contingent, collaborative communication. Acquiring the capacity for integrating coherence comes from dyadic communication. Emotional attunement, reflective dialogue, co-construction of narrative, memory talk, and the interactive repair of disruptions in connection are all fundamental elements of secure attachment and of effective interpersonal relationships.

Connections between minds therefore involve a dyadic form of resonance in which energy and information are free to flow across two brains. When such a process is in full activation, the vital feeling of connection is exhilarating. When interpersonal communication is "fully engaged"—when the joining of minds is in full force—there is an overwhelming sense of immediacy, clarity, and authenticity. It is in these heightened moments of engagement, these dyadic states of resonance, that one can appreciate the power of relationships to nurture and to heal the mind.

Notes

Preface
1. Kandel (1998).
2. Stoller (1985, p. x).

Chapter 1
1. *Webster's New World College Dictionary* (1997, p. 1085).
2. Kandel and Schwartz (1992); Milner, Squire, and Kandel (1998); Eisenberg (1995).
3. See Eccles (1990); Andreasen (1997).
4. See Posner (1990).
5. Post and Weiss (1997); Post et al. (1998).
6. Kandel and Schwartz (1992); Nieuwenhuys, (1994).
7. Fuster (1989); Tucker et al. (1995); Rolls (1995).
8. Kandel and Schwartz (1992).
9. Green et al. (1998, p. 427).
10. Hockfield and Lombroso (1998); Barnes et al. (1995); Kempermann et al. (1997).
11. Wiesel and Hubel (1963).
12. Bowlby (1969, 1988).
13. Thelen (1989).
14. Baldrini et al. (1998).
15. Hubel (1967).
16. Schuman (1997).
17. Kagan (1992); Nelson (1994).
18. See Kandel (1998); Hur and Bouchard (1995).
19. Benedersky and Lewis (1994); Coe et al. (1992); Goldsmith et al. (1997); Kendler and Eaves (1986); Rosenblum et al. (1994); Rutter et al. (1997); Gunnar (1992); Teicher et al. (1997); Rakic et al. (1994).
20. Kandel (1998).
21. Kandel (1989, 1998); Post and Weiss (1997).

22. Rutter (1989).
23. Schore (1997, p. 616).
24. Thelen (1989).
25. Rutter et al. (1997).
26. Pike and Plomin (1996); Plomin (1990).
27. Plomin et al. (1991); Dunn and McGuire (1994).
28. Kandel (1998).
29. Kandel (1998); Schore (1997); Post and Weiss (1997).
30. M. Lewis (1992); Gunnar (1990).
31. Kagan (1994a).
32. Perry (1997).
33. Kagan (1994a).
34. Gottman and Declaire (1997); Baumrind (1993); van den Boom (1994, 1995).
35. Ainsworth et al. (1978); Fonagy et al. (1991b); Pederson et al. (1998).
36. Fonagy and Target (1997).

Chapter 2

1. Milner et al. (1998).
2. Johnson-Laird (1983); Ingvar (1985); Bechara et al. (1994).
3. Tucker (1992); Rolls and Treves (1994).
4. McClelland et al. (1995).
5. Morris (1989).
6. Kandel and Abel (1995); Martin and Kandel (1996).
7. Milner et al. (1998).
8. Milner et al. (1998, p. 463).
9. Bailey and Kandel (1995).
10. Hebb (1949, p. 70).
11. Hebb (1949, p. 70).
12. Kosslyn (1994).
13. Perner (1991).
14. Wheeler et al. (1997).
15. Kapur et al. (1995); Buckner (1996).
16. Schacter (1996).
17. Squire (1992); Schacter (1992).
18. Schacter (1996).
19. Bauer (1996); Schacter (1996); Emde et al. (1991); Fivush and Hudson (1990).
20. Squire et al. (1993).
21. Stern (1985).
22. Johnson-Laird (1983).
23. See Freyd (1987).
24. Ingvar (1985).
25. Pinker (1997).
26. Jensen and Hoagwood (1997).
27. Main (1995).
28. Schore (1994); Hofer (1994).
29. Perry et al. (1995).
30. Squire and Zola-Morgan (1991); Perner and Ruffman (1995); Tulving (1993); Schacter et al. (1996).
31. Edelman (1992); Bauer (1996).

32. Squire (1987).
33. Wheeler et al. (1997).
34. Bauer and Dow (1994); K. Nelson (1993a).
35. Wheeler et al. (1997).
36. Wheeler et al. (1997).
37. K. Nelson (1993b); Myers et al. (1987).
38. Miller et al. (1990); Ochs and Capps (1996); McCabe and Peterson (1991).
39. Fivush (1998); Bauer et al. (1998).
40. Moscovitch (1995); Squire et al. (1993).
41. Baddeley (1992); Andreasen et al. (1995a).
42. Andreasen et al. (1995a); D'Esposito et al. (1995).
43. Bailey and Kandel (1995).
44. Incisa della Rochetta and Milner (1993); Gershberg and Shimamura (1995).
45. Milner et al. (1998); Schacter (1996).
46. Kandel (1989).
47. Winson (1993); Karni et al. (1992).
48. Milner et al. (1998).
49. Schacter (1992).
50. Wheeler et al. (1997).
51. Fink et al. (1996).
52. Wheeler et al. (1997).
53. Wheeler et al. (1997).
54. Buckner (1996).
55. Tucker et al. (1995).
56. Wheeler et al. (1997).
57. Schore (1997); Stecklis and Kling (1985).
58. Tucker et al. (1995).
59. Damasio (1994).
60. Baron-Cohen (1995).
61. Schacter (1996); Wheeler et al. (1997).
62. Tulving (1993).
63. Wheeler et al. (1997).
64. Bjork (1989).
65. Buckner et al. (1995).
66. Freud (1895/1966); Christianson and Lindholm (1998).
67. Rovee-Collier (1993); Newcombe and Fox (1994); Meltzoff (1995).
68. Perner and Ruffman (1995); Bachevalier (1992); Howe (1998); Nelson and Carver (1998).
69. K. Nelson (1993a); Bauer and Dow (1994).
70. Bauer (1996).
71. Bauer et al. (1995).
72. Bauer et al. (1998).
73. Wheeler et al. (1997); Perner and Ruffman (1995).
74. Bauer (1996).
75. Bauer and Wewerka (1995).
76. Reese and Fivush (1993); McCabe and Peterson (1991); Dunn and Brown (1991).
77. Bauer et al. (1998, p. 677).
78. Bretherton (1993); C. A. Nelson (1993).
79. Oppenheim et al. (1997); Fivush (1996).

80. C. A. Nelson and Carver (1998, pp. 798–799).
81. Bjork (1989).
82. Christianson (1992).
83. Diamond and Rose (1994); Zola-Morgan et al. (1991).
84. Siegel (1995a).
85. McGaugh (1992); Leichtman et al. (1992); Edelman (1992).
86. Edelman (1992).
87. McGaugh (1992, pp. 261, 262).
88. Milner et al. (1998).
89. Post et al. (1998, p. 849).
90. McEwen (1999); Lombroso and Sapolsky (1998).
91. Bremner and Narayan (1998).
92. Howe (1998).
93. Bower and Sivers (1998, p. 631).
94. Siegel (1995a).
95. Siegel (1995a, 1996a); Terr (1998).
96. Koopman et al. (1994); Yehuda and McFarlane (1995); van der Kolk and van der Hart (1989).
97. Bremner et al. (1995).
98. van der Kolk et al. (1996); Perry (1997).
99. Felitti et al. (1998).
100. Siegel (1995a, 1996a).
101. Hobson (1992).
102. Tulving et al. (1994); Wheeler et al. (1997).
103. Kinsbourne (1972).
104. Winson (1993).
105. Siegel (1995a).
106. Rauch et al. (1996); Schiffer et al. (1995).
107. Teicher et al. (1997).
108. Bremner et al. (1995).
109. van der Kolk et al. (1996); Williams (1995); Freyd (1996); Herman (1992).
110. Rauch et al. (1996).
111. Terr (1993).
112. Schumacher (1991); Bartlett (1932).
113. Ceci and Bruch (1993).
114. Cicchetti and Toth (1998).
115. Fivush (1998, p. 713).
116. Christianson and Lindholm (1998, pp. 774, 776).
117. Karr-Morse and Wiley (1997); Perry (1997).
118. Lynch and Cicchetti (1998a, p. 744).
119. Lynch and Cicchetti (1998a, pp. 756–757).
120. Bremner and Narayan (1998, pp. 881–882).
121. Ochs and Capps (1996); Coles (1989).
122. K. Nelson (1989); Cohler (1982).
123. Squire (1992).
124. Ochs and Capps (1996).
125. Vygotsky (1986).
126. Britton and Pellegrini (1990); Bruner (1986, 1990); White and Epston (1990).

127. Baron-Cohen (1995); Baron-Cohen and Ring (1994); Capps et al. (1992).
128. Baddeley (1994).
129. Neisser and Fivush (1994).
130. Reed (1994, p. 278).

Chapter 3
1. Bowlby (1969).
2. Hofer (1994).
3. Ainsworth et al. (1978).
4. Bowlby (1988); Sroufe (1996).
5. Bowlby (1969, 1988).
6. Main (1995); Main et al. (1985); Fox et al. (1994); Oppenheim and Waters (1995).
7. Main (1996).
8. Bowlby (1973).
9. Main (1995).
10. Jones et al. (1996); Atkinson and Zucker (1997).
11. Rutter (1987, 1997).
12. Parkes et al. (1991).
13. Trevarthen (1993).
14. Trevarthen (1993).
15. Stern (1985); Haft and Slade (1989).
16. Ainsworth et al. (1978); de Wolff and van IJzendoorn (1997); Ward and Carlson (1995).
17. Hofer (1984).
18. Schore (1994).
19. Schore (1994); Oppenheim et al. (1997).
20. Trevarthen (1993).
21. Stern (1985).
22. Ainsworth et al. (1978); Dunn (1996).
23. Schore (1994).
24. Bowlby (1969); George and Solomon (1996).
25. Main (1995).
26. Bowlby (1969); Bretherton (1992a).
27. Bretherton (1992a); Ainsworth et al. (1978).
28. Ainsworth et al. (1978).
29. Ainsworth et al. (1978).
30. Ainsworth et al. (1978).
31. Main and Solomon (1986).
32. Sroufe (1996); Main (1996); E. Carlson and Sroufe (1995).
33. Sroufe and Jacobvitz (1989).
34. Bowlby (1988).
35. van den Boom (1995); Nachmias et al. (1996); Juffer et al. (1997); Moss and Gotts (1998); Ramey et al. (1984); Schweinhart and Weikart (1992); Korfmacher et al. (1997); Bakermans-Kranenburg et al. (1998).
36. Main (1995).
37. Main (1991).
38. Ainsworth et al. (1978).
39. van IJzendoorn and Bakermans-Kranenburg (1996).

40. Main (1995).
41. Ainsworth et al. (1978).
42. Main and Solomon (1990).
43. Main and Hesse (1990).
44. V. Carlson et al. (1989); Lyons-Ruth et al. (1991); Ogawa et al. (1997).
45. Main (1995).
46. Main and Hesse (1990).
47. G. Liotti (1992); Main and Morgan (1996).
48. Main et al. (1985).
49. C. George et al. (1996).
50. C. George et al. (1984, 1985, 1996).
51. van IJzendoorn (1995); Hesse (1999).
52. Main and Goldwyn (1998); see Main (1995); Hesse (1999).
53. van IJzendoorn and Bakermans-Kranenburg (1996); Waters et al. (1996).
54. Hesse (1999); DeHass et al. (1994).
55. Hesse (1999).
56. Ogawa et al. (1997); Hesse (1999); E. Carlson (1998).
57. .Main (1996).
58. Main and Goldwyn (1998); Bakermans-Kranenburg and van IJzendoorn (1993).
59. Bakermans-Kranenburg and van IJzendoorn (1993); Benoit and Parker (1994); Sagi et al. (1994); Hesse (1999).
60. Bakermans-Kranenburg and van IJzendoorn (1993); Rosenstein and Horowitz (1996); Sagi et al. (1994); Steele and Steele (1994).
61. Sagi et al. (1994); Bakermans-Kranenburg and van IJzendoorn (1993).
62. van IJzendoorn (1995).
63. C. George et al. (1996); Hesse (1999).
64. Main and Goldwyn (1998).
65. Main and Goldwyn (1998).
66. Main and Goldwyn (1998).
67. C. George et al. (1996).
68. Hesse (1996).
69. Grice (1975).
70. Main and Goldwyn (1998, p. 46).
71. Main and Goldwyn (1998).
72. Hesse (1996).
73. van IJzendoorn (1995).
74. Main (1995).
75. van IJzendoorn (1992, 1995); Sagi et al. (1994); Hesse (1999).
76. Fonagy et al. (1991a); van IJzendoorn (1995).
77. Benoit and Parker (1994); Main (1995); van IJzendoorn (1995); van IJzendoorn and Bakermans-Kranenburg (1996); M. Main (personal communication, 1998, regarding unpublished reports); Hesse (1999). See discussion in Fonagy (1998).
78. Ogawa et al. (1997); Main (1995); Main and Goldwyn (1998); Fagot and Pears (1996); E. Carlson (1998).
79. Main (1995); Steele et al. (1996); Cohn et al. (1992).
80. Fonagy et al. (1991a); Hesse (1999); Radojevic (1994); Benoit and Parker (1994); Ward and Carlson (1995).

81. Steele et al. (1996).
82. Vaughn et al. (1992).
83. Plomin et al. (1994a, 1994b); Kendler (1996); J. Cohen (1996).
84. Sagi et al. (1997).
85. Palaez-Nogueras et al. (1994); National Institute of Child Health and Human Development (NICHD) Early Child Care Research Network (1997); Hossain et al. (1994).
86. van IJzendoorn and Bakermans-Kranenburg (1996).
87. Lichtenstein et al. (1998).
88. Main (1995); Benoit et al. (1992); Crowell et al. (1992); Greenberg et al. (1997).
89. Main (1995); Sroufe (1996); Colin (1996); Cassidy and Shaver (1999); Bretherton (1992a); Zeanah (1993).
90. Cicchetti and Rogosch (1997b); Ogawa et al. (1997); E. Carlson (1998); Schuengel et al. (in press).
91. Atkinson and Zucker (1997); Cowan et al. (1996); Crowell et al. (1988); Fonagy et al. (1996); Manassis et al. (1994); Pianta et al. (1996); Rosenstein and Horowitz (1997); Sroufe (1997); Greenberg et al. (1993); Adam et al. (1996); Bretherton (1996); Zeanah et al. (1997); Routh et al. (1995); Constantino (1996); Allen et al. (1996).
92. Ogawa et al. (1997); E. Carlson (1998).
93. Ogawa et al. (1997); E. Carlson (1998); Yehuda and McFarlane (1995).
94. Lyons-Ruth et al. (1993); E. Carlson (1998); Herstgaard et al. (1995); Solomon et al. (1995).
95. Lieberman (1991); Moss and Gotts (1998); Butterfield (1996); Durlak and Wells (1997); Erickson et al. (1992); Zeanah et al. (1997a); Minde and Hesse (1996).
96. Main (1995).
97. Post and Weiss (1997); Rosenblum et al. (1994).
98. Kraemer (1992); Sigman and Siegel (1992).
99. Post and Weiss (1997).
100. Kandel (1998).
101. Brodsky and Lombroso (1998, pp. 2, 3).
102. Goldsmith et al. (1997).
103. Perry (1997); Teicher et al. (1997).
104. Schore (1997, p. 618).
105. Perry (1997); Karr-Morse and Wiley (1997).
106. Calkins and Fox (1994); Kagan (1997); Kendler and Eaves (1986); Rothbart and Ahadi (1994); Thomas and Chess (1977); Bouchard (1994).
107. Merzenich et al. (1991); Merzenich and Sameshima (1993).
108. Perry (1997); Karr-Morse and Wiley (1997); Rutter (1997).
109. Fonagy (1998).
110. Atkinson and Zucker (1997); Cowan et al. (1996); Crowell et al. (1988); Fonagy et al. (1996); Manassis et al. (1994); Pianta et al. (1996); Rosenstein and Horowitz (1996); Sroufe (1997); Greenberg et al. (1993).
111. Schuengel et al. (in press); see also Schuengel et al. (1997).
112. van IJzendoorn and Bakermans-Kranenburg (1997).
113. Main (1995).
114. Main (1995, p. 451).

115. Schore (1997).
116. Ainsworth et al. (1978); de Wolff and van IJzendoorn (1997).
117. Field (1985); Beebe and Lachman (1988).
118. Fonagy et al. (1991b); Fonagy and Target (1997).
119. Trevarthen (1993).
120. See Stern (1985).
121. Beebe and Lachman (1994).
122. Field (1985); Hofer (1984); Trvarthen (1993); Stern (1985).
123. Hofer (1994).
124. Lieberman (1997).
125. Bauer et al. (1995); Bauer and Wewerka (1995); Fivush (1996).
126. Main and Goldwyn (1998).
127. Hesse (1996).
128. Fonagy et al. (1997); Fonagy and Target (1997).
129. Morton and Frith (1995).
130. Main (1995).
131. Main and Goldwyn (1998); Lichtenstein Phelps et al. (1998).
132. M. Main (personal communication, 1990); Pearson et al. (1994).
133. Pearson et al. (1994); Lichtenstein Phelps et al. (1998).
134. Steele and Steele (1994); Sagi et al. (1997); Lyons-Ruth et al. (1990).
135. Ainsworth et al. (1978).
136. Spangler and Grossmann (1993).
137. Ainsworth et al. (1978).
138. Crowell et al. (1988); Beebe and Lachman (1988, 1994).
139. Main (1995).
140. Fonagy et al. (1997).
141. Main and Goldwyn (1998).
142. Bowlby (1969).
143. Spangler and Grossmann (1993); Dozier et al. (1994).
144. Fonagy et al. (1991b).
145. Main (1995).
146. See van IJzendoorn and Bakermanns-Kranenburg (1996).
147. Ogawa et al. (1997); E. Carlson (1998).
148. Dozier et al. (1994).
149. Wheeler et al. (1997); Damasio (1994); Schore (1994); Baron-Cohen (1995); Tucker et al. (1995).
150. Singer and Salovey (1993); Neisser and Fivush (1994).
151. Schacter (1996); Rubin (1987).
152. Wheeler et al. (1997).
153. Wheeler et al. (1997); Kinsbourne (1972).
154. M. Main and Hesse (personal communication, 1999).
155. Christianson (1992).
156. Damasio (1994); Edelman (1992).
157. Ochs and Capps (1996).
158. Main (1996).
159. Ainsworth et al. (1978).
160. Main (1995).
161. Fonagy et al. (1997).
162. Aitken and Trevarthen (1997).
163. Stern (1985).

164. Main (1991); Bowlby (1973).
165. Main (1991).
166. Main and Goldwyn (1998).
167. Main and Goldwyn (1998).
168. Lyons-Ruth and Jacobwitz (1999); Hesse (1999).
169. Schacter and Buckner (1998); NcNally et al. (1994).
170. Bowers (1987).
171. Hesse (1996).
172. Bretherton (1992b); Walden (1991).
173. Main and Solomon (1990).
174. Main and Solomon (1990); Spangler et al. (1996).
175. G. Liotti (1992); Main and Hesse (1990).
176. Main and Hesse (1990); Hesse and Main (1999, in press).
177. Main (1995); Hesse (1999).
178. Lyons-Ruth et al. (1991); V. Carlson et al. (1989); Lyons-Ruth and Jacobwitz (1999).
179. Main and Morgan (1996).
180. Perry et al. (1995).
181. Main and Hesse (1990).
182. Ogawa et al. (1997); E. Carlson (1998).
183. See Lyons-Ruth et al. (1993), Ogawa et al. (1997), van IJzendoorn (in press), and E. Carlson (1998).
184. Lyons-Ruth and Jacobwitz (1999).
185. Siegel (1995a).
186. Siegel (1996a).
187. Main and Hesse (1999).
188. van IJzendoorn (1995).
189. Main and Goldwyn (1998).
190. Main and Goldwyn (1998); Hesse (1996).
191. Siegel (1996a).
192. Hesse (1996); Main and Morgan (1996).
193. Ainsworth and Eichberg (1991); Hesse (1999).
194. Siegel (1995).
195. Hesse and Main (1999).
196. Lyons-Ruth et al. (1993); Cicchetti and Toth (1995); Yehuda and McFarlane (1995); E. Carlson (1998).
197. Main and Hesse (1990).
198. Hesse (1996).
199. Siegel (1996).
200. Main and Hesse (1990); Hesse and Main (1999, in press).
201. Lyons-Ruth and Jacobwitz (1999).
202. Schuengel et al. (in press); Main and Hesse (1990).
203. Hesse and van IJzendoorn (1998).
204. Siegel (1995~a); van der Kolk et al. (1996); Zeitlin and McNally (1991).
205. Siegel (1996a).
206. Perry et al. (1995).
207. Lyons-Ruth and Jacobwitz (1999).
208. Yehuda and McFarlane (1995).
209. Lyons-Ruth and Jacobwitz (1999); Karr-Morse and Wiley (1997).
210. Post and Weiss (1997).

Chapter 4
1. Bretherton (1992b); Walden (1991).
2. Bowers et al. (1993).
3. Etcoff and Magee (1992); Ortony and Turner (1990).
4. Kagan (1994b); Davidson (1992b); Dodge and Garber (1991); Holstege et al. (1994).
5. LeDoux (1996); Harr, (1986).
6. Brothers (1997).
7. LeDoux (1996); Brothers (1997).
8. Watt (1998); Stein and Trabasso (1992).
9. Brothers (1997); Ciompi (1991); Harr, (1986).
10. LeDoux (1996).
11. Ortony and Turner (1990).
12. Ekman (1992b).
13. Garber and Dodge (1991); Fox (1994a); Cicchetti et al. (1991).
14. Dodge (1991, p. 159).
15. Sroufe (1996, p. 15).
16. Izard and Kobak (1991).
17. Barbas (1995); LeDoux (1990).
18. Rolls (1995); Barbas (1995); Lewis (1996).
19. Edelman (1992).
20. Davidson et al. (1990).
21. Sroufe (1996).
22. Thompson (1994).
23. Davidson et al. (1990).
24. Dawson (1994b); Heller (1993).
25. Kagan (1994a).
26. Dunn and Brown (1991).
27. Kagan (1994).
28. Izard (1991); M. Lewis and Haviland (1993).
29. Darwin (1872/1965).
30. Ekman (1992a).
31. Izard (1992); Ekman (1992b).
32. Doi (1973).
33. Stern (1985).
34. Sroufe (1996); Camras (1992).
35. R. Feldman and Greenbaum (1997); Field et al. (1990); Winnicott (1965).
36. Rubinow and Post (1992).
37. M. S. George et al. (1997).
38. Dawson (1994a); Field (1995); Lyons-Ruth et al. (1990).
39. Schore (1998); LeDoux (1996).
40. Halgren (1992).
41. Allman and Brothers (1994).
42. Porges et al. (1994).
43. Price et al. (1994); Schore (1997).
44. Porges et al. (1994).
45. Watts (1998).
46. Spence et al. (1996); M. D. Lewis (1995); Damasio (1994).
47. Davis (1992).
48. LeDoux et al. (1991).

49. Gazzaniga (1988); Crick (1994); Rolls (1995); Marcel and Bisach (1988); Greenwald (1992).
50. Baddeley (1992,).
51. Goldman-Rakic (1993).
52. Crick (1994); Llinas (1990).
53. Dennett (1991).
54. Tononi and Edelman (1998).
55. LeDoux (1996); Rolls (1995).
56. Damasio (1994).
57. James (1884); Panksepp (1982).
58. Edelman (1992).
59. Leichtman et al. (1992); McGaugh (1992).
60. Damasio (1998).
61. Main and Hesse (1990).
62. Lyons-Ruth and Jacobwitz (1999).
63. Allman and Brothers (1994).
64. Pinker (1997).
65. Thelen (1989).
66. Damasio (1994).
67. Damasio (1994).
68. Schore (1994).
69. Baron-Cohen (1995).
70. Wheeler et al. (1997).
71. Baron-Cohen (1995).
72. LeDoux (1996); Rolls (1995).
73. Brothers (1997).
74. Izard (1991).
75. Nobre et al. (1999, p. 12).
76. Freedman et al. (1998).
77. Mesulam (1998, p. 1013).
78. Main (1991, 1995, 1996, in press).
79. Hesse (1996).
80. Watt (1998); LeDoux (1996).
81. Schore (1994, 1997).
82. Brothers (1997).
83. Damasio (1994); Rolls (1996); Fuster (1985).
84. Porges et al. (1994); Ehlers and Margraf (1987).
85. Larsen et al. (1992).
86. Schiff et al. (1992).
87. Damasio (1994).
88. Schore (1994).
89. Damasio (1994).
90. Gilligan (1996); Benenson (1996).
91. Gilligan (1997).
92. Brothers (1997).
93. Brothers (1997).
94. Brothers (1997); Ekman (1992a); Dawson (1994b).
95. Adolphs et al. (1994); Hornak et al. (1996); Haxby et al. (1996).
96. Schuman (1997).
97. Ali and Cimino (1997); Ross (1984); Tucker (1981).

98. Porges et al. (1994).
99. Springer and Deutsch (1993); Nass and Koch (1991).
100. Otto et al. (1987).
101. Davidson (1992a); Dawson (1994a).
102. Ross et al. (1994).
103. Schore (1997); Ross et al. (1994); Porges et al. (1994); Cutting (1992); Wittling and Schweiger (1993).
104. Heller et al. (1995); Ross et al. (1994).
105. Fox (1994b).
106. Field (1994); Dawson (1994b); Calkins (1994).
107. Dawson (1994b).
108. Springer and Deutsch (1993).
109. Springer and Deutsch (1993); Wittling and Roschmann (1993).
110. Schore (1997).
111. Halgren and Markinovic (1995).
112. Ornstein (1997).
113. M. D. Lewis (1995); Fox (1994b).
114. Ross et al. (1994).
115. Fonagy and Target (1997).
116. Toth et al. (1997).
117. Garber and Dodge (1991); Fox (1994a); Sroufe (1996).
118. Sroufe (1996, p. 159).
119. Calkins (1994).

Chapter 5

1. Trevarthen (1996).
2. Pinker (1997).
3. Eggermont (1998).
4. Perner (1991); Eggermont (1998).
5. Pinker (1997).
6. Edelman (1992); Posner (1990); Perner (1991).
7. Edelman (1992).
8. Wheeler et al. (1997).
9. Perner and Ruffman (1995).
10. Buckner (1996).
11. Pinker (1997).
12. Hamann and Squire (1997); Shevrin (1992).
13. Trevarthen (1990b, p. 357).
14. Trevarthen (1996).
15. Trevarthen (1996, p. 583).
16. M. Liotti and Tucker (1992); Trevarthen (1996).
17. Tucker et al. (1995, pp. 233–234).
18. Tucker et al. (1995, p. 222).
19. Tucker et al. (1995, p. 223).
20. Springer and Deutsch (1993); Zaidel et al. (1990).
21. Springer and Deutsch (1993).
22. Trevarthen (1996).
23. Ornstein et al. (1979).
24. Trevarthen (1996).

25. Ornstein (1997); Rotenberg (1994).
26. Gazzaniga et al. (1996).
27. Gazzaniga (1996).
28. Jaynes (1976); Joseph (1992).
29. Damasio (1994).
30. Johnson and Hugdahl (1991); Sergent et al. (1992).
31. Semrud-Clikeman and Hynd (1990).
32. Damasio (1994).
33. Schore (1994).
34. Zaidel et al. (1995).
35. Schore (1997).
36. Davidson (1992).
37. Davidson et al. (1990).
38. Trevarthen (1996).
39. Ross et al. (1994).
40. Ekman (1992a).
41. Ali and Cimino (1997); Heller et al. (1995); Zaidel et al. (1995).
42. Zaidel et al. (1995).
43. Zaidel et al. (1990).
44. Dawson (1994a); Field et al. (1995).
45. Field (1995); Hossain et al. (1994); Palaez-Nougueras et al. (1994).
46. Bavellier et al. (1998).
47. Neville (1998); Neville and Bavellier (1998).
48. Thatcher et al. (1987); Chiron et al. (1997).
49. Schore (1997).
50. Thatcher (1994, 1997); Thatcher et al. (1987).
51. Haft and Slade (1989).
52. Fonagy et al. (1991b, 1997); Fonagy and Target (1997).
53. Fonagy and Target (1997); Fonagy et al. (1997).
54. Aitken and Trevarthen (1997, pp. 653–654).
55. Greenspan and Benderly (1997).
56. Aitken and Trevarthen (1997, pp. 655, 664).
57. Beebe and Lachman (1988).
58. Springer and Deutsch (1993).
59. Trevarthen (1996); Friede and Weinstock (1988).
60. Springer and Deutsch (1993).
61. Trevarthen (1996).
62. Levy (1969).
63. Trevarthen (1996).
64. Levy (1969).
65. Thatcher et al. (1987).
66. C. A. Nelson and Bloom (1997).
67. Pons (1996).
68. Springer and Deutsch (1993).
69. Hubel (1967).
70. Schuman (1997).
71. Bowlby (1988); Colin (1996).
72. Merzenich et al. (1991).
73. Post and Weiss (1997, p. 925).

74. Nass and Koch (1991); Wheeler et al. (1993); Gunnar (1992); Davidson et al. (1990).
75. Davidson (1992a).
76. Tucker et al. (1995).
77. Kagan (1992).
78. Levy (1969).
79. Kelley et al. (1998).
80. Schacter (1996, p. 141).
81. Goldberg and Costa (1981).
82. Edwards (1989).
83. Zaidel et al. (1990).
84. Aitken and Trevarthen (1997).
85. Oznoff and Miller (1996).
86. Fonagy and Target (1997, pp. 690–691).
87. Sigman and Capps (1997).
88. Baron-Cohen (1995).
89. Fonagy and Target (1997).
90. Fonagy and Target (1997).
91. M. Main, personal communication (January, 1999).
92. Hesse (1999).

Chapter 6
1. Morris (1989).
2. Eggermont (1998).
3. Perry et al. (1995); Horowitz (1987, 1991).
4. Fuster (1989).
5. van der Kolk et al. (1996).
6. Skinner et al. (1992); Robertson and Combs (1995); Prigogine and Stengers (1984); Taylor (1994).
7. van Pelt et al. (1994).
8. Robertson and Combs (1995).
9. Boldrini et al. (1998); Cicchetti and Rogosch (1997b).
10. Gleick (1987).
11. Skinner et al. (1992).
12. Doebeli (1993).
13. Pinker (1997).
14. Corner (1994).
15. McClelland and Rumelhart (1986).
16. Globus and Arpaia (1993); Jeffery and Reid (1997).
17. Hagler and Goda (1998).
18. Black (1998).
19. Milner et al. (1998).
20. Robertson and Combs (1995).
21. Boldrini et al. (1998 p. 25).
22. Globus and Arpaia (1993).
23. Thelen (1989).
24. Post and Weiss (1997, p. 911; emphasis added).
25. Fogel et al. (1997).
26. Cicchetti and Rogosch (1997a).

27. Fogel et al. (1997); Globus and Arpaia (1993); Chamberlain (1995); Jackson (1991); March and Mulle (1998).
28. L. J. Cohen et al. (1997).
29. Robertson and Combs (1995); Globus and Arpaia (1993).
30. Aitken and Trevarthen (1997).
31. Fonagy and Target (1997).
32. Main and Hesse (1990).
33. Beebe and Lachman (1988, 1994).
34. M. D. Lewis (1995).
35. Fogel et al. (1997); Fogel and Branco (1997).
36. Schore (1997, p. 600).
37. Shinbrot et al. (1993).
38. Boldrini et al. (1998, p. 25).
39. Otto et al. (1987); Coffey (1987); Rubinow and Post (1992); M. S. George et al. (1997).
40. Hofer (1990, p. 74).
41. Harter (1988); Harter et al. (1997).
42. Harter et al. (1997).
43. Sroufe (1996).
44. Sroufe (1990).
45. Harter et al. (1997).
46. Harter et al. (1997).
47. Harter et al. (1997).
48. Yawkey and Johnson (1988); Fonagy and Target (1997); Harter et al. (1997).
49. Noam and Fischer (1996).
50. Cicchetti and Rogosch (1997a).
51. O'Donohue (1997).
52. Chamberlain (1995).

Chapter 7
1. Ciompi (1991).
2. Sroufe (1996).
3. Hofer (1994).
4. Sroufe (1996).
5. Tronick (1989); Kraemer (1992).
6. Sroufe (1996).
7. Lieberman (1993).
8. Damasio (1998, p. 84).
9. Rutter (1991); Calkins (1994); Cole et al. (1994); Feeney and Kirkpatrick (1996); Fox et al. (1996).
10. Sroufe (1996); Schore (1994); Fox (1994a); Garber and Dodge (1991); Cicchetti and Tucker (1994).
11. Cicchetti and Rogosch (1997b); Schore (1997).
12. Post and Weiss (1997).
13. Ogawa et al. (1997); E. Carlson (1998).
14. Cole et al. (1994).
15. Goleman (1995).
16. Baxter et al. (1992).
17. Fox (1994a); Garber and Dodge (1991); Schore (1994); Olds et al. (1998).

18. Kagan (1994a); Calkins and Fox (1994).
19. Sroufe (1996).
20. Rolls (1995); Fox (1994a); Garber and Dodge (1991); Halgren and Marinkovic (1995). See also Epstein (1995).
21. LeDoux (1990); Porges et al. (1994); Lewis (1997); Lyra and Winegar (1997).
22. Dawson (1994b).
23. Dawson (1994a).
24. Stern (1985); Field (1994).
25. Sroufe (1996).
26. Schore (1996).
27. Schore (1994).
28. Schacter and Buckner (1998).
29. Perry (1997); Post et al. (1998).
30. LeDoux (1996).
31. Sroufe (1996).
32. Camras (1992).
33. Malatesta-Magai (1991).
34. Cassidy (1994); Dunn and Brown (1991).
35. M. Lewis and Haviland (1993); Izard (1991).
36. Goleman (1995).
37. Schore (1994).
38. Kihlstrom (1987).
39. Tononi and Edelman (1998).
40. Mesulam (1998); Peterson (1998); Shimamura (1995); Posner and Rothbart (1998).
41. Nobre et al. (1999, p. 12).
42. Dunn and Brown (1991).
43. Metcalfe and Shimamura (1989).
44. Edelman (1992).
45. Malatesta-Magai (1991).
46. LeDoux (1996).
47. LeDoux (1996); Allman and Brothers (1994); Ekman (1992b); Etcoff and Magee (1992); Johnson and Hugdahl (1991).
48. Harter et al. (1997).
49. M. S. George et al. (1997); Rubinow and Post (1992).

Chapter 8
1. Hofer (1994).
2. Sapolsky (1997).
3. McCraty et al. (1998).
4. Sroufe (1996).
5. Schore (1994, 1996, 1997).
6. Porges et al. (1994).
7. Schore (1994).
8. Schore (1997).
9. Sroufe (1996).
10. Schore (1994).
11. Schore (1994).
12. Schore (1994).

13. Stern (1985).
14. Field (1985); Schore (1994).
15. Schore (1996).
16. Cassidy (1994).
17. Cassidy (1994).
18. Schore (1996, 1997).
19. Siegel (1995b).
20. Walden (1991).
21. Pearson et al. (1994); Lichtenstein Phelps et al. (1998).
22. Main and Goldwyn (1998).
23. Edwards (1989).
24. Edwards (1989).
25. G. Liotti (1992).
26. Siegel (1996b).
27. Liu et al. (1997); Perry (1997); Hofer (1996).
28. Post and Weiss (1997); Post et al. (1998).
29. Bowlby (1980).

Chapter 9
1. Tucker et al. (1995, p. 214).
2. Tucker et al. (1995).
3. Trevarthen (1996).
4. Trevarthen (1990a, p. 49).
5. Tucker et al. (1995, p. 218).
6. Wise et al. (1996).
7. Calvin (1993).
8. Mesulam (1998); Nobre et al. (1999).
9. van Ooyen and van Pelt (1994, pp. 245, 246).
10. Freeman (1994).
11. Trevarthen (1996, pp. 571–572; emphasis in original).
12. Mesulam (1998); Posner et al. (1997).
13. Damasio (1998, p. 83).
14. Benes (1994).
15. Benes (1998, p. 1489).
16. Yawkey and Johnson (1988).
17. Harter et al. (1997).
18. Baynes et al. (1998); Trevarthen (1990a, 1990b).
19. Ciompi (1991).
20. Main and Goldwyn (1998).
21. Fonagy and Target (1997).
22. Pearson et al. (1994, p. 360).
23. Main and Goldwyn (1998).
24. Lichtenstein Phelps et al. (1998).
25. Harter et al. (1997).
26. Harter et al. (1997).
27. Sroufe et al. (1990); Feeney and Kirkpatrick (1996); Howes et al. (1998).
28. Cicchetti and Rogosch (1997a).
29. Ogawa et al. (1997 p. 871), paraphrasing Loevinger (1976).
30. Ogawa et al. (1997, pp. 871–872).

31. Schore (1997, p. 607).
32. Main (1991).
33. Schore (1997).
34. G. Liotti (1991).
35. Ogawa et al. (1997); E. Carlson (1998).
36. Yehuda and McFarlane (1995).
37. Ogawa et al. (1997, p. 856).
38. Putnam (1989); D. O. Lewis and Putnam (1996); Bernstein and Putnam (1986); Spiegel (1996); Waller et al. (1996); Putnam (1997).
39. American Psychiatric Association (1994).
40. Krystal et al. (1994).
41. Corner (1994); Mesulam (1998).
42. Ross (1996).
43. Siegel (1996a).
44. A quote from the bulletin board of the First Presbyterian Church Preschool, Los Angeles.
45. Csikszentmihalyi (1990).
46. Snow (1990); Wolf (1990); Haden et al. (1997); K. Nelson (1989).
47. Wolf (1990 p. 185).
48. Wolf (1990, p. 183).
49. Haden et al. (1997); Snow (1990); Wolf (1990); Fivush (1996).
50. Hilgard (1977).
51. Schacter (1996).
52. Putnam (1989).
53. Vandenberg (1998, pp. 265, 266).
54. Vygotsky (1934/1986).
55. Gazzaniga et al. (1996).
56. Schacter (1996); Gazzaniga (1995).
57. Bost et al. (1998); Bagwell et al. (1998); Howes et al. (1994a, 1994b); Booth et al. (1998); Sroufe et al. (1990).
58. Sroufe et al. (1990).
59. Elder (1998, p. 9).
60. Pinker (1997); Brothers (1997).
61. Edelman (1992).
62. Fuster (1989); Edelman (1992).
63. Tulving et al. (1994).
64. Wheeler et al. (1997).
65. Winson (1993).
66. Milner et al. (1998).
67. Trevarthen (1990b).
68. Cicchetti and Rogosch (1997a).
69. Beebe and Lachman (1994).
70. Ross (1996).
71. Sroufe (1996, p. 17).

References

Abel, T., Martin, K. C., Bartsch, D., & Kandel, E. R. (1998). Memory suppressor genes: Inhibitory constraints on the storage of long-term memory. *Science, 279,* 338–341.

Adam, K. S., Sheldon-Keller, A. E., & West, M. (1996). Attachment organization and history of suicidal behavior in adolescents. *Journal of Consulting and Clinical Psychology, 674,* 264–292.

Adolphs, R., Tranel, D., Damasio, H., & Damasio, A. (1994). Impaired recognition of emotion in facial expressions following bilateral damage to the human amygdala. *Nature, 372,* 669–672.

Ainsworth, M. D. S., Blehar, M. C., Waters, E., & Wall, S. (1978). *Patterns of attachment: A psychological study of the Strange Situation.* Hillsdale, NJ: Erlbaum.

Ainsworth, M. D. S., & Eichberg, C. (1991). Effects on infant–mother attachment of mother's unresolved loss of an attachment figure, or other traumatic experience. In C. M. Parkes, J. Stevenson-Hinde, & P. Marris (Eds.), *Attachment across the life cycle* (pp. 160–186). London: Routledge.

Aitken, K. J., & Trevarthen, C. (1997). Self–other organization in human psychological development. *Development and Psychopathology, 9,* 653–678.

Ali, N., & Cimino, C. R. (1997). Hemispheric lateralization of perception and memory for emotional verbal stimuli in normal individuals. *Neuropsychology, 11,* 114–125.

Allen, J. P., Hauser, S. T., & Borman-Spurrell, E. (1996). Attachment theory as a framework for understanding sequelae of severe adolescent psychopathology: An eleven-year follow-up study. *Journal of Consulting and Clinical Psychology, 64,* 254–263.

Allman, J., & Brothers, L. (1994). Faces, fear and the amygdala. *Nature, 372,* 613–614.

American Psychiatric Association. (1994). *Diagnostic and statistical manual of mental disorders* (4th ed.). Washington, DC: Author.

Andreasen, N. C. (1997). Linking mind and brain in the study of mental illnesses: A project for a scientific psychopathology. *Science, 275,* 1586–1593.

Andreasen, N. C., O'Leary, D. S., Arndt, S., Cizaldo, T., Hurtig, R., Rezai, K., Watkins, G. L., Ponto, L. L. B., & Hichwa, R. D. (1995a). Short-term and long-

357

term verbal memory: A positron emission tomography study. *Proceedings of the National Academy of Sciences USA, 92,* 5111–5115.

Andreasen, N. C., O'Leary, D. S., Arndt, S., Cizaldo, T., Hurtig, R., Rezal, K., Watkins, G. L., Ponto, L. L. B., & Hichwa, R. D. (1995b). Remembering the past: Two facets of episodic memory explored with positron emission tomography. *American Journal of Psychiatry, 152,* 1576–1585.

Atkinson, L., & Zucker, K. J. (Eds.). (1997). *Attachment and psychopathology.* New York: Guilford Press.

Bachevelier, J. (1992). Cortical versus limbic immaturity: Relationship to infantile amnesia. In M. R. Gunnar & C. A. Nelson (Eds.), *Minnesota Symposia on Child Psychology: Vol. 24. Developmental Behavioral Neuroscience* (pp. 129–154). Hillsdale, NJ: Erlbaum.

Baddeley, A. (1992). Working memory. *Science, 255,* 556–559.

Baddeley, A. (1994). The remembered self and the enacted self. In U. Neisser & R. Fivush (Eds.), *The remembering self: Construction and accuracy in the self-narrative* (pp. 236–242). Cambridge, UK: Cambridge University Press.

Bagwell, C. L., Newcomb, A. F., & Bukowski, W. M. (1998). Preadolescent friendship and peer rejection as predictors of adult adjustment. *Child Development, 69,* 140–153.

Bailey, C. H., & Kandel, E. R. (1995). Molecular and structural mechanisms underlying long-term memory. In M. S. Gazzaniga (Ed.), *The cognitive neurosciences* (pp. 19–36). Cambridge, MA: MIT Press.

Bakermans-Kranenburg, M. J., Juffer, F., & van IJzendoorn, M. H. (1998). Intervention with video feedback and attachment discussions: Does type of maternal insecurity make a difference? *Infant Mental Health Journal, 19,* 202–219.

Bakermans-Kranenburg, M. J., & van IJzendoorn, M. H. (1993). A psychometric study of the Adult Attachment Interview: Reliability and discriminant validity. *Developmental Psychology, 29,* 870–879.

Barbas, H. (1995). Anatomic basis of cognitive–emotional interactions in the primate prefrontal cortex. *Neuroscience and Biobehavioral Reviews, 19,* 499–510.

Barnes, C. A., Erickson, C. A., Davis, S., & McNaughton, B. L. (1995). Hippocampal synaptic enhancement as a basis for learning and memory: A selected review of current evidence from behaving animals. In J. L. McGaugh, N. M. Weinberger, & G. Lynch (Eds.), *Brain and memory: Modulation and mediation of neuroplasticity* (pp. 259–276). New York: Oxford University Press

Baron-Cohen, S. (1995). *Mindblindness: An essay on autism and theory of mind.* Cambridge, MA: MIT Press.

Baron-Cohen, S., & Ring, H. (1994). A model of the mind-reading system: Neuropsychological and neurobiological perspectives. In P. Mitchell & C. Lewis (Eds.), *Origins of an understanding of mind* (pp. 183–207). Hillsdale, NJ: Erlbaum.

Bartlett, F. C. (1932). *Remembering: A study in experimental and social psychology.* Cambridge, UK: Cambridge University Press.

Bauer, P. J. (1996). What do infants recall of their lives?: Memory for specific events by one- to two-year-olds. *American Psychologist, 51,* 29–41.

Bauer, P. J., & Dow, G. A. (1994). Episodic memory in sixteen- and twenty-month-old children: Specifics are generalized but not forgotten. *Developmental Psychology, 30,* 403–417.

Bauer, P. J., Hertsgaard, L. A., & Dow, G. A. (1994). After eight months have passed: Long-term recall of events by one- and two-year-old children. *Memory, 2,* 353–382.

Bauer, P. J., Hertsgaard, L. A., & Wewerka, S. S. (1995). Effects of experience and reminding on long-term recall in infancy: Remembering not to forget. *Journal of Experimental Child Psychology, 59,* 260–298.

Bauer, P. J., Kroupina, M. G., Schwade, J. A., Dropik, P. L., & Saeger Wewerka, S. (1998). If memory serves, will language? Later verbal accessibility of early memories. *Development and Psychopathology, 10,* 655–680.

Bauer, P. J., & Wewerka, S. S. (1995). One- to two-year-olds' recall of events: The more expressed, the more impressed. *Journal of Experimental Child Psychology, 59,* 475–496.

Baumrind, D. (1993). The average expectable environment is not good enough: A response to Scarr. *Child Development, 64,* 1299–1317.

Bavellier, D., Corina, D. P., & Neville, H. J. (1998). Brain and language: A perspective from sign language. *Neuron, 21,* 275–278.

Baxter, L. R., Schwartz, J. M., Bergman, K. S., Szuba, M. P., Guze, B. H., Mazziotta, J. C., Alazraki, A., Selin, C. E., Fering, H. K., & Munford, P. (1992). Caudate glucose metabolic rate changes with both drug and behavior therapy for obsessive–compulsive disorder. *Archives of General Psychiatry, 49,* 681–689.

Baynes, K., Eliassen, J. C., Lutsep, H. L., & Gazzaniga, M. S. (1998). Modular organization of cognitive systems masked by interhemispheric integration. *Science, 280,* 902–905.

Bechara, A., Damasio, A. R., Damasio, H., & Anderson, S. W. (1994). Insensitivity to future consequences following damage to human prefrontal cortex. *Cognition, 50,* 7–15.

Beebe, B., & Lachman, F. M. (1988). Mother–infant mutual influence and precursors of psychic structure. In A. Goldberg (Ed.), *Progress in self psychology* (Vol. 3, pp. 3–25). Hillsdale, NJ: Analytic Press.

Beebe, B., & Lachman, F. M. (1994). Representation and internalization in infancy: Three principles of salience. *Psychoanalytic Psychology, 11,* 127–166.

Belsky, J., & Cassidy, J. (1994). Attachment : Theory and evidence. In M. Rutter & D. F. Hay (Eds.), *Development through life: A handbook for clinicians* (pp. 373–402). Oxford: Blackwell.

Benedersky, M., & Lewis, M. (1994). Environmental risks, biological risks, and developmental outcome. *Developmental Psychology, 30,* 484–494.

Benenson, J. F. (1996). Gender differences in the development of relationships. In G. G. Noam & K. W. Fischer (Eds.), *Development and vulnerability in close relationships* (pp. 263–286). Hillsdale, NJ: Erlbaum.

Benes, F. M. (1994). Development of the corticolimbic system. In G. Dawson & K. W. Fischer (Eds.), *Human behavior and the developing brain* (pp. 176–206). New York: Guilford Press.

Benes, F. M. (1998). Human brain growth spans decades. *American Journal of Psychiatry, 155,* 1489.

Benoit, D., & Parker, K. C. H. (1994). Stability and transmission of attachment across three generations. *Child Development, 65,* 1444–1456.

Benoit, D., Zeanah, C. H., Boucher, C., Minde, K. K. (1992). Sleep disorders in early childhood: Association with insecure maternal attachment. *Journal of the American Academy of Child and Adolescent Psychiatry, 31,* 86–93.

Bernstein, E., & Putnam, R. (1986). Development, reliability and validity of a dissociation scale. *Journal of Nervous and Mental Disease, 174,* 727–735.

Bjork, R. (1989). Retrieval inhibition as an adaptive mechanism in human memory. In H. L. Roediger & F. I. M. Craik (Eds.), *Varieties of memory and consciousness: Essays in honor of Endel Tulving* (pp. 283–288). Chichester, UK: Wiley.

Black, I. B. (1998). Genes, brain, and mind: The evolution of cognition. *Neuron, 20,* 1073–1080.

Boldrini, M., Placidi, G. P. A., & Marazziti, D. (1998). Applications of chaos theories to psychiatry: A review and future perspectives. *International Journal of Neuropsychiatric Medicine, 3,* 22–29.

Booth, C. L., Rubin, K. H., & Rose-Krasnor, L. (1998). Perceptions of emotional support from mother and friend in middle childhood: Links with social-emotional adaptation and preschool attachment security. *Child Development, 69,* 427–442.

Bost, K. K., Vaughn, B. E., Washington, W. N., Cielinski, K. L., & Bradbard, M. R. (1998). Social competence, social support, and attachment: Demarcation of construct domains, measurement, and paths of influence for preschool children attending Head Start. *Child Development, 69,* 192–218.

Bouchard, T. J. (1994). Genes, environment, and personality. *Science, 264,* 1700–1701.

Bower, G. H. (1987). Commentary on mood and memory. *Behaviour Research and Therapy, 25,* 443–456.

Bower, G. H., & Sivers, H. (1998). Cognitive impact of traumatic events. *Development and Psychopathology, 10,* 625–654.

Bowers, D., Bauer, R. M., & Heilman, K. M. (1993). The nonverbal affect lexicon: Theoretical perspectives from neuropsychological studies of affect perception. *Neuropsychology, 7,* 433–444.

Bowlby, J. (1969). *Attachment and loss: Vol. 1. Attachment.* New York: Basic Books.

Bowlby, J. (1973). *Attachment and loss: Vol. 2. Separation and anger.* New York: Basic Books.

Bowlby, J. (1980). *Attachment and loss: Vol. 3. Loss: Sadness and depression.* New York: Basic Books.

Bowlby, J. (1988). *A secure base: Parent–child attachment and healthy human development.* New York: Basic Books.

Bremner, J. D., & Narayan, M. (1998). The effects of stress on memory and the hippocampus throughout the life cycle: Implications for childhood development and aging. *Development and Psychopathology, 10,* 871–888.

Bremner, J. D., Randall, P., Scott, T. M., Bronen, R. A., Seibyl, J. P., Southwick, S. M., Delaney, R. C., McCarthy, G., Charney, D. S., & Innis, R. B. (1995). M-based measures of hippocampal volume in patients with PTSD. *American Journal of Psychiatry, 152,* 973–981.

Bretherton, I. (1992a). The origins of attachment theory: John Bowlby and Mary Ainsworth. *Developmental Psychology, 28,* 759–775.

Bretherton, I. (1992b). Social referencing, intentional communication, and the interfacing of minds in infancy. In S. Feinman (Ed.), *Social referencing and the social construction of reality in infancy* (pp. 57–77). New York: Plenum Press.

Bretherton, I. (1993). From dialogue to internal working models: The co-construction of self in relationships. In C. A. Nelson (Ed.), *Minnesota Symposia on Child Psychology: Vol. 26. Memory and affect in development* (pp. 237–264). Hillsdale, NJ: Erlbaum.

Bretherton, I. (1996). Internal working models of attachment relationships as related to resilient coping. In G. G. Noam & K. W. Fischer (Eds.), *Development and vulnerability in close relationships* (pp. 3–28). Hillsdale, NJ: Erlbaum.

Britton, B. K., & Pellegrini, A. D. (1990). *Narrative thought and narrative language.* Hillsdale, NJ: Erlbaum.

Broadwell, R. D. (Ed.). (1995). *Decade of the brain* (Vol. 1). Washington, DC: U.S. Government Printing Office.

Brodsky, M., & Lombroso, P. J. (1998). Molecular mechanisms of developmental disorders. *Development and Psychopathology, 10,* 1–20.

Brothers, L. (1997). *Friday's footprint: How society shapes the human mind.* New York: Oxford University Press.

Bruner, J. (1986). *Actual minds, possible worlds.* Cambridge, MA: Harvard University Press.

Bruner, J. (1990). *Acts of meaning.* Cambridge, MA: Harvard University Press.

Buckner, R. L. (1996). Beyond HERA: Contributions of specific prefrontal brain areas to long-term memory retrieval. *Psychonomic Bulletin, 3,* 149–158.

Buckner, R. L., Petersen, S. E., Ojemann, J. G., Miezin, F. M., Squire, L. R., & Raichle, M. E. (1995). Functional anatomical studies of explicit and implicit memory retrieval tasks. *Journal of Neuroscience, 15,* 12–29.

Butterfield, P. M. (1996). The Partners in Parenting Education Program: A new option for parent education. *Zero to Three, 17,* 3–10.

Calkins, S. D. (1994). Origins and outcomes of individual differences in emotion regulation. In N. A. Fox (Ed), The development of emotion regulation: Biological and behavioral considerations. *Monographs of the Society for Research in Child Development, 59*(2–3, Serial No. 240), 53–72.

Calkins, S. D., & Fox, N. A. (1994). Individual differences in the biological aspects of temperament. In J. E. Bates & T. D. Wachs (Eds.), *Temperament: Individual differences at the interface of biology and behavior* (pp. 199–217). Washington, DC: American Psychological Association.

Calvin, W. H. (1993). The unitary hypothesis: A common neural circuitry for novel manipulations, language, plan-ahead, and throwing? In K. R. Gibson & T. Ingold (Eds.), *Tools, language and cognition in human evolution* (pp. 230–250). Cambridge, UK: Cambridge University Press.

Camras, L. A. (1992). Expressive development and basic emotions. *Cognition and Emotion, 3,* 269–283.

Carlson, E. A. (1998). A prospective longitudinal study of disorganized/disoriented attachment. *Child Development, 69,* 1107–1128.

Carlson, E., & Sroufe, L. A. (1995). Contribution of attachment theory to developmental psychopathology. In D. Cicchetti & D. J. Cohen (Eds.), *Developmental psychopathology: Vol. 1. Theory and methods* (pp. 581–617). New York: Wiley.

Carlson, V., Cicchetti, D., Barnett, D., & Braunwald, K. (1989). Disorganized/disoriented attachment relationships in maltreated infants. *Developmental Psychology, 25,* 525–531.

Carnegie Task Force on Meeting the Needs of Young Children. (1994). *Starting points: Meeting the needs of our youngest children.* New York: Carnegie Corporation of New York.

Carter, C. S., Krener, P., Chaderjan, M., Northcutt, C., & Wolfe, V. (1995). Asymmetrical visual–spatial attentional performance in ADHD: Evidence for a right hemisphere deficit. *Biological Psychiatry, 37,* 789–797.

Cassidy, J. (1994). Emotion regulation: Influences of attachment relationships. In N. Fox (Ed.), Biological and behavioral foundations of emotion regulation. *Monographs of the Society for Research in Child Development, 59*(2–3, Serial No. 240), 228–249.

Cassidy, J., & Shaver, P. R. (Eds.). (1999). *Handbook of attachment: Theory, research, and clinical applications.* New York: Guilford Press.

Ceci, S., & Bruch, M. (1993). Suggestibility of the child witness: A historical review and synthesis. *Psychological Bulletin, 113,* 403–439.

Chamberlain, L. (1995). Strange attractors in patterns of family interaction. In R. Robertson & A. Combs (Eds.), *Chaos theory in psychology and the life sciences* (pp. 267–273). Hillsdale, NJ: Erlbaum.

Chiron, C., Jambaque, I., Nabbot, R., Lounes, R., Syrota, A., & Dulac, O. (1997). The right brain is dominant in human infants. *Brain, 120,* 1057–1065.

Christianson, S. A. (Ed.). (1992). *Handbook of emotion and memory.* Hillsdale, NJ: Erlbaum.

Christianson, S. A., & Lindholm, T. (1998). The fate of traumatic memories in childhood and adulthood. *Development and Psychopathology, 10,* 761–780.

Cicchetti, D., Ganiban, J., & Barnett, D. (1991). Contributions from the study of high-risk populations to understanding emotion regulation. In J. Garber & K. A. Dodge (Eds.), *The development of emotion regulation and dysregulation* (pp. 15–48). Cambridge, UK: Cambridge University Press.

Cicchetti, D., & Lynch, M. (1993). Toward an ecological/transactional model of community violence and child maltreatment: Consequences for children's development. *Psychiatry, 53,* 96–118.

Cicchetti, D., & Rogosch, F. A. (1997a). The role of self-organization in the promotion of resilience in maltreated children. *Development and Psychopathology, 9,* 797–816.

Cicchetti, D., & Rogosch, F. A. (Eds.). (1997b). Self-organization [Special issue]. *Development and Psychopathology, 9*(4).

Cicchetti, D., & Toth, S. (1995). A developmental psychology perspective on child abuse and neglect. *Journal of the American Academy of Child and Adolescent Psychiatry, 34,* 541–565.

Cicchetti, D., & Toth, S. (Eds.). (1998). Risk, trauma, and memory [Special issue]. *Development and Psychopathology, 10*(4).

Cicchetti, D., & Tucker, D. (1994). Development and self-regulatory structures of the mind. *Development and Psychopathology, 6,* 533–549.

Ciompi, L. (1991). Affects as central organising and integrating factors: A new psychosocial/biological model of the psyche. *British Journal of Psychiatry, 159,* 97–105.

Coe, C. L., Lubach, G. R., Schneider, M. L., Dierschke, D. J., & Ershler, W. B. (1992). Early rearing conditions alter immune responses in the developing infant primate. *Pediatrics, 90,* 505–509.

Coffey, C. E. (1987). Cerebral laterality and emotion: The neurology of depression. *Comprehensive Psychiatry, 28,* 197–219.

Cohen, J. (1996). Does nature drive nurture? *Science, 273,* 577–578.

Cohen, L. J., Stein, D., Galynker, E., & Hollander, E. (1997). Towards an integration of psychological and biological models of obsessive–compulsive disorder: Phylogenetic considerations. *International Journal of Neuropsychiatric Medicine, 2,* 26–44.

Cohler, B. J. (1982). Personal narrative and the life course. In P. B. Bates & O. G. Brim (Eds.), *Life-span development and behavior* (Vol. 4, pp. 205–241). New York: Academic Press.

Cohn, D. A., Cowan, P. A., Cowan, C. P., & Pearson, J. (1992). Mothers' and fathers' working models of childhood attachment relationships, parenting styles, and child behavior. *Development and Psychopathology, 4,* 417–431.

Cole, P. M., Michael, M. K., & O'Donnell-Teti, L. (1994). The development of emotion regulation and dysregulation: A clinical perspective. In N. A. Fox (Ed.), *The development of emotion regulation: Biological and behavioral considerations. Monographs of the Society for Research in Child Development, 59*(2–3, Serial No. 240), 250–283.

Coles, R. (1989). *The call of stories: Teaching and the moral imagination.* Boston: Houghton-Mifflin.

Colin, V. L. (1996). *Human attachment.* New York: McGraw-Hill.

Constantino, J. N. (1996). Intergenerational aspects of the development of aggression: A preliminary report. *Journal of Developmental and Behavioral Pediatrics, 17,* 176–182.

Corner, M. A. (1994). Reciprocity of structure–function relations in developing neural networks: The odyssey of a self-organizing brain through research fads, fallacies and prospects. *Progress in Brain Research, 102,* 3–32.

Cowan, P. A., Cohn, D. A., Cowan, C. P., & Pearson, J. L. (1996). Parents' attachment histories and children's externalizing and internalizing behaviors: Exploring family systems models of linkage. *Journal of Consulting and Clinical Psychology, 64,* 53–63.

Crick, F. (1994). *The astonishing hypothesis.* New York: Scribners.

Crittenden, P. M. (1985). Maltreated infants: Vulnerability and resilience. *Journal of Child Psychology and Psychiatry, 26,* 85–96.

Crittenden, P. M., Partridge, M. F., & Clausen, A. H. (1991). Family patterns of relationship in normative and dysfunctional families. *Development and Psychopathology, 3,* 491–513.

Crowell, J. A., & Feldman, S. S. (1995). A review of adult attachment measures: Implications for theory and research. *Social Development, 4,* 294–327.

Crowell, J. A., Feldman, S. S., & Ginsberg, N. (1988). Assessment of mother–child interaction in preschoolers with behavior problems. *Journal of the American Academy of Child and Adolescent Psychiatry, 27,* 303–311.

Crowell, J. A., O'Connor, E., Wollmers, G., Sprafkin, J., & Rao, U. (1992). Mothers' conceptualizations of parent–child relationships: Relation to mother–child interaction and child behavior problems. *Development and Psychopathology, 3,* 431–444.

Csikszentmihalyi, M. (1990). *Flow.* New York: HarperCollins.

Cutting, J. (1992). The role of the right hemisphere in psychiatric disorders. *British Journal of Psychiatry, 160,* 583–588.

Damasio, A. R. (1994). *Descartes' error: Emotion, reason, and the human brain.* New York: Grosset/Putnam.

Damasio, A. R. (1998). Emotion in the perspective of an integrated nervous system. *Brain Research Reviews, 26,* 83–86.

Darwin, C. (1965). *The expression of the emotions in man and animals.* Chicago: University of Chicago Press. (Original work published 1872)

Davidson, R. J. (1992a). Anterior cerebral asymmetry and the nature of emotion. *Brain and Cognition, 20,* 125–151.

Davidson, R. J. (1992b). Prolegomenon to the structure of emotion: Gleanings from neuropsychology. *Cognition and Emotion, 6,* 245–268.

Davidson, R. J., Ekman, P., Saron, C., Senulis, J., & Friesen, W. (1990). Approach–withdrawal and cerebral asymmetry: I. Emotion expression and brain physiology. *Journal of Personality and Social Psychology, 58,* 330–341.

Davis, M. (1992). The role of the amygdala in fear and anxiety. *Annual Review of Neuroscience, 15,* 353–375.

Dawson, G. (1994a). Frontal electroencephalographic correlates of individual differences in emotion expression in infants: A brain systems perspective on emotion. In N. A. Fox (Ed.), The development of emotion regulation: Biological and behavioral considerations. *Monographs of the Society for Research in Child Development, 59* (2–3, Serial No. 240), 135–151.

Dawson, G. (1994b). Development of emotional expression and emotion regulation in infancy. Contributions of the frontal lobe. In G. Dawson & K. W. Fischer (Eds.), *Human behavior and the developing brain* (pp. 346–379). New York: Guilford Press.

Dawson, G., & Fischer, K. W. (Eds.). (1994). *Human behavior and the developing brain.* New York: Guilford Press.

DeHass, M., Bakermans-Kranenburg, M., & van IJzendoorn, M. H. (1994). The Adult Attachment Interview and questionnaires for attachment style, temperament and memories of parental behavior. *Journal of Genetic Psychology, 155,* 471–486.

Dennett, D. C. (1991). *Consciousness explained.* Boston: Little, Brown.

D'Esposito, M., Detre, J., Alsop, D. Shin, R., Atlas, S., & Grossman, M. (1995). The neural basis of the central executive system of working memory. *Nature, 378,* 279–281.

de Wolff, M. S., & van IJzendoorn, M. H. (1997). Sensitivity and attachment: A meta-analysis of parental antecedents of infant attachment. *Child Development, 68,* 571–591.

Diamond, D. M., & Rose, G. (1994). Stress impairs LTP and hippocampal-dependent memory. *Annals of the New York Academy of Sciences, 746,* 411–414.

Dias, R., Robbins, T. W., & Roberts, A. C. (1996). Dissociation in prefrontal cortex of affective and attentional shifts. *Nature, 380,* 69–72.

Dodge, K. A. (1991). Emotion and social information processing. In J. Garber & K. A. Dodge (Eds.), *The development of emotion regulation and dysregulation* (pp. 159–181). Cambridge, UK: Cambridge University Press.

Dodge, K. A. (1993). Social-cognitive mechanisms in the development of conduct disorder and depression. *Annual Review of Psychology, 44,* 559–584.

Dodge, K. A., & Garber, J. (1991). Domains of emotion regulation. In J. Garber & K. A. Dodge (Eds.), *The development of emotion regulation and dysregulation* (pp. 3–14). Cambridge, UK: Cambridge University Press.

Doebeli, M. (1993). The evolutionary advantage of controlled chaos. *Proceedings of the Royal Society of London: Series B. Biological Sciences, 254,* 281–285.

Doi, T. (1973). *The anatomy of dependence.* Tokyo: Kodansha International Press.

Dozier, M., Cue, K. L., & Barnett, L. (1994). Clinicians as caregivers: Role of attachment organization in treatment. *Journal of Consulting and Clinical Psychology, 62,* 793–800.

Dozier, M., & Kobak, R. R. (1992). Psychophysiology in attachment interviews: converging evidence for deactivating strategies. *Child Development, 63,* 1473–1480.

Dunn, J. (1996). The Emanuel Miller Memorial Lecture 1995. Children's relationships: Bridging the divide between cognitive and social development. *Journal of Child Psychology and Psychiatry, 37,* 508–518.

Dunn, J., & Brown, J. (1991). Relationships, talk about feelings, and the development of affect regulation in early childhood. In J. Garber & K. A. Dodge (Eds.), *The development of emotion regulation and dysregulation* (pp. 89–110). Cambridge, UK: Cambridge University Press.

Dunn, J., & McGuire, S. (1994). Young children's nonshared experiences: A summary of studies in Colorado and Cambridge. In E. M. Hetherington, D. Reiss, & R. Plomin (Eds.), *Separate social worlds of siblings: The impact of nonshared environment on development* (pp. 111–128). Hillsdale, NJ: Erbaum.

Durlak, J. A., & Wells, A. M. (1997). Primary prevention mental health programs for children and adolescents: A meta-analytic review. *American Journal of Community Psychology, 25,* 115–152.

Eccles, J. C. (1990). A unitary hypothesis of mind–brain interaction in the cerebral cortex. *Proceedings of the Royal Society of London: Series B. Biological Sciences, 240,* 433–451.

Edelman, G. (1992). *Bright air, brilliant fire.* New York: Basic Books.

Edwards, B. (1989). *Drawing on the right side of the brain* (rev. ed.). New York: Tarcher/Putnam.

Eggermont, J. J. (1998). Is there a neural code? *Neuroscience and Biobehavioral Reviews, 22,* 355–370.

Ehlers, A., & Margraf, J. (1987). Anxiety induced by false heart rate feedback in patients with panic disorder. *Behaviour Research and Therapy, 26,* 1–11.

Eiden, R. D., Teti, D. M., & Corns, K. M. (1995). Maternal working models of attachment, marital adjustment and the parent–child relationship. *Child Development, 66,* 1504–1518.

Eisenberg, L. (1995). The social construction of the human brain. *American Journal of Psychiatry, 152,* 1563–1575.

Ekman, P. (1992a). Facial expressions of emotion: New findings, new questions. *Psychological Science, 3,* 34–38.

Ekman, P. (1992b). An argument for basic emotions. *Cognition and Emotion, 6,* 169–200.

Elder, G. H. (1998). The life course as developmental theory. *Child Development, 69,* 1–12.

Emde, R. N. (1990). Mobilizing fundamental modes of development: Empathic availability and therapeutic action. *Journal of the American Psychoanalytic Association, 38,* 881–913.

Emde, R. N., Zeynep, B., Clyman, R. B., & Oppenheim, D. (1991). The moral self of infancy: Affective core and procedural knowledge. *Developmental Review, 11,* 251–270.

Epstein, J. (1995, December 19). *Emotional processes* (Grand Rounds). The Toronto Hospital, Toronto, Canada.

Erickson, M. F., Korfmacher, J., & Egeland, B. (1992). Attachments past and present: Implications for therapeutic intervention with mother–infant dyads. *Development and Psychopathology, 4,* 495–507.

Etcoff, N., & Magee, J. (1992). Categorical perception of facial expressions. *Cognition, 44,* 227–240.

Fagot, B. I., & Pears, K. C. (1996). Changes in attachment during the third year: Consequences and predictions. *Development and Psychopathology, 8,* 325–344.

Feeney, B. C., & Kirkpatrick, L. A. (1996). Effects of adult attachment and presence of romantic partners on physiological responses to stress. *Journal of Personality and Social Psychology, 70,* 255–270.

Feldman, D. E., & Knudsen, E. I. (1998). Experience-dependent plasticity and the maturation of glutamatergic synapses. *Neuron, 20,* 1067–1071.

Feldman, R., & Greenbaum, C. W. (1997). Affect regulation and synchrony in mother–infant play as precursors to the development of symbolic competence. *Infant Mental Health Journal, 18,* 4–23.

Felitti, V. J., Anda, R. F., Nordenberg, D., Williamson, D. F., Spitz, A. M., Edwards, V., Koss, M. P., & Marks, J. S. (1998). Relationship of childhood abuse and household dysfunction to many of the leading causes of death in adults: The Adverse Childhood Experiences (ACE) Study. *American Journal of Preventive Medicine, 14,* 245–258.

Field, T. (1985). Attachment as psychobiological attunement: Being on the same wavelength. In M. Reite & T. Field (Eds.), *The psychobiology of attachment and separation* (pp. 415–454). Orlando, FL: Academic Press.

Field, T. (1994). The effects of mother's physical and emotional unavailability on emotion regulation. In N. A. Fox. (Ed.), The development of emotion regulation: Biological and behavioral considerations. *Monographs of the Society for Research in Child Development, 59*(2–3, Serial No. 240), 208–227.

Field, T. (1995). Infants of depressed mothers. *Infant Behavior and Development, 18,* 1–13.

Field, T., Fox, N. A., Pickens, J., & Nawrocki, T. (1995). Relative right frontal EEG activation in 3- to 6-month-old infants of "depressed" mothers. *Developmental Psychology, 31,* 358–363.

Field, T., Healy, B., Goldstein, S., & Gutherz, M. (1990). Behavior state matching in mother–infant interactions of non-depressed versus depressed mother–infant dyads. *Developmental Psychology, 26,* 7–14.

Fink, G. R., Markowowitsch, H. J., Reinkemeier, M., Bruckbauer, T., Kessler, J., & Wolf-Dieter, H. (1996). Cerebral representation of one's own past: Neural networks involved in autobiographical memory. *Journal of Neuroscience, 16,* 4275–4282.

Fivush, R. (1996). Constructing narrative, emotion, and self in parent–child conversations about the past. In U. Neisser & R. Fivush (Eds.), *The remembering self: Construction and accuracy in the self-narrative* (pp. 136–157). Cambridge, UK: Cambridge University Press.

Fivush, R. (1998). Children's recollections of traumatic and nontraumatic events. *Development and Psychopathology, 10,* 699–716.

Fivush, R., & Hudson, J. A. (Eds.). (1990). *Knowing and remembering in young children.* New York: Cambridge University Press.

Flavell, J. H., Green, F. L., & Flavell, E. R. (1986). Development of knowledge about the appearance–reality distinction. *Monographs of the Society for Research in Child Development, 51*(1–68, Serial No. 212).

Flavell, J. H., Miller, P. H., & Miller, S. A. (1993). *Cognitive development* (3rd ed.). Englewood Cliffs, NJ: Prentice-Hall.

Flor-Henry, P., & Gruzelier, J. (Eds.). (1983). *Laterality and psychopathology.* New York: Elsevier Science.

Fogel, A., & Branco, A. U. (1997). Metacommunication as a source of indeterminism in relationship development. In A. Fogel, M. C. D. P. Lyra, & J. Valsiner (Eds.), *Dynamics and indeterminism in developmental and social processes* (pp. 65–92). Mahwah, NJ: Erlbaum.

Fogel, A., Lyra, M. C. D. P., & Valsiner, J. (Eds.). (1997). *Dynamics and indeterminism in developmental and social processes.* Mahwah, NJ: Erlbaum.

Fonagy, P. (1998). *Early influences on development and social inequalities: Paper for Sir Donald Acheson's independent inquiry into inequalities in health.* Unpublished manuscript.

Fonagy, P., Leigh, T., Steele, M., Steele, H., Kennedy, G., Mattoon, M., Target, M., & Gerber, A. (1996). The relation of attachment status, psychiatric classification and response to psychotherapy. *Journal of Consulting and Clinical Psychology, 64,* 22–31.

Fonagy, P., Steele, H., & Steele, M. (1991a). Maternal representations of attachment during pregnancy predict the organization of infant–mother attachment at one year of age. *Child Development, 62,* 891–905.

Fonagy, P., Steele, M., Steele, H., Moran, G. S., & Higgitt, A. C. (1991b). The capacity for understanding mental states: The reflective self in parent and child and its significance for security of attachment. *Infant Mental Health Journal, 12,* 201–218.

Fonagy, P., & Target, M. (1997). Attachment and reflective function: Their role in self-organization. *Development and Psychopathology, 9,* 679–700.

Fonagy, P., Target, M., Steele, M., Steele, H., Leigh, T., Levinson, A., & Kennedy, R. (1997). Crime and attachment: Morality, disruptive behavior, borderline personality disorder, crime and their relationship to security of attachment. In L. Atkinson & K. J. Zucker (Eds.), *Attachment and psychopathology* (pp. 223–274). New York: Guilford Press.

Fox, N. A. (Ed.). (1994a). The development of emotion regulation: Biological and behavioral considerations. *Monographs of the Society for Research in Child Development, 59*(2–3, Serial No. 240).

Fox, N. A. (1994b). Dynamic cerebral processes underlying emotion regulation. In N. A. Fox (Ed.), *The development of emotion regulation: Biological and behavioral considerations. Monographs of the Society for Research in Child Development, 59*(2–3, Serial No. 240), 152–166.

Fox, N. A., Calkins, S. D., & Bell, M. A. (1994). Neural plasticity and development in the first two years of life: Evidence from cognitive and socioemotional domains of research. *Development and Psychopathology, 6,* 677–696.

Fox, N. A., Kimmerly, N. L., & Schafer, W. D. (1991). Attachment to mother/attachment to father: A meta-analysis. *Child Development, 62,* 210–225.

Fox, N. A., Schmidt, L. A., Calkins, S. D., Rubin, K. H., & Coplan, R. J. (1996). The role of frontal activation in the regulation and dysregulation of social behavior during the preschool years. *Development and Psychopathology, 8,* 89–102.

Freedman, M., Black, S., Ebert, P., & Binns, M. (1998). Orbitofrontal function, object alternation and perseveration. *Cerebral Cortex, 8,* 18–27.

Freeman, W. J. (1994). Role of chaotic dynamics in neural plasticity. *Progress in Brain Research, 102,* 319–333.

Freud, S. (1966). Project for a scientific psychology. In J. Strachey (Ed. and Trans.), *The standard edition of the complete psychological works of Sigmund Freud* (Vol. 1, pp. 281–397). London: Hogarth Press. (Original work published 1895)

Freyd, J. J. (1987). Dynamic mental representations. *Psychological Review, 94*, 427–438.

Freyd, J. J. (1996). *Betrayal trauma: The logic of forgetting childhood abuse.* Cambridge, MA: Harvard University Press.

Friede, E., & Weinstock, M. (1988). Prenatal stress increases anxiety related bahavior and alters cerebral lateralization of dopamine activity. *Life Sciences, 42*, 1059–1065.

Fuster, J. M. (1985). *The prefrontal cortex and temporal integration.* In A. Peters & E. G. Jones (Eds.), *Cerebral cortex: Vol. 4. Association and auditory cortices* (pp. 151–171). New York: Plenum Press.

Fuster, J. M. (1989). *The prefrontal cortex: Anatomy, physiology, and neuropsychology of the frontal lobe* (2nd ed.). New York: Raven Press.

Garber, J., & Dodge, K. A. (Eds.). (1991). *The development of emotion regulation and dysregulation.* Cambridge, UK: Cambridge University Press.

Gazzaniga, M. S. (1988). Brain modularity: Towards a philosophy of conscious experience. In A. J. Marcel & E. Bisach (Eds.), *Consciousness in contemporary science.* Oxford: Clarendon Press.

Gazzaniga, M. S. (Ed.). (1995). *The cognitive neurosciences.* Cambridge, MA: MIT Press.

Gazzaniga, M. S. (1996, January 11). *Cognitive neuroscience and the future of psychiatry.* Plenary address to the American Association of Directors of Psychiatric Residency Training, San Francisco.

Gazzaniga, M. S., Eliassen, J. C., Nisenson, L., Wessinger, C. M., & Baynes, K. B. (1996). Collaboration between the hemispheres of a callosotomy patient: Emerging right hemisphere speech and the left brain interpreter. *Brain, 119*, 1255–1262.

George, C., Kaplan, N., & Main, M. (1994) *An Adult Attachment Interview: Interview protocol.* Unpublished manuscript, University of California at Berkeley.

George, C., Kaplan, N., & Main, M. (1995) *An Adult Attachment Interview: Interview protocol.* (2nd ed.). Unpublished manuscript, University of California at Berkeley.

George, C., Kaplan, N., & Main, M. (1996). *An Adult Attachment Interview: Interview protocol* (3rd ed.). Unpublished manuscript, University of California at Berkeley.

George, C., & Solomon, J. (1996). Representational models of relationships: Links between caregiving and attachment. *Infant Mental Health Journal, 17*, 198–216.

George, M. S., Ketter, T. A., Parekh, P. I., Gill, D. S., Marangell, L., Pazzaglia, P. J., Herscovitch, P., & Post, R. M. (1997). Depressed subjects have decreased rCBF activation during facial emotion recognition. *International Journal of Neuropsychiatric Medicine, 2*, 45–55.

Gershberg, F. B., & Shimamura, A. P. (1995). The role of the frontal lobes in the use of organizational strategies in free recall. *Neuropsychologia, 13*, 1305–1333.

Gilligan, C. (1996). The centrality of relationship in human development: A puzzle, some evidence, and a theory. In G. G. Noam & K. W. Fischer (Eds.), *Development and vulnerability in close relationships* (pp.237–262). Hillsdale, NJ: Erlbaum.

Gilligan, C. (1997). Remembering Iphigenia: Voice, resonance, and a talking cure. In B. S. Mark & J. A. Incorvaia (Eds.), *The handbook of infant, child, and adolescent psychotherapy: Vol. 2. New directions in integrative treatment* (pp. 169–194). Northvale, NJ: Jason Aronson.

Gleick, J. (1987). *Chaos: Making a new science.* New York: Viking.

Globus, G., & Arpaia, J. P. (1993). Psychiatry and the new dynamics. *Biological Psychiatry 35*, 352–364.

Goerner, S. (1995). Chaos, evolution, and deep ecology. In R. Robertson & A. Combs (Eds.), *Chaos theory in psychology and the life sciences* (pp. 17–38). Hillsdale, NJ: Erlbaum.

Goldberg, E., & Costa, L. D. (1981). Hemispheric differences in the acquisition and use of descriptive systems. *Brain and Language, 14,* 144–173.

Goldberg, S., Muir, R., & Kerr, J. (Eds.). (1995). *Attachment theory: Social, developmental, and clinical perspectives.* Hillsdale, NJ: Analytic Press.

Goldman-Rakic, P. S. (1993). Working memory and the mind. In *Mind and brain readings from* Scientific American *magazine, September* (pp. 66–77). New York: Freeman.

Goldsmith, H. H., Gottesman, I. I., & Lemery, K. S. (1997). Epidgenetic approaches to developmental psychopathology. *Development and Psychopathology, 9,* 365–288.

Goleman, D. (1995). *Emotional intelligence.* New York: Bantam.

Gottman, J. M., & Declaire, J. (1997). *The heart of parenting: Raising an emotionally intelligent child.* New York: Simon & Schuster.

Gottman, J. M., Guralnick, M. J., Wilson, B., Swanson, C. C., & Murray, J. D. (1997). What should be the focus of emotion regulation in children?: A nonlinear dynamic mathematical model of children's peer interaction in groups. *Development and Psychopathology, 9,* 421–452.

Green, T., Neinemann, S. F., & Gusella, J. F. (1998). Molecular neurobiology and genetics: Investigation of neural function and dysfunction. *Neuron, 20,* 427–444

Greenberg, M. T., DeKlyen, M., Speltz, M. L., & Endriga, M. C. (1997). The role of attachment processes in externalizing psychopathology in young children. In L. Atkinson & K. J. Zucker (Eds.), *Attachment and psychopathology* (pp. 196–222). New York: Guilford Press.

Greenberg, M. T., Speltz, M. L., & DeKlyen, M. (1993). The role of attachment in the early development of disruptive behavior problems. *Development and Psychopathology, 5,* 191–214.

Greenough, W. T., & Black, J. E. (1992). Induction of brain structure by experience: Substrates for cognitive development. In M. R. Gunnar & C. A. Nelson (Eds.), *Minnesota Symposia on Child Psychology: Vol. 24. Developmental behavioral neuroscience* (pp. 155–200). Hillsdale, NJ: Erlbaum.

Greenspan, S. I., & Benderly, B. L. (1997). *The growth of the mind and the endangered origins of intelligence.* Reading, MA: Addison-Wesley.

Greenwald, A. G. (1992). New Look 3: Unconscious cognition reclaimed. *American Psychologist, 47,* 766–779.

Grice, H. P. (1975). Logic and conversation. In P. Cole & J. L. Moran (Eds.), *Syntax and semantics III: Speech acts* (pp. 41–58). New York: Academic Press.

Gross-Tsur, V., Shalev, R. S., Manor, O., & Amir, N. (1995). Developmental right-hemisphere syndrome: Clinical spectrum of the nonverbal learning disability. *Journal of Learning Disabilities, 28,* 80–86.

Gunnar, M. R. (1990). The psychobiology of infant temperament. In J. Colombo & J. Fagen (Eds.), *Individual differences in infancy: Reliability, stability, prediction* (pp. 387–409). Hillsdale, NJ: Erlbaum.

Gunnar, M. R. (1992). Reactivity of the hypothalamic–pituitary–adrenocortical system to stressors in normal infants and children. *Pediatrics, 90,* 491–497.

Haden, C. A., Haine, R. A., & Fivush, R. (1997). Developing narrative structure in parent–child reminiscing across the preschool years. *Developmental Psychology, 33,* 295–307.

Haft, W. L., & Slade, A. (1989). Affect attunement and maternal attachment: A pilot study. *Infant Mental Health Journal, 10,* 157–172.

Hagler, D. J., & Goda, Y. (1998). Synaptic adhesion: The building blocks of memory? *Neuron, 20,* 1059–1062.

Halgren, E. (1992). Emotional neurophysiology of the amygdala within the context of human cognition. In J. Aggleton (Ed.), *The amygdala: Neurobiological aspects of emotion, memory, and mental dysfunction* (pp. 191–228). New York: Wiley-Liss.

Halgren, E., & Marinkovic, K. (1995). Neurophysiological networks integrating human emotions. In M. S. Gazzaniga (Ed.), *The cognitive neurosciences* (pp. 1137–1151). Cambridge, MA: MIT Press.

Hamann, S. B., & Squire, L. R. (1997). Intact perceptual memory in the absence of conscious memory. *Behavioral Neuroscience, 4,* 850–854.

Harr,, R. (1986). *The social construction of emotions.* New York: Blackwell.

Harter, S. (1988). Developmental processes in the construction of the self. In T. D. Yawkey & J. E. Johnson (Eds.), *Integrative processes and socialization: Early to middle childhood* (pp. 45–78). Hillsdale, NJ: Erlbaum.

Harter, S., Bresnick, S., Bouchey, H. A., & Whitsell, N. R. (1997). The development of multiple role-related selves during adolescence. *Development and Psychopathology, 9,* 835–854.

Haxby, J. V., Ungerleider, L. G., Horwitz, B., Maisog, J. M., Rapoport, S. L., & Grady, C. L. (1996). Face encoding and recognition in the human brain. *Proceedings of the National Academy of Sciences USA, 93,* 922–927.

Hebb, D. O. (1949). *The organization of behavior: A neuropsychological theory.* New York: Wiley.

Heller, W. (1993). Neuropsychological mechanisms of individual differences in emotion, personality, and arousal. *Neuropsychology, 7,* 476–489.

Heller, W., Etienne, M. A., & Miller, G. A. (1995). Patterns of perceptual asymmetry in depression and anxiety: Implications for neuropsychological models of emotion and psychopathology. *Journal of Abnormal Psychology, 104,* 327–333.

Herman, J. L. (1992). *Trauma and recovery.* New York: Basic Books.

Herstgaard, L., Gunnar, M., Erickson, M. F., & Nachmias, M. (1995). Adrenocortical responses to the Strange Situation in infants with disorganized/disoriented attachment relationships. *Child Development, 61,* 1100–1106.

Hesse, E. (1996). Discourse, memory and the Adult Attachment Interview: A note with emphasis on the emerging cannot classify category. *Infant Mental Health Journal, 17,* 4–11.

Hesse, E. (1999). The adult attachment interview: Historical and current perspectives. In J. Cassidy & P. R. Shaver (Eds.), *Handbook of attachment: Theory, research, and clinical applications* (pp. 395–433). New York: Guilford Press.

Hesse, E., & Main, M. (1999). Unresolved/disorganized responses to trauma in non-maltreating parents: Previously unexamined risk factor for offspring. *Psychoanalytic Inquiry, 19,* 4– .

Hesse, E., & Main, M. (in press). Disorganization in infant and adult attachment: Descriptions, correlates and implications for developmental psychopathology. *Journal of the American Psychoanalytic Association.*

Hesse, E., & van IJzendoorn, M. H. (1998). Parental loss of close family members and propensities towards absorption in offspring. *Developmental Science, 1,* 299–305.

Hilgard, E. R. (1977). *Divided consciousness: Multiple controls in human thought and action.* New York: Wiley.

Hobson, J. (1992). The brain as a dream machine: An activation–synthesis hypothesis of dreaming. In M. Lansky (Ed.), *Essential papers on dreams* (pp. 452–473). New York: New York University Press.

Hockfield, S., & Lombroso, P. J. (1998). Development of the cerebral cortex IX: Cortical development and experience—II. *Journal of the American Academy of Child and Adolescent Psychiatry, 37,* 1103–1105.

Hofer, M. A. (1984). Relationships as regulators: A psychobiologic perspective on bereavement. *Psychosomatic Medicine, 46,* 183–197.

Hofer, M. (1990). Early symbiotic processes: Hard evidence from a soft place. In R. A. Glick & S. Bone (Eds.), *Pleasure beyond the pleasure principle* (pp. 55–78). New Haven: Yale University Press.

Hofer, M. A. (1994). Hidden regulators in attachment, separation, and loss. In N. A. Fox (Ed.), The development of emotion regulation: Biological and behavioral considerations. *Monographs of the Society for Research in Child Development, 59*(2–3, Serial No. 240), 192–207.

Hofer, M. A. (1996). On the nature and consequences of early loss. *Psychosomatic Medicine, 58,* 570–581.

Holstege, G., Bandler, R., & Saper, C. B. (1994). The emotional motor system. *Progress in Brain Research, 107,* 3–8.

Hornak, J., Rolls, E. T., & Wade, D. (1996). Face and voice expression identification in patients with emotional and behavioral changes following ventral frontal lobe damage. *Neuropsychologia, 34,* 247–261.

Horowitz, M. J. (1987). *States of mind* (2nd ed.). New York: Plenum Press.

Horowitz, M. J. (Ed.). (1991). *Person schemas and maladaptive interpersonal patterns.* Chicago: University of Chicago Press.

Hossain, Z., Field, R., Gonzalez, T., Malphurs, J., & Del Valle, C. (1994). Infants of "depressed" mothers interact better with their nondepressed fathers. *Infant Mental Health Journal, 15,* 348–357.

Howe, M. L. (1998). Individual differences in factors that modulate storage and retrieval of traumatic memories. *Development and Psychopathology, 10,* 681–698.

Howes, C., Hamilton, C. E., & Matheson, C. C. (1994a). Children's relationships with peers: Differential associations with aspects of the teacher–child relationship. *Child Development, 65,* 253–263.

Howes, C., Hamilton, C. E., & Philipsen, L. C. (1998). Stability and continuity of child–caregiver and child–peer relationships. *Child Development, 69,* 418–426.

Howes, C., Matheson, C. C., & Hamilton, C. E. (1994b). Maternal, teacher, and child care history correlates of children's relationships with peers. *Child Development, 65,* 264–273.

Hubel, D. H. (1967). Effects of distortion of sensory input on the visual cortex and the influence of the environment. *Physiologist, 10,* 17–45.

Hur, Y. M., & Bouchard, T. J. (1995). Genetic influences on perceptions of childhood family environment: A reared apart twin study. *Child Development, 66,* 330–345.

Incisa della Rochetta, A., & Milner, B. (1993). Strategic search and retrieval inhibition: The role of the frontal lobes. *Neuropsychologia, 31,* 503–524.

Ingvar, D. H. (1985). "Memory of the future": An essay on the temporal organization of conscious awareness. *Human Neurobiology, 4,* 127–136.

Izard, C. E. (1991). *The psychology of emotions.* New York: Plenum Press.

Izard, C. E. (1992). Basic emotions, relations among emotions, and emotion–cognition relations. *Psychological Review, 99,* 561–565.

Izard, C. E., & Kobak, R. R. (1991). Emotions system functioning and emotion regulation. In J. Garber & K. A. Dodge (Eds.), *The development of emotion regulation and dysregulation* (pp. 303–322). Cambridge, UK: Cambridge University Press.

Jackson, E. A. (1991). Controls of dynamic flows with attractors. *Physical Review A, 44,* 4389–4853.

James, W. (1884). What is an emotion? *Mind, 9,* 188–205.

James, W. (1890). *The principles of psychology.* New York: Henry Holt.

Jaynes, J. (1976). *The origin of consciousness in the breakdown of the bicameral mind.* Boston: Houghton Mifflin.

Jeffery, K. J., & Reid, I. C. (1997). Modifiable neuronal connections: An overview for psychiatrists. *American Journal of Psychiatry, 154,* 156–164.

Jensen, P. S., & Hoagwood, K. (1997). The book of names: DSM-IV in context. *Development and Psychopathology, 9,* 231–249.

Johnson, B. H., & Hugdahl, K. (1991). Hemispheric asymmetry in conditioning to facial emotional expressions. *Psychophysiology, 28,* 154–162.

Johnson-Laird, P. N. (1983). *Mental models: Towards a cognitve science of language, inference, and consciousness.* Cambridge, MA: Harvard University Press.

Jones, E., Main, M., & Del Carman, R. (Eds.). (1996). Attachment and psychopathology [Special section]. *Journal of Consulting and Clinical Psychology, 64*(2).

Joseph, R. (1992). *The right brain and the unconscious: Discovering the stranger within.* New York: Plenum Press.

Juffer, F., van IJzendoorn, M. H., & Bakermans-Kranenburg, M. J. (1997). Intervention in transmission of insecure attachment: A case study. *Psychological Reports, 80,* 531–543.

Kagan, J. (1992). Behavior, biology, and the meanings of temperamental constructs. *Pediatrics, 90,* 510–513.

Kagan, J. (1994a). *Galen's prophecy: Temperament in human nature.* New York: Basic Books.

Kagan, J. (1994b). On the nature of emotion. In N. A. Fox (Ed.), The development of emotion regulation: Biological and behavioral considerations. *Monographs of the Society for Research in Child Development, 59*(2–3, Serial No. 240), 7–24.

Kagan, J. (1997). Conceptualizing psychopathology: The importance of developmental profiles. *Development and Psychopathology, 9,* 321–334.

Kandel, E. R. (1989). Genes, nerve cells, and the remembrance of things past. *Journal of Neuropsychiatry and Clinical Neurosciences, 1,* 103–125.

Kandel, E. R. (1998). A new intellectual framework for psychiatry. *American Journal of Psychiatry, 155,* 457–469.

Kandel, E. R., & Abel, T. (1995). Neuropeptides, adenylyl cyclase, and memory storage. *Science, 268,* 825–826.

Kandel, E. R., & Schwartz, H. (Eds.). (1992). *Principles of neural science* (2nd ed.). New York: Elsevier.

Kapur, S., Craik, F. I. M., Jones, C., Brown, G. M., Houle, S., & Tulving. E. (1995). Functional role of the prefrontal cortex in retrieval of memories: A PET study. *NeuroReport, 6,* 1880–1884.

Karni, A., Tanne, D., Rubenstein, B. S., Askenasi, J. J., & Sagi, D. (1992). No dreams, no memory: The effect of REM sleep deprivation on learning a new perceptual skill. *Society for Neuroscience Abstracts, 18,* 387.

Karr-Morse, R., & Wiley, M. S. (1997). *Ghosts from the nursery: Tracing the roots of violence.* New York: Atlantic Monthly Press.

Kelley, W. M., Miezin, F. M., McDermott, K. B., Buckner, R. L., Raichle, M. E., Cohen, N. J., Ollinger, J. M., Akbudak, E., Conturo, T. E., Snyder, A. Z., & Petersen, S. E. (1998). Hemispheric specialization in human dorsal frontal cortex and medial temporal lobe for verbal and nonverbal memory encoding. *Neuron, 20,* 927–936.

Kempermann, G., Kuhn, H. G., & Gage, F. H. (1997). More hippocampal neurons in adult mice living in an enriched environment. *Nature, 386,* 493–495.

Kendler, K. S. (1996). Parenting: A genetic–epidemiologic perspective. *American Journal of Psychiatry, 153,* 11–20.

Kendler, K. S., & Eaves, L. S. (1986). Models for the joint effect of genotype and environment on liability to psychiatric illness. *American Journal of Psychiatry, 143,* 279–289.

Kihlstrom, J. F. (1987). The cognitive unconscious. *Science, 237,* 1445–1452.

Kinsbourne, M. (1972). Eye and head turning indicates cerebral lateralization. *Science, 176,* 539–541.

Koopman, C., Classen, C., & Spiegel, D. (1994). Predictors of posttraumatic stress symptoms among survivors of the Oakland/Berkeley, California firestorm. *American Journal of Psychiatry, 151,* 888–894.

Korfmacher, J., Adam, E., Ogawa, J., & Egland, B. (1997). Adult attachment: Implications for the therapeutic process in a home intervention. *Applied Developmental Science, 1,* 43–52.

Kosslyn, S. M. (1994). *Image and brain The resolution of the imagery debate.* Cambridge, MA: MIT Press.

Kraemer, G. W. (1992). A psychobiological theory of attachment. *Behavioral and Brain Sciences, 15,* 493–541.

Krystal, J. H., Karper, L. P., Seibyl, J. P., Freeman, G. K., Delaney, R., Bremner, J. D., Haninger, G. R., Bowers, M. B., & Charney, D. S. (1994). Subanaesthetic effects of the noncompetitive NMDA antagonist ketamine in humans: Psychotomimetic, perceptual, cognitive and neuroendocrine responses. *Archives of General Psychiatry, 51,* 199–213.

Larsen, R. J., Kasimatis, M., & Frey, K. (1992). Facilitating the furrowed brow: An unobtrusive test of the facial feedback hypothesis applied to unpleasant affect. *Cognition and Emotion, 6,* 321–338.

LeDoux, J. E. (1990). Information flow from sensation to emotion: Plasticity of the neural computation of stimulus value. In M. Gabriel & J. Moore (Eds.), *Learning and computational neuroscience: Foundations of adaptive networks* (pp. 3–51). Cambridge, MA: MIT Press.

LeDoux, J. E. (1996). *The emotional brain: The mysterious underpinning of emotional life.* New York: Simon & Schuster.

LeDoux, J. E., Romanski, L., & Xagoraris, A. (1991). Indelibility of subcortical emotional memories. *Journal of Cognitive Neuroscience, 1,* 238–243.

Leichtman, M. D., Ceci, S., & Ornstein, P. A. (1992). The influence of affect on memory: Mechanism and development. In S. A. Christianson (Ed.), *Handbook of emotion and memory* (pp. 181–199). Hillsdale, NJ: Erlbaum.

Levy, J. (1969). Possible basis for the evolution of the human brain. *Nature, 224,* 614–615.

Lewis, D. O., & Putnam, F. W. (1996). Dissociative identity disorder/multiple personality disorder. *Child and Adolescent Clinics of North America, 5*(2), 263–541.

Lewis, M. (1992). Individual differences in response to stress. *Pediatrics, 90,* 487–490.

Lewis, M., & Haviland, J. M. (Eds.). (1993). *Handbook of emotions.* New York: Guilford Press.

Lewis, M. D. (1995). Cognition–emotion feedback and the self-organization of developmental paths. *Human Development, 38,* 71–102.

Lewis, M. D. (1996). Self-organising cognitive appraisals. *Cognition and Emotion, 10,* 1–25.

Lewis, M. D. (1997). Personality self-organization: Cascading constraints on cognition–emotion interaction. In A. Fogel, M. C. D. P. Lyra, & J. Valsiner (Eds.), *Dynamics and indeterminism in developmental and social processes* (pp. 193–216). Mahwah, NJ: Erlbaum.

Lichtenstein Phelps, J., Belsky, J., & Crnic, K. (1998). Earned security, daily stress, and parenting: A comparison of five alternative models. *Development and Psychopathology, 10,* 21–38.

Lieberman, A. F. (1991). Attachment theory and infant–parent psychotherapy: Some conceptual, clinical and research considerations. In D. Cicchetti & S. L. Toth (Eds.), *Rochester Symposium on Developmental Psychopathology: Vol. 3. Modes and integrations* (pp. 261–287). Rochester, NY: University of Rochester Press.

Lieberman, A. F. (1993). *The emotional life of the toddler.* New York: Free Press.

Lieberman, A. F. (1997). Toddlers' internalization of maternal attributions as a factor in quality of attachment. In L. Atkinson & K. J. Zucker (Eds.), *Attachment and psychopathology* (pp. 277–291). New York: Guilford Press.

Llinas, R. R. (1990). Intrinsic electrical properties of mammalian neurons and CNS function. *Fidia Research Foundation Neuroscience Award Lectures, 4,* 175–194.

Liotti, G. (1992). Disorganized/disoriented attachment in etiology of dissociative disorders. *Dissociation, 5,* 196–204.

Liotti, M., & Tucker, D. M. (1992). Right hemisphere sensitivity to arousal and depression. *Brain and cognition, 18,* 138–151.

Liu, D., Dioria, J., Tannenbaum, B., Caldji, C., Francis, D., Freedman, A., Sharma, S., Pearson, D., Plotsky, P. M., & Meaney, M. J. (1997). Maternal care, hippocampal glucocorticoid receptors, and hypothalamic–pituitary–adrenal responses to stress. *Science, 277,* 1659–1662.

Loevinger, J. (1976). *Ego development.* San Francisco: Jossey-Bass.

Lombroso, P. J., & Sapolsky, R. (1998). Development of the cerebral cortex XII: Stress and brain development—I. *Journal of the American Academy of Child and Adolescent Psychiatry, 37,* 1337–1339.

Lynch, M., & Cicchetti, D. (1998a). Trauma, mental representation, and the organization of memory for mother-referent material. *Development and Psychopathology, 10,* 739–760.

Lynch, M., & Cicchetti, D. (1998b). An ecological-transactional analysis of children and contexts: The longitudinal interplay among maltreatment, community violence, and children's symptomatology. *Development and Psychopathology, 10,* 235–257.

Lyons-Ruth, K. (1995). Broadening our conceptual frameworks: Can we re-introduce relational strategies and implicit representational systems to the study of psychopathology? *Developmental Psychology, 31,* 432–436.

Lyons-Ruth, K., Alpern, L., & Repacholi, B. (1993). Disorganized infant attachment classification and maternal psychosocial problems as predictors of hostile–aggressive behavior in the preschool classroom. *Child Development, 64,* 572–585.

Lyons-Ruth, K., Connell, D. B., & Grunebaum, H. U. (1990). Infants at social risk: Maternal depression and family support services as mediators of infant development and security of attachment. *Child Development, 61,* 85–98.

Lyons-Ruth, K., & Jacobwitz, D. (1999). Attachment disorganization: Unresolved loss, relational violence, and lapses in behavioral and attentional strategies. In J. Cassidy & P. R. Shaver (Eds.), *Handbook of attachment: Theory, research, and clinical applications* (pp. 520–554). New York: Guilford Press.

Lyons-Ruth, K., Repacholi, B., McLeod, S., & Silva, E. (1991). Disorganized attachment behavior in infancy: Short-term stability, maternal and infant correlates, and risk-related subtypes. *Development and Psychopathology, 3,* 397–412.

Lyra, M. C. D. P., & Winegar, L. T. (1997). Processual dynamics of interaction through time: Adult–child interactions and process of development. In A. Fogel, M. C. D. P. Lyra, & J. Valsiner (Eds.), *Dynamics and indeterminism in developmental and social processes* (pp. 93–109). Mahwah, NJ: Erlbaum.

MacMillan, H. L., MacMillan, J. H., Offord, D. R., Griffith, L., & MacMillan, A. (1994). Primary prevention of child physical abuse and neglect: A critical review. Parts I and II. *Journal of Child Psychology and Psychiatry, 35,* 835–856, 857–876.

Main, M. (1991). Metacognitive knowledge, metacognitive monitoring, and singular (coherent) versus multiple (incoherent) models of attachment: Findings and directions for future research. In C. M. Parkes, J. Stenson-Hinde, & P. Marris (Eds.), *Attachment across the life cycle* (pp. 127–159). London: Routledge.

Main, M. (1993). Discourse, prediction, and recent studies in attachment: Implications for psychoanalysis. *Journal of the American Psychoanalytic Association, 41,* 209–244.

Main, M. (1995). Attachment: Overview, with implications for clinical work. In S. Goldberg, R. Muir, & J. Kerr (Eds.), *Attachment theory: Social, developmental, and clinical perspectives* (pp. 407–474). Hillsdale, NJ: Analytic Press.

Main, M. (1996). Introduction to the special section on attachment and psychopathology: 2. Overview of the field of attachment. *Journal of Consulting and Clinical Psychology, 64,* 237–243.

Main, M. (in press). The Adult Attachment Interview: Fear, attention, safety and discourse processes. *Journal of the American Psychoanalytic Association.*

Main, M., & Goldwyn, R. (1984). *Adult attachment scoring and classification system.* Unpublished manuscript, University of California at Berkeley.

Main, M., & Goldwyn, R. (1998). *Adult attachment scoring and classification systems* (Version 6.3). Unpublished manuscript, University of California at Berkeley.

Main, M., & Hesse, E. (1990). Parents' unresolved traumatic experiences are related to infant disorganized status: Is frightened and/or frightening parental behavior the linking mechanism? In M. T. Greenberg, D. Cicchetti, & E. M. Cummings (Eds.), *Attachment in the preschool years: Theory, research, and intervention* (pp. 161–182). Chicago: University of Chicago Press.

Main, M., Kaplan, N., & Cassidy, J. (1985). Security in infancy, childhood, and adulthood: A move to the level of representation. In I. Bretherton & E. Waters (Eds.), Growing points of attachment theory and research. *Monographs of the Society for Research in Child Development, 50*(2–3, Serial No. 209), 66–104.

Main, M., & Morgan, H. (1996). Disorganization and disorientation in infant Strange Situation behavior: Phenotypic resemblance to dissociative states. In L. K. Michelson & W. J. Ray (Eds.), *Handbook of dissociation: Theoretical, empirical, and clinical perspectives* (pp. 107–138). New York: Plenum Press.

Main, M., & Solomon, J. (1986). Discovery of an insecure–disorganized/disoriented attachment pattern. In T. B. Brazelton & M. Yogman (Eds.), *Affective development in infancy* (pp. 95–124). Norwood, NJ: Ablex.

Main, M., & Solomon, J. (1990). Procedures for identifying infants as disorganized/disoriented during the Ainsworth Strange Situation. In M. T. Greenberg, D. Cicchetti, & E. M. Cummings (Eds.), *Attachment in the preschool years: Theory, research, and intervention* (pp. 121–160). Chicago: University of Chicago Press.

Malatesta-Magai, C. (1991). Development of emotion expression during infancy: General course and patterns of individual difference. In J. Garber & K. A. Dodge (Eds.), *The development of emotion regulation and dysregulation* (pp. 49–68). Cambridge, UK: Cambridge University Press.

Manassis, K., Bradley, S. Goldberg, S., Hood, J., & Swinson, R. P. (1994). Attachment in mothers with anxiety disorders and their children. *Journal of the American Academy of Child and Adolescent Psychiatry, 33,* 1106–1113.

Marcel, A., & Bisiach, E. (Eds.). (1988). *Consciousness in contemporary science.* Oxford: Clarendon Press.

March, J. S., & Mulle, K. (1998). *OCD in children and adolescents: A cognitive-behavioral treatment manual.* New York: Guilford Press.

Martin, K. C., & Kandel, E. R. (1996). Cell adhesion molecules, CREB, and the formation of new synaptic connections [Comment]. *Neuron. 4,* 567–570.

McCabe, A., & Peterson, C. (1991). Getting the story: A longitudinal study of parental styles in eliciting narratives and developing narrative skill. In A. McCabe & C. Peterson (Eds.), *Developing narrative structure* (pp. 217–253). Hillsdale, NJ: Erlbaum.

McClelland, J. L., McNaughton, B. L., & O'Reilly, R. C. (1995). Why there are complementary learning systems in the hippocampus and neocortex: Insights from the successes and failures of connectionist models of learning and memory. *Psychological Review, 102,* 419–457.

McClelland, J. L., & Rumelhart, D. E. (Eds.). (1986). *Parallel distributed processing: Explorations in the microstructure of cognition* (Vols. 1 and 2). Cambridge, MA: MIT Press.

McCraty, R., Atkinson, M., Tomasion, D., & Tiller, W. A. (1998). The electricity of touch: Detection and measurement of cardiac energy exchange between people. In K. H. Pribram & J. King (Eds.), *Brain and values: Is a biological science of values possible?* (pp. 359–379). Hillsdale, NJ: Erlbaum.

McEwen, B. (1999). Development of the cerebral cortex XIII: Stress and brain development—II. *Journal of the American Academy of Child and Adolescent Psychiatry, 38,* 101–103.

McGaugh, J. L. (1992). Affect, neuromodulatory systems, and memory storage. In S. A. Christianson (Ed.), *Handbook of emotion and memory* (pp. 245–268). Hillsdale, NJ: Erlbaum.

McNally, R. J., Litz, B. T., Prassas, A., Shin, L. M., & Weathers, F. W. (1994). Emotional priming of autobiographical memory in post-traumatic stress disorder. *Cognition and Emotion. 8,* 351–367.

Meltzoff, A. N. (1995). What infant memory tells us about infantile amnesia: Long-term recall and deferred imitation. *Journal of Experimental Child Psychology, 59,* 497–515.

Merzenich, M. M., Grajski, K. A., Jenkins, W. M., Recanzone, G. H., & Peterson, B. (1991). Functional cortical plasticity: Cortical network origins of representations changes. *Cold Spring Harbor Symposium on Quantitative Biology, 55,* 873–887.

Merzenich, M. M., & Sameshima, K. (1993). Cortical plasticity and memory. *Current Opinion in Neurobiology, 3,* 187–196.

Mesulam, M. M. (1998). Review article: From sensation to cognition. *Brain, 121,* 1013–1052.

Metcalfe, J., & Shimamura, A. P. (1989). *Metacognition: Knowing about knowing.* Cambridge, MA: MIT Press.

Mikulincer, M. (1995). Attachment style and the mental representation of self. *Journal of Personality and Social Psychology, 69,* 1203–1215.

Mikulincer, M., & Orbach, I. (1995). Attachment styles and repressive defensiveness: The accessibility and architecture of affective memories. *Journal of Personality and Social Psychology, 68,* 917–925.

Miller, P. J., Potts, R., Fung, H., Hoogstra, L., & Mintz, J. (1990). Narrative practices and the social construction of self in childhood. *American Ethnologist, 17,* 292–311.

Milner, B., Petrides, M., & Smith, M. L. (1985). Frontal lobes and the temporal organization of memory. *Human Neurobiology, 4,* 137–142.

Milner, B., Squire L. R., & Kandel, E. R. (1998). Cognitive neuroscience and the study of memory. *Neuron, 20,* 445–468.

Minde, K., & Hesse, E. (1996). The role of the Adult Attachment Interview in parent–infant psychotherapy: A case presentation. *Infant Mental Health Journal, 17,* 115–126.

Morris, R. G. M. (Ed.). (1989). *Parallel distributed processing: Implications for psychology and neurobiology.* Oxford: Clarendon Press.

Morton, J., & Frith, U. (1995). Causal modeling: A structural approach to developmental psychology. In D. Cicchetti & D. J. Cohen (Eds.), *Developmental psychopathology: Vol. 1. Theory and methods* (pp. 357–390). New York: Wiley.

Moscovitch, M. (1995). Recovered consciousness: A hypothesis concerning modularity and episodic memory. *Journal of Clinical and Experimental Neuropsychology, 17,* 276–290.

Moss, B., & Gotts, E. A. (1998). Relationship-based early childhood intervention: A progress report from the trenches. *Zero to Three, 18,* 24–32.

Myers, N. A., Clifton, R. K., & Clarkson, M. G. (1987). When they were very young: Almost-threes remember two years ago. *Infant Behavior and Development, 10,* 123–132.

Nachmias, M., Gunnar, M. R., Mangelsdorf, S., Parritz, R. H., & Buss, K. (1996). Behavioral inhibition and stress reactivity: Moderating role of attachment security. *Child Development, 67,* 508–522.

Nass, R., & Koch, D. (1991). Innate specialization for emotion: Temperament differences in children with left versus right brain damage. In N. Amir, I. Rapin, & D. Branski (Eds.), *Pediatric neurology: Vol. 1. Behavior and cognition of the child with brain dysfunction* (pp. 1–17). Basel: Karger.

National Institute of Child Health and Human Development (NICHD) Early Child Care Research Network. (1996). Characteristics of infant child care: Factors contributing to positive caregiving. *Early Childhood Research Quarterly, 11,* 269–306.

National Institute of Child Health and Human Development (NICHD) Early Child Care Research Network. (1997). The effects of infant child care on infant–mother attachment security: Results of the NICHD study of early child care. *Child Development, 68,* 860–879.

Neisser, U., & Fivush, R. (Eds.). (1994). *The remembering self: Construction and accuracy in the self-narrative.* Cambridge, UK: Cambridge University Press.

Nelson, C. A. (Ed.). (1993). *Minnesota Symposia on Child Psychology: Vol. 26. Memory and affect in development.* Hillsdale, NJ: Erlbaum.

Nelson, C. A. (1994). Neural bases of infant temperament. In J. E. Bates & T. D. Wachs (Eds.), *Temperament: Individual differences at the interface of biology and behavior* (pp. 47–82). Washington, DC: American Psychological Association.

Nelson, C. A., & Bloom, F. E. (1997). Child development and neuroscience. *Child Development, 68,* 970–987.

Nelson, C. A., & Carver, L. J. (1998). The effects of stress and trauma on brain and memory: A view from developmental cognitive neuroscience. *Development and Psychopathology, 10,* 793–810.

Nelson, K. (Ed.). (1989). *Narratives from the crib.* Cambridge, MA: Harvard University Press.

Nelson, K. (1993a). Events, narratives, memory: What develops? In C. A. Nelson (Ed.), *Minnesota Symposia on Child Psychology: Vol. 26. Memory and affect in development* (pp. 1–24). Hillsdale, NJ: Erlbaum.

Nelson, K. (1993b). The psychological and social origins of autobiographical memory. *Psychological Science 2,* 1–8.

Neville, H. J. (1998, November 9). *Specificity and plasticity in human brain development.* Special lecture of the 28th annual meeting of the Society for Neuroscience, Los Angeles, California.

Neville, H. J., & Bavellier, D. (1998). Neural organization and plasticity of language. *Current Opinion in Neurobiology, 8*(2), 254–258.

Newcombe, N., & Fox, N. A. (1994). Infantile amnesia: Through a glass darkly. *Child Development, 65,* 31–40.

Nieuwenhuys, R. (1994). The greater limbic system, the emotional motor system and the brain. *Progress in Brain Research, 107,* 551–582.

Noam, G. G., & Fischer, K. W. (Eds.). (1996). *Development and vulnerability in close relationships.* Hillsdale, NJ: Erlbaum.

Nobre, A. C., Coull, J. T., Frith, C. D., & Mesulam, M. M. (1999). Orbitofrontal cortex is activated during breaches of expectation in tasks of visual attention. *Nature Neuroscience, 2,* 11–12.

Oatley, K., & Duncan, E. (1994). The experience of emotions in everyday life. *Cognition and Emotion, 8,* 369–381.

Ochs, E., & Capps, L. (1996). Narrating the self. *Annual Review of Anthropology, 25,* 19–43.

O'Donohue, J. (1997). *Anam cara: A book of celtic wisdom.* New York: HarperCollins.

Ogawa, J. R., Sroufe, L. A., Weinfeld, N. S., Carlson, E. A., & Egeland, B. (1997). Development and the fragmented self: Longitudinal study of dissociative symptomatology in a nonclinical sample. *Development and Psychopathology, 9,* 855–880.

Olds, D., Henderson, C. R., Jr., Cole, R., Eckenrode, J., Kitzman, H., Luckey, D., Pettitt, L., Sidora, K., Morris, P., & Powers, J. (1998). Long-term effects of nurse home visitation on children's criminal and antisocial behavior: 15-year follow-up of a randomized controlled trial. *Journal of the American Medical Association, 280,* 1238–1244.

Oppenheim, D., Nir, A., Warren, S., & Emde, R. N. (1997). Emotion regulation in mother–child narrative co-construction: Associations with children's narratives and adaptation. *Developmental Psychology, 33,* 284–294.

Oppenheim, D., & Waters, H. (1995). Narrative processes and attachment representations: Issues of development and assessment. In E. Waters, B. E. Vaughn, G. Posada, & K. Kondo-Ikemura (Eds.), Caregiving, cultural, and cognitive perspectives on secure-base behavior and working models: New growing points of attachment theory and research. *Monographs of the Society for Research in Child Development, 60*(2–3, Serial No. 244), 197–215.

Ornstein, R. (1997). *The right mind: Making sense of the hemispheres.* New York: Harcourt Brace.

Ornstein, R., Herron, J., Johnstone, J., & Swencionis, C. (1979). Differential right hemisphere involvement in two reading tasks. *Psychophysiology 16,* 398–401.

Ortony, A., & Turner, T. (1990). What's basic about basic emotions? *Psychological Review, 97,* 315–331.

Otto, M. W., Yeo, R. A., & Dougher, M. J. (1987). Right hemisphere involvement in depression: Toward a neuropsychological theory of negative affective experience. *Biological Psychiatry, 22,* 1201–1215.

Oznoff, S., & Miller, J. N. (1996). An exploration of right-hemisphere contributions to the pragmatic impairments of autism. *Brain and Language, 52,* 411–434.

Palaez-Nogueras, M., Field, T., Cigales, M., Gonzalez, A., & Clasky, S. (1994). Infants of depressed mothers show less "depressed" behavior with a familiar caregiver. *Infant Mental Health Journal, 15,* 358–367.

Panksepp, J. (1982). Toward a general psychobiological theory of emotions. *Behavioral and Brain Sciences, 5,* 407–467.

Parkes, C. M., Stevenson-Hinde, J., & Marris, P. (Eds.). (1991). *Attachment across the life cycle.* London: Routledge.

Pearson, J. L., Cohn, D. A., Cowan, P. A., & Cowan, C. P. (1994). Earned and continuous security in adult attachment: Relation to depressive symptomatology and parenting style. *Development and Psychopathology, 6,* 259–373.

Pederson, D. R., Gleason, E., Moran, G., & Bento, S. (1998). Maternal attachment representations, maternal sensitivity and the infant-mother relationship. *Developmental Psychology, 34,* 925–933.

Pennebaker, J. W., Kiecolt-Glaser, J. K., & Glaser, R. (1988). Disclosure of traumas and immune function: Health implications for psychotherapy. *Journal of Consulting and Clinical Psychology, 56,* 239–245.

Perner, J. (1991). *Understanding the representational mind.* Cambridge, MA: MIT Press.

Perner, J., & Ruffman, T. (1995). Episodic memory and autonoetic consciousness: Developmental evidence and a theory of childhood amnesia. *Journal of Experimental Child Psychology, 59,* 516–548.

Perry, B. D. (1997). Incubated in terror: Neurodevelopmental factors in the "cycle of violence." In J. Osofsky (Ed.), *Children in a violent society* (pp. 124–149). New York: Guilford Press.

Perry, B. D., Pollard, R. A., Blakely, T. L. Baker, W. L., & Vigilante, D. (1995). Childhood trauma, the neurobiology of adaptation, and "use-dependent" development of the brain: How states become traits. *Infant Mental Health Journal, 16,* 271–291.

Peterson, B. S. (1998, October). *Functional neuroimaging of impulse control circuits.* Symposium on the Interface of Psychodynamics, Cognitive Science and Neurobiology at the 45th annual meeting of the American Academy of Child and Adolescent Psychiatry, Anaheim, CA.

Pianta, R. C., Egeland, B., & Adam, E. K. (1996). Adult attachment classification and self-reported psychiatric symptomatology as assessed by the Minnesota Multiphasic Personality Inventory—2. *Journal of Consulting and Clinical Psychology, 64,* 273–281.

Pike, A., & Plomin, R. (1996). Importance of nonshared environmental factors for childhood and adolescent psychopathology. *Journal of the American Academy of Child and Adolescent Psychiatry, 35,* 560–570.

Pinker, S. (1997). *How the mind works.* New York: W. W. Norton.

Plomin, R. (1990). *Nature and nurture: An introduction to human behavioral genetics.* Pacific Grove, CA: Brooks/Cole.

Plomin, R., & Daniels, D. (1987). Why are children in the same family so different from each other? *Behavioral and Brain Sciences, 10,* 1–16.

Plomin, R., Owen, M. J., & McGuffin, P. (1994a). The genetic basis of complex human behaviors. *Science, 264,* 1733–1739.

Plomin, R., Reiss, D., Hetherington, E. M., & Howe, G. W. (1994b). Nature and nurture: Genetic contributions to measures of the family environment. *Developmental Psychology, 30,* 32–43.

Plomin, R., Rende, R., & Rutter, M. (1991). Quantitative genetics and developmental psychopathology. In D. Cicchetti & S. L. Toth (Eds.), *Rochester symposium on Developmental Psychopathology: Vol. 2. Internalizing and externalizing expressions of dysfunction* (pp. 155–202). Hillsdale, NJ: Erlbaum.

Pons, T. (1996). Novel sensations in the congenitally blind. *Nature, 380,* 479–480.

Porges, S. W., Doussard-Roosevelt, J. A., & Maiti, A. K. (1994). Vagal tone and the physiological regulation of emotion. In N. A. Fox. (Ed.), The development of emotion regulation: Biological and behavioral considerations. *Monographs of the Society for Research in Child Development, 59*(2–3, Serial No. 240), 167–188.

Posner, M. I. (1990). *Foundations of cognitive science.* Cambridge, MA: MIT Press.

Posner, M. I., DiGirolamo, G. J., & Fernandez-Duque, D. (1997). Brain mechanisms of cognitive skills. *Consciousness and Cognition, 6,* 267–290.

Posner, M. I., & Rothbart, M. K. (1998). Attention, self-regulation and consciousness. *Philosophical Transactions of the Royal Society of London: Series B. Biological Sciences, 353* (1377), 1915–1927.

Post, R. M., & Weiss, S. R. B. (1997). Emergent properties of neural systems: How focal molecular neurobiological alterations can affect behavior. *Development and Psychopathology, 9,* 907–930.

Post, R. M., Weiss, S. R. B., Li, H., Smith, M. A., Zhang, L. X., Xing, G., Osuch, E. A., & McCann, U. D. (1998). Neural plasticity and emotional memory. *Development and Psychopathology, 10,* 829–856.

Price, J. L., Carmichael, S. T., & Drevets, W. C. (1994). Networks related to the orbital and medial prefrontal cortex: A substrate for emotional behavior? *Progress in Brain Research, 107,* 523–536.

Prigogine, I., & Stengers, I. (1984). *Order out of chaos.* New York: Bantam.

Putnam, F. W. (1989). *Diagnosis and treatment of multiple personality disorder.* New York: Guilford Press.

Putnam, F. W. (1997). *Dissociation in children and adolescents: A developmental perspective.* New York: Guilford Press.

Radojevic, M. (1994). Mental representations of attachment among prospective Australian fathers. *Australian and New Zealand Journal of Psychiatry, 28,* 505–511.

Rakic, P., Bourgeois, J. P., & Goldman-Rakic, P. S. (1994). Synaptic development of the cerebral cortex: Implications for learning memory and mental illness. *Progress in Brain Research, 102,* 227–243.

Ramey, C. T., Yeates, K. O., & Short, E. J. (1984). The plasticity of intellectual development: Insights from preventative intervention. *Child Development, 55,* 1913–1925.

Rauch, S. L., van der Kolk, B. A., Fisler, R. E., Alpert, N. M., Orr, S. P., Savage, C. R., Fischman, A. J., Jenike, M. A., & Pitman, R. K. (1996). A symptom provocation study of posttraumatic stress disorder using positron emission tomography and script-driven imagery. *Archives of General Psychiatry, 53,* 380–387.

Reed, E. S. (1994). Perception is to self as memory is to selves. In U. Neisser & R. Fivush (Eds.), *The remembering self: Construction and accuracy in the self-narrative* (pp. 278–292). Cambridge, UK: Cambridge University Press.

Reese, E., & Fivush, R. (1993). Parental styles of talking about the past. *Developmental Psychology, 29,* 596–606.

Robertson, R., & Combs, A. (Eds.). (1995). *Chaos theory in psychology and the life sciences.* Hillsdale, NJ: Erlbaum.

Rolls, E. T. (1995). A theory of emotion and consciousness, and its application to understanding the neural basis of emotion. In M. S. Gazzaniga (Ed.), *The cognitive neurosciences* (pp. 1091–1106). Cambridge, MA: MIT Press.

Rolls, E. T. (1996). The orbitofrontal cortex. *Philosophical Transactions of the Royal Society of London: Series B. Biological Sciences, 351,* 1433–1444.

Rolls, E. T., & Treves, A. (1994). Neural networks in the brain involved in memory and recall. *Progress in Brain Research, 102,* 335–341.

Rosenblum, L. A., Coplan, J. D., Friedman, S., Basoff, T., Gorman, J. M., & Andrews, M. W. (1994). Adverse early experiences affect noradrenergic and serotonergic functioning in adult primates. *Biological Psychiatry, 35,* 221–227.

Rosenstein, D., & Horowitz, H. A. (1996). Adolescent attachment and psychopathology. *Journal of Consulting and Clinical Psychology, 64,* 244–253.

Ross, E. D. (1984). Right hemisphere's role in language, affective behavior and emotion. *Trends in Neuroscience, 7,* 342–346.

Ross, E. D. (1996). Hemispheric specialization for emotions, affective aspects of language and communication and the cognitive display behaviors in humans. *Progress in Brain Research, 107,* 583–594.

Ross, E. D., Homan, R. W., & Buck, R. (1994). Differential hemispheric lateralization of primary and social emotions: Implications for developing a comprehensive neurology of emotions, repression, and the subconscious. *Neuropsychiatry, Neuropsychology, and Behavioral Neurology, 7,* 1–19.

Rotenberg, V. S. (1994). An integrative psychophysiological approach to brain hemisphere functions in schizophrenia. *Neuroscience and Biobehavioral Reviews, 18,* 487–495.

Rothbart, M. K., & Ahadi, S. A. (1994). Temperament and the development of personality. *Journal of Abnormal Psychology, 103,* 55–66.

Routh, C. P., Hill, J. W., Steele, H., Elliott, C. E., & Dewey, E. W. (1995). Maternal attachment status, psychosocial stressors and problem behavior: Follow-up after parent training courses for conduct disorder. *Journal of Child Psychology and Psychiatry, 36,* 1179–1198.

Rovee-Collier, C. (1993). The capacity for long-term memory in infancy. *Current Directions in Psychological Science, 2,* 130–135.

Rubin, D. C. (1986). *Autobiographical memory.* Cambridge, UK: Cambridge University Press.

Rubinow, D. R., & Post, R. M. (1992). Impaired recognition of affect in facial expression in depressed patients. *Biological Psychiatry, 31,* 947–953.

Rutter, M. (1987). Psychosocial resilience and protective mechanisms. *American Journal of Orthopsychiatry, 57,* 316–331.

Rutter, M. (1989). Temperament: Conceptual issues and implications. In G. A. Kohstamm, J. E. Bates, & M. K. Rothbart (Eds.), *Temperament in childhood* (pp. 362–479). New York: Wiley.

Rutter, M. (1991). Age changes in depressive disorders: Some developmental considerations. In J. Garber & K. A. Dodge (Eds.), *The development of emotion regulation and dysregulation* (pp. 273–302). Cambridge, UK: Cambridge University Press.

Rutter, M. (1997). Clinical implications of attachment concepts: Retrospect and prospect. In L. Atkinson & K. J. Zucker (Eds.), *Attachment and psychopathology* (pp. 17–46). New York: Guilford Press.

Rutter, M., Dunn, J., Plomin, R., Simonoff, E., Pickles, A., Maughan, B., Ormel, J., Meyer, J., & Eaves, L. (1997). Integrating nature and nurture: Implications of person–environment correlations and interactions in developmental psychopathology. *Development and Psychopathology, 9,* 335–364.

Sagi, A., van IJzendoorn, M. H., Scharf, M., Joels, T., Koren-Karie, N., Mayseless, O., & Aviezer, O. (1997). Ecological constraints for intergenerational transmission of attachment. *International Journal of Behavioral Development, 20,* 287–299.

Sagi, A., van IJzendoorn, M. H. Scharf, M. H., Koren-Karie, N., Joels, T., & Mayseless, O. (1994). Stability and discirminant validity of the Adult Attachment Interview: A psychometric study in young Israeli adults. *Developmental Psychology, 30,* 771–777.

Sapolsky, R. M. (1997). The importance of a well-groomed child. *Science, 277,* 1620–1621.

Schacter D. L. (1992). Understanding implicit memory: A cognitive neuroscience approach. *American Psychologist, 47,* 559–569.

Schacter, D. L. (1996). *Searching for memory: The brain, the mind, and the past.* New York: Basic Books.

Schacter, D. L., Alpert, N. M., Savage, C. R., Rauch, S. L., & Albert, M. S. (1996). Conscious recollection and the human hippocampal formation: Evidence from positron emission tomography. *Proceedings of the National Academy of Sciences USA, 93,* 321–325.

Schacter, D. L., & Buckner, R. L. (1998). Priming and the brain. *Neuron, 20,* 185–195.

Schiff, B. B., Esses, V. M., & Lamon, M. (1992). Unilateral facial contractions produce mood effect on social cognitive judgements. *Cognition and Emotion 6,* 357–368.

Schiffer, F., Teicher, M. H., & Papanicolaou, A. C. (1995). Evoked potential evidence for right brain activity during recall of traumatic memories. *Journal of Neuropsychiatry, 7,* 187–250.

Schore, A. N. (1994). *Affect regulation and the origin of the self: The neurobiology of emotional development.* Hillsdale, NJ: Erlbaum.

Schore, A. N. (1996). The experience-dependent maturation of a regulatory system in the orbital prefrontal cortex and the origin of developmental psychopathology. *Development and Psychopathology, 8,* 59–87.

Schore, A. N. (1997). Early organization of the nonlinear right brain and development of a predisposition to psychiatric disorders. *Development and Psychopathology 9,* 595–631.

Schore, A. N. (1998). The experience-dependent maturation of an evaluative system in the cortex. In K. H. Pribram & J. King (Eds.), *Brain and values: Is a biological science of values possible?* (pp. 337–358). Mahway, NJ: Erlbaum.

Schuengel, C., Bakermans-Kranenburg, M. J., & van IJzendoorn, M. H. (in press). Attachment and loss: Frightening maternal behavior linking unresolved loss and disorganized infant attachment. *Journal of Consulting and Clinical Psychology.*

Schuengel, C., van IJzendoorn, M. H., Bakermans-Kranenburg, M. J., & Blom, M. (1997). *Frightening, frightened, and dissociated behavior, unresolved loss and infant disorganization.* Paper presented at the biennial meeting of the Society for Research in Child Development, Washington, DC.

Schumacher, J. F. (1991). *Human suggestibility: Advances in theory, research and applications.* New York: Routledge.

Schuman, J. (1997). *The neurobiology of affect in language.* Malden, MA: Blackwell.

Schweinhart, J. L., & Weikart, D. P. (1992). High/Scope Perry Preschool Program outcomes. In J. McCord & R. E. Tremblay (Eds.), *Preventing antisocial behavior: Interventions from birth through adolescence* (pp. 67–86). New York: Guilford Press.

Semrud-Clikeman, M., & Hynd, G. W. (1990). Right hemisphere dysfunction in nonverbal learning disabilities: Social, academic, and adaptive functioning in adults and children. *Psychological Bulletin, 107,* 196–209.

Sergent, J., Ohta, S., & MacDonald, B. (1992). Functional neuroanatomy of face and object processing. *Brain, 115,* 15–36.

Shapiro, F. (1995). *Eye movement desensitization and reprocessing: Basic principles, protocols, and procedures.* New York: Guilford Press.

Shevrin, H. (1992). Subliminal perception, memory, and consciousness: Cognitive and dynamic perspectives. In R. F. Bornstein & T. S. Pittman (Eds.), *Perception without awareness: Cognitive, clinical, and social perspectives* (pp. 123–142). New York: Guilford Press.

Shimamura, A. P. (1995). Memory and frontal lobe function. In M. S. Gazzaniga (Ed.), *The cognitive neurosciences* (pp. 803–814). Cambridge, MA: MIT Press.

Shinbrot, T., Grebogi, C., Ott, E., & Yorke, J. A. (1993). Using small perturbations to control chaos. *Nature, 363,* 411–417.

Siegel, D. J. (1995a). Memory, trauma, and psychotherapy: A cognitive science view. *Journal of Psychotherapy Practice and Research, 4,* 93–122.

Siegel, D. J. (1995b). Perception and cognition. In B. Kaplan & W. Sadock (Eds.), *Comprehensive textbook of psychiatry* (Vol. 6, pp. 277–291). Baltimore: Williams & Wilkins.

Siegel, D. J. (1996a). Cognition, memory, and dissociation. *Child and Adolescent Psychiatric Clinics of North America, 5,* 509–536.

Siegel, D. J. (1996b). Dissociation, psychotherapy and the cognitive sciences. In J. Spira (Ed.), *The treatment of dissociative identity disorder* (pp. 39–80). San Francisco: Jossey-Bass.

Sigman, M., & Capps, L. (1997). *Children with autism: A developmental perspective.* Cambridge, MA: Harvard University Press.

Sigman, M., & Siegel, D. J. (1992). The interface between the psychobiological and cognitive models of attachment. Behavioral and Brain Sciences, 15, 523.

Singer, J. A., & Salovey, P. (1993). *The remembered self: Emotion and memory in personality.* New York: Free Press.

Skinner, J. E., Molnar, M., Vybiral, T., & Mitra, M. (1992). Application of chaos theory to biology and medicine. *Integrative Physiological and Behavioral Science, 27,* 43–57.

Snow, C. E. (1990). Building memories: The ontogeny of autobiography. In D.

Cicchetti & M. Beeghly (Eds.), *The self in transition* (pp. 213–242). New York: Academic Press.

Solomon, J., George, C., & de Jong, A. (1995). Children classified as controlling at age six: Evidence for disorganized representational strategies and aggression at home and at school. *Development and Psychopathology, 7,* 447–463.

Spangler, G., & Grossmann, K. E. (1993). Biobehavioral organization in securely and insecurely attached infants. *Child Development, 64,* 1439–1450.

Spangler, G., Fremmer-Bombik, E., & Grossmann, K. (1996). Social and individual determinants of infant attachment security and disorganization. *Infant Mental Health Journal, 17,* 127–139.

Spence, S., Shapiro, D., & Zaidel, E. (1996). The role of the right hemisphere in the physiological and cognitive components of emotional processing. *Psychophysiology, 33,* 112–122.

Spiegel, D. (1996). Dissociative disorders. In R. E. Hales & S. C. Yudofsky (Eds.). *American Psychiatric Press synopsis of psychiatry* (pp. 583–604). Washington, DC: American Psychiatric Press.

Springer, S. P., & Deutsch, G. (1993). *Left brain, right brain* (4th ed.). New York: Freeman.

Squire, L. R. (1987). *Memory and brain.* New York: Oxford University Press.

Squire, L. R. (1992). Declarative and non-declarative memory: Multiple brain systems supporting learning and memory. *Journal of Cognitive Neuroscience, 4,* 232–243.

Squire, L. R., Knowlton, B., & Musen, G. (1993). The structure and organization of memory. *Annual Review of Psychology, 44,* 453–495.

Squire, L. R., & Zola-Morgan, S. (1991). The medial temporal lobe memory system. *Science, 153,* 2380–2386.

Sroufe, L. A. (1990). An organizational perspective on the self. In D. Cicchetti & M. Beeghly (Eds.), *The self in transition: Infancy to childhood* (pp. 281–307). Chicago: University of Chicago Press.

Sroufe, L. A. (1996). *Emotional development: The organization of emotional life in the early years.* New York: Cambridge University Press.

Sroufe, L. A. (1997). Psychopathology as an outcome of development. *Development and Psychopathology, 9,* 251–268.

Sroufe, L. A., Egeland, B., & Kreutzer, T. (1990). The fate of early experience following developmental change: Longitudinal approaches to individual adaptation in childhood. *Child Development, 61,* 1363–1373.

Sroufe, L. A., & Jacobvitz, D. (1989). Diverging pathways, developmental transformations, multiple etiologies, and the problem of continuity in development. *Human Development, 32,* 196–203.

Stansbury, K., & Gunnar, M. R. (1994). Adrenocortical activity and emotion regulation. In N. A. Fox (Ed.), The development of emotion regulation: Biological and behavioral considerations. *Monographs of the Society for Research in Child Development, 59*(2–3, Serial No. 240), 108–134.

Stecklis, H. D., & Kling, A. (1985). Neurobiology of affiliative behavior in nonhuman primates. In M. Reite & T. Field (Eds.), *The psychobiology of attachment and separation* (pp. 93–134). Orlando, FL: Academic Press.

Steele, H., & Steele, M. (1994). Intergenerational patterns of attachment. In K. Bartholomew & D. Perlman (Eds.), *Advances in personal relationships: Vol. 5. Attachment processes in adulthood (pp 93–120).* London: Jessica Kingsley.

Steele, H., Steele, M., & Fonagy, P. (1996). Associations among attachment classifications in mothers, fathers and their infants: Evidence for a relationship-specific perspective. *Child Development, 67,* 541–555.

Stein, N. L., & Trabasso, T. (1992). The organization of emotional experience: Creating links among emotion, thinking, language, and intentional action. *Cognition and Emotion, 6,* 225–244.

Stern, D. N. (1985). *The interpersonal world of the infant.* New York: Basic Books.

Stoller, R. J. (1985). *Observing the erotic imagination.* New Haven, CT: Yale University Press.

Taylor, J. G. (1994). Non-linear dynamics in neural networks. *Progress in Brain Research, 102,* 371–382.

Teicher, M. H., Ito, Y., Glod, C. A., Andersen, S. L., Dumont, N., & Ackerman, E. (1997). Preliminary evidence for abnormal cortical development in physically and sexually abused children using EEG coherence and MRI. *Annals of the New York Academy of Sciences, 821,* 160–175.

Terr, L. C. (1988). What happens to early memories of trauma? *Journal of the American Academy of Child and Adolescent Psychiatry, 27,* 96–104.

Terr, L. C. (1991). Childhood traumas: An outline and overview. *American Journal of Psychiatry, 148,* 10–20.

Terr, L. (1993). *Unchained memories.* New York: Basic Books.

Thatcher, R. W. (1994). Cyclical cortical reorganization: Origins of human cognitive development. In G. Dawson & K. W. Fischer (Eds.), *Human behavior and the developing brain* (pp. 232–266). New York: Guilford Press.

Thatcher, R. W. (1997). Human frontal lobe development: A theory of cyclical cortical reorganization. In N. A. Krasnegor, G. Reid-Lyon, & P. S. Goldman-Rakic (Eds.), *Development of the prefrontal cortex: Evolution, neurobiology, and behavior* (pp. 85–113). Baltimore: Brookes.

Thatcher, R. W., Walker, R. A., & Guidice, S. (1987). Human cerebral hemispheres develop at different rates and ages. *Science, 236,* 1110–1113.

Thelen, E. (1989). Self-organization in developmental processes: Can systems approaches work? In M. Gunnar & E. Thelen (Eds.), *Minnesota Symposium on Child Psychology: Vol. 22. Systems and development* (pp. 77–117). Hillsdale, NJ: Erlbaum.

Thomas, A., & Chess, S. (1977). *Temperament and development.* New York: Brunner/Mazel.

Thompson, R. A. (1994). Emotion regulation: A theme in search of definition. In N. A. Fox. (Ed.), The development of emotion regulation: Biological and behavioral considerations. *Monographs of the Society for Research in Child Development, 59*(2–3, Serial No. 240), 25–52.

Tononi, G., & Edelman, G. M. (1998). Consciousness and complexity. *Science 282,* 1896–1851.

Toth, S. L., Cicchetti, D., Macfie, J., & Emde R. (1997). Representations of self and other in the narratives of neglected, physically abused and sexually abused preschoolers. *Development and Psychopathology, 9,* 781–796.

Trevarthen, C. (1990a). Integrative functions of the cerebral commissures. In F. Boller & J. Grafman (Eds.), *Handbook of neurospsychology* (Vol. 4, pp. 49–83). Amsterdam, Netherlands: Elsevier Sciences.

Trevarthen, C. (1990b). Growth and education of the hemispheres. In C. Trevarthen (Ed.), *Brain circuits and functions of the mind: Essays in honour of Roger W. Sperry* (pp. 334–363). New York: Cambridge University Press.

Trevarthen C. (1993). The self born in intersubjectivity: The psychology of infant communicating. In U. Neisser (Ed.), *The perceived self: Ecological and interpersonal sources of self-knowledge* (pp. 121–173). New York: Cambridge University Press.

Trevarthen, C. (1996). Lateral asymmetries in infancy: Implications for the development of the hemispheres. *Neuroscience and Biobehavioral Reviews, 20,* 571–586.

Tronick, E. Z. (1989). Emotions and emotional communication in infants. *American Psychologist, 44,* 112–119.

Tucker, D. M. (1981). Lateral brain function, emotion, and conceptualization. *Psychological Bulletin, 89,* 19–46.

Tucker, D. M. (1992). Developing emotions and cortical networks. In M. R. Gunnar & C. Nelson (Eds.), *Minnesota Symposia on Child Psychology: Vol. 24. Developmental behavioral neuroscience* (pp. 75–128). Hillsdale, NJ: Erlbaum.

Tucker, D. M., Luu, P., & Pribram, K. H. (1995). Social and emotional self-regulation. *Annals of the New York Academy of Sciences, 769,* 213–239.

Tulving, E. (1993). Varieties of consciousness and levels of awareness in memory. In A. Baddeley & L. Weiskrantz (Eds.), *Attention, selection, awareness and control: A tribute to Donald Broadbent* (pp. 283–299). London: Oxford University Press.

Tulving, E., Kapur, S., Craik, F. I. M., Moscovitch, M., & Houle, S. (1994). Hemispheric encoding/retrieval asymmetry in episodic memory: Positron emission tomography findings. *Proceedings of the National Academy of Sciences USA, 91,* 2016–2020.

Vandenberg, B. (1998). Hypnosis and human development: Interpersonal influence of intrapersonal processes. *Child Development, 69,* 262–267.

van den Boom, D. C. (1994). The influence of temperatment and mothering on attachment and exploration: An experimental manipulation of sensitive responsiveness among lower-class mothers with irritable infants. *Child Development, 65,* 1449–1469.

van den Boom, D. C. (1995). Do first-year intervention effects endure? Follow-up during toddlerhood of a sample of Dutch irritable infants. *Child Development, 66,* 1798–1816.

van der Kolk, B. A., McFarlane, A. C., & Weisaeth, L. (Eds.). (1996). *Traumatic stress: The effects of overwhelming experience on mind, body, and society.* New York: Guilford Press.

van der Kolk, B. A., & van der Hart, O. (1989). Pierre Janet and the breakdown of adaptation in psychological trauma. *American Journal of Psychiatry, 146,* 1530–1540.

van IJzendoorn, M. H. (1992). Intergenerational transmission of parenting: A review of studies in nonclinical populations. *Developmental Review, 12,* 76–99.

van IJzendoorn, M. H. (1995). Adult attachment representations, parental responsiveness, and infant attachment: A meta-analysis on the predictive validity of the Adult Attachment Interview. *Psychological Bulletin, 117,* 387–403.

van IJzendoorn, M. H., & Bakermans-Kranenburg, M. J. (1996). Attachment representations in mothers, fathers, adolescents and clinical groups: A meta-analytic search for normative data. *Journal of Consulting and Clinical Psychology, 64,* 8–21.

van IJzendoorn, M. H., & Bakermans-Kranenburg, M. J. (1997). Intergenerational transmission of attachment: A move to the contextual level. In L. Atkinson & K. J. Zucker (Eds.), *Attachment and psychopathology* (pp. 135–170). New York: Guilford Press.

van Ooyen, A., & van Pelt, J. (1994). Activity-dependent neurite outgrowth and neural network development. *Progress in Brain Research, 102,* 245–259.

van Pelt, J., Corner, M. A., Uylings, H. B. M., & Lopes Da Silva, F. H. (Eds.). (1994). The self-organizing brain: From growth cones to functional networks. *Progress in Brain Research, 102,* 1–446.

Vaughn, B. E., Stevenson-Hinde, J., Waters, E., Kotsaftis, A., Lefever, G. B., Shouldice, A., Trudel, M., & Belsky, J. (1992). Attachment security and temperament in infancy and childhood: Some conceptual clarifications. *Developmental Psychology, 28,* 463–473.

Vygotsky, L. (1986). *Thought and language* (Ed. A. Kozulin). Cambridge, MA: MIT Press. (Original work published 1934)

Walden, T. A. (1991). Infant social referencing. In J. Garber & K. A. Dodge (Eds.), *The development of emotion regulation and dysregulation* (pp. 69–88). Cambridge, UK: Cambridge University Press.

Waller, N., Putnam, F. W., & Carlson, E. B. (1996). Types of dissociation and dissociative types: A taxometric analysis of dissociative experiences. *Psychological Methods, 1,* 300–321.

Ward, M. J., & Carlson, E. A. (1995). Associations among adult attachment representation, maternal sensitivity, and infant–mother attachment in a sample of adolescent mothers. *Child Development 66,* 69–79.

Waters, E., Crowell, J., Treboux, D., O'Connor, E., Posada, G., & Golby, B. (1996). Discriminant validity of the Adult Attachment Interview. *Child Development, 67,* 2584–2599.

Watt, D. F. (1998). Affect and the limbic system: Some hard problems. *Journal of Neuropsychiatry and Clinical Neurosciences, 10,* 113–116.

Webster's New World Dictionary (3rd ed.). (1997). New York: Simon & Schuster/Macmillan.

Weinberger, N. M. (1995). Retuning the brain by fear conditioning. In M. S. Gazzaniga (Ed.), *The cognitive neurosciences* (pp. 1071–1089). Cambridge, MA: MIT Press.

Wheeler, M. A., Stuss, D. T., & Tulving, E. (1997). Toward a Theory of episodic memory: The frontal lobes and autonoetic consciousness. *Psychological Bulletin, 121,* 331–354.

Wheeler, R. E., Davidson, R. J., & Tomarken, A. J. (1993). Frontal brain asymmetry and emotional reactivity: A biological substrate of affective style. *Psychophysiology, 30,* 82–89.

White, M., & Epston D. (1990). *Narrative means to therapeutic ends.* New York: Norton.

Wiesel, T. N., & Hubel, D. H. (1963). Single cell responses in striate cortex of kittens deprived of vision in one eye. *Journal of Neurophysiology, 26,* 1003–1007.

Williams, L. M. (1995). Recovered memories of abuse in women with documented child sexual victimization histories. *Journal of Traumatic Stress, 8,* 649–674.

Winnicott, D. W. (1965). *The maturational processes and the facilitating environment: Studies in the theory of emotional development.* New York: International Universities Press.

Winson, J. (1993). The biology and function of rapid eye movement sleep. *Current Opinion in Neurobiology 3,* 243–248.

Wise, S. P., Murray, E. A., & Gerfen, C. R. (1996). The frontal cortex–basal ganglia system in primates. *Critical Reviews in Neurobiology, 10,* 317–356.

Wittling, W., & Roschmann, R. (1993). Emotion-related hemisphere asymmetry: Subjective emotional responses to laterally presented films. *Cortex, 29,* 431–448.

Wittling, W., & Schweiger, E. (1993). Neuroendocrine brain asymmetry and physical complaints. *Neuropsychologia, 31,* 591–608.

Wolf, D. P. (1990). Being of several minds: Voices and versions of the self in early childhood. In D. Cicchetti & M. Beeghly (Eds.), *The self in transition: Infancy to childhood* (pp. 183–212). Chicago: University of Chicago Press.

Yawkey, T. D., & Johnson, J. E. (Eds.). (1988). *Integrative processes and socialization: Early to middle childhood.* Hillsdale, NJ: Erlbaum.

Yehuda, R., & McFarlane, A. C. (1995). Conflict between current knowledge about posttraumatic stress disorder and its original conceptual basis. *American Journal of Psychiatry, 152,* 1705–1713.

Zaidel, D. W., Hugdahl, K., & Johnsen, B. H. (1995). Physiological responses to verbally inaccessible pictorial information in the left and right hemispheres. *Neuropsychology, 9, 52–57.*

Zaidel, E. Clarke, J. M., & Suyenobu, B. (1990). Hemispheric independence: A paradigm case for cognitive neuroscience. In A. B. Scheibel & A. F. Wechsler (Eds.), *Neurobiology of higher cognitive function* (pp. 297–355). New York: Guilford Press.

Zeanah, C. H. (Ed.). (1993). *Handbook of infant mental health.* New York: Guilford Press.

Zeanah, C. H., Boris, N. W., & Larrieu, J. A. (1997a). Infant development and developmental risk: A review of the past 10 years. *Journal of the American Academy of Child and Adolescent Psychiatry, 36,* 165–178.

Zeanah, C. H., Finely-Belgrad, E., & Benoit, D. (1997b). Intergenerational transmission of relationship psychopathology: A mother–infant case study. In L. Atkinson & K. J. Zucker (Eds.), *Attachment and psychopathology* (pp 292–318). New York: Guilford Press.

Zeitlin, S. B., & McNally, R. J. (1991). Implicit and explicit memory bias for threat in post-traumatic stress disorder. *Behaviour Research and Therapy, 29,* 451–457

Zola-Morgan, S., Squire, L. R., Alvarez-Royo, P., & Clower, R. P. (1991). Independence of memory functions and emotional behavior: Separate contributions of the hippocampal formation and the amygdala. *Hippocampus, 1,* 207–220.

Index

Abuse. *See* Trauma
Activity-dependent process and brain development, 14
Adult Attachment Interview (AAI), 77–83, 89–92, 107
Adults
  attachment figures and, 68
  state of mind with respect to attachment, 74, 79–80, 81, 83
    dismissing, 94–100, 161–162, 287–290
    preoccupied, 103–107
    secure/autonomous, 89–92
    unresolved/disorganized, 110–116
Affect. *See* Vitality affects
Ainsworth, Mary, 72–73
Alignment, 280–281
Ambivalent attachment
  in adulthood, 103–107
  complexity theory and, 293
  description of, 74, 76, 100–103
  parenting and, 283–284
  self-organization and, 224
  states of mind in, 237–238
American Sign Language and brain asymmetry, 186–187
Amnesia, 38, 43–47
Amygdala
  appraisal of meaning and, 48, 49, 131
  face-recognition cells in, 138
  fight-or-flight response and, 132–133, 249
  function of, 10, 132
  intrinsic motive formation and, 174
  stress and, 50
Anatomy of brain
  cerebral asymmetry and, 178–181
  "hard-wiring" of, 137–138, 149–150
  interconnections of, 13
  as open and dynamic system, 16–17
  See also specific structures of the brain (i.e., Amygdala, Anterior cingulate)

Anterior cingulate, 10, 131, 132, 265
Anterior commissures, 12, 178, 303
Anterograde amnesia, 38
Anticipation of future, 30–31, 305, 328, 330
Appraisal system
  emotion and, 124–125, 264–265
  emotion as value system for, 6, 136–139, 158, 278
  feedback mechanism of process of, 132–133
  limbic system and, 131
  sensitivity and modifications in, 248
  somato-sensory data and, 143–144
  specificity of, 250–253
"Approach" behavior and left hemisphere, 175
Arousal
  autonomic nervous system and, 278–279
  emotion and, 124–125, 158, 264–265
  suspended cortical processing and, 258–262
"As-if" somatic marker, 144, 146
Associational linkages, 27
Asymmetrical relationships, 88–89
Asymmetry of brain
  anticipation and, 305
  assertive versus acceptive states, 175
  attachment, mental representational processes, and, 185–190
  consciousness and, 154, 184–185
  dorsal versus ventral pathways, 175–176, 178
  emotion and, 150–155, 181–184
  gender and, 190–192
  implications of, 196–199
  infants and, 173–175
  influence of experience on, 193–196
  integration and, 326–327
  overview of, 7, 17–18

387